FIVE WAYS OF DOING
QUALITATIVE ANALYSIS

Five Ways of Doing
Qualitative Analysis

Phenomenological Psychology, Grounded Theory, Discourse Analysis, Narrative Research, and Intuitive Inquiry

Frederick J. Wertz,
Kathy Charmaz, Linda M. McMullen, Ruthellen Josselson,
Rosemarie Anderson, and Emalinda McSpadden

THE GUILFORD PRESS
New York   London

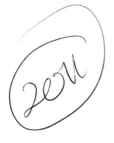

Library of Congress Cataloging-in-Publication Data

Five ways of doing qualitative analysis: phenomenological psychology, grounded
theory, discourse analysis, narrative research, and intuitive inquiry / Frederick J.
Wertz ... [et al.].
   p. cm.
  Includes bibliographical references and index.
  ISBN 978-1-60918-142-0 (pbk.: alk. paper)
  ISBN 978-1-60918-143-7 (hbk.: alk. paper)
  1. Psychology–Qualitative research. 2. Qualitative research. I. Wertz,
Frederick J. (Frederick Joseph), 1951–
  BF76.5.F545 2011
  150.72–dc22

                                            2010052862

*To those who dedicate themselves
to learning and doing qualitative research
in the 21st century*

Acknowledgments

W e would like to thank our significant others and families for their understanding, sharing of our work, and selfless support.

We also extend thanks to our doctoral students and colleagues at Fordham University, Sonoma State University, the University of Saskatchewan, Fielding Graduate University, and the Institute of Transpersonal Psychology for their support, encouragement, and common vision. Special thanks go to the students in the graduate class, Qualitative Research Methods for Psychology, at Fordham University, who shaped the project that provided data for our analyses.

Heartfelt thanks go to Kamla Modi, the person who provided the written description and participated in the secondary interview, as well as to the two interviewers, Frank Williams and Tameeka Jordan, whose data collection has formed the basis of this project. Emily Maynard deserves commendation for her meticulous editing of the manuscript.

We are especially grateful for all the help given to us by C. Deborah Laughton, Publisher, Methodology and Statistics, at The Guilford Press. Accompanying us as a colleague, she has consistently offered encouragement, constructive criticism, and invaluable advice.

We also thank the following reviewers for their helpful and insightful comments: Jeanne Marecek, Department of Psychology at Swarthmore College; Mark A. Hector, Department of Psychology at the University of Tennessee, Knoxville; Suzanne Wilson, Department of Teacher Education at Michigan State University; and graduate students: Heidi Mattilla and Kat Tighe at

Fielding Institute; Sarah Kamens at Fordham University; and Melanie Bayly at the University of Saskatchewan.

Finally, we thank those who have made contributions of so many sorts, including understanding dialogue, offering public forums, brainstorming ideas, giving guidance, and working with our manuscripts: Judy Abbott, Richard Bargdill, Bob Bennett, Jayne Bigelsen, Scott Churchill, Lester Embree, Linda Finlay, Celia Fisher, Mark Freeman, Ken Gergen, Andy Giorgi, Barbara Held, Matt James, Sarah Kamens, Sheila Katz, Daniel Malpica, Doyle McCarthy, Donna Mertens, David Rennie, David Rigney, Linda Silka, Katherine Unthank, Mary Watkins, and Tryon Woods. Last but not least, we would like to thank the Society for Humanistic Psychology of the American Psychological Association for providing a forum and conversation space for the development of this project over the years.

Contents

3. Contemporary Movement, Methodological Pluralism, and Challenges **75**

Institutionalization of Qualitative Methods as Normal Science 76
Journals 76
Professional Organizations and Conferences 77
The Spread of Qualitative Research through Subfields 78
Key Issues in Qualitative Research 79
Philosophy and Human Science 79
The Qualitative–Quantitative Debate 81
The Generative Tensions of Pluralism 82
Reflexivity and Standpoint 84
Ethics, Power, and Politics 84
Education in Research Methodology and Praxis 86
Criteria and Guidelines for Best Practices 86
The Typical Organization of the Qualitative Research Project 87
Formulation of a Research Problem 87
Participants, Situations, and Data 89
Analytic Methods 91
Report of Findings 93
Delineating the Implications of Research 94
Contributions of Qualitative Research Methods to Psychology 94
The Five Ways Project 95
References 96

II. FIVE APPROACHES TO QUALITATIVE DATA ANALYSIS

4. The Teresa Texts: Thick Description of Living through Misfortune **103**

Written Description 104
Interviewer's Introduction 108
Interview Transcript 108

5. A Phenomenological Psychological Approach to Trauma and Resilience **124**
Frederick J. Wertz

The Phenomenological Approach 124
The Phenomenological Attitude: Focus on Lived Experience 125
Phenomenological Method: Intentional and Eidetic Analysis 126
The Phenomenological Movement 128
Philosophical and Transdisciplinary Directions 128
Phenomenological Psychology 129
Learning Phenomenology 130
Psychological Research Method Using Lifeworld Descriptions 131
General Analytic Procedures 131
Applications and Exemplary Studies 134
Limits and Critical Evaluation 134
Personal Appeal 135

— ethnographic?

III. PLURALISM, PARTICIPATION, AND UNITY IN QUALITATIVE RESEARCH

Introduction

T his book is about an adventure. One of the great challenges facing the human sciences and service professions is the choice and application of research methods that respect the uniqueness, complexity, and meanings of human experience. Qualitative research methods have made seminal contributions to psychology over the past century, employed by such eminent researchers as William James, Sigmund Freud, Jean Piaget, Lawrence Kohlberg, Abraham Maslow, and Nobel Prize awardees Herbert Simon and Daniel Kahneman. Only in the most recent decades has a rich and diverse plurality of such methods become formalized and made available in the academic curriculum for training researchers. Since the 1970s, qualitative methods have had an increasing presence in education settings, in funded research, and in professional conferences and journals. This movement has been characterized as "the qualitative revolution" (Denzin & Lincoln, 1994). Nevertheless, although textbooks and graduate courses currently introduce various approaches to students and scholars, there has been little focused and systematic comparison of the various methods past and present. Students and even seasoned researchers seeking to expand their methodological competence to include qualitative practice are often baffled by similarities and differences of such methods and may be at a loss in choosing analytic methods that are most relevant for their purposes. This volume contributes to the emerging interest in qualitative research methods by focusing on the historical background, contemporary context, concrete demonstrations, and comparisons of five leading approaches to qualitative analysis: phenomenological psychology, grounded theory, discourse analysis, narrative research, and intuitive inquiry. The goal of this book is to assist novice and seasoned researchers in achieving more rigorous qualitative *praxis*, the reflective application of qualitative analyses.

1

The Nature and Importance
of Qualitative Research Methods

Qualitative research addresses the question of "what?" Knowing *what* something is entails a conceptualization of the matter under investigation as a whole and in its various parts, the way these parts are related and organized as a whole, and how the whole is similar to and different from other things. Knowing *what something is* may also involve the conceptualization of its "how"—its process and temporal unfolding in time. Qualitative knowledge may also include an understanding of the context, the consequences/outcomes, and even the significance of what is investigated in the larger world. The construction of theories, hypothetical explanation, prediction, and measurement of a subject matter presupposes qualitative knowledge—that is, knowledge of the basic characteristics of the subject matter. Knowledge of the "what" may be implicit or explicit, uncritically assumed or carefully established, and informally or formally acquired. In the history of the sciences that concern human mental life, great attention has been devoted to the rigorous specification of procedures for measurement and quantitative analysis, and the qualitative/descriptive procedures have received far less attention. However, in and of itself, measurement tells us only *magnitude*, and even when many measurements are made with the finest instruments and rationally analyzed with the most sophisticated statistical procedures, they do not themselves provide *qualitative knowledge of what is being measured*. Therefore, a different kind of research and analysis—research about *what a subject matter is* in all its real-world complexity—is a necessary foundation and complement to quantitative research.

Qualitative knowledge is easily taken for granted. We are already familiar with "what things are" through ordinary experience in everyday life. However, important basic qualitative work has always been done in the physical sciences—for instance, in charting the stars and planets in astronomy, developing classification systems for plants in botany, describing the structure and functions of organ systems, and the stages of embryonic development in biology. Perhaps such human phenomena as learning, intelligence, emotion, the family, education, democracy, and the Cold War era are so close to us that we can theorize, measure, explain, and even sometimes successfully predict and control them without undertaking any methodical qualitative investigations of them. However, given that qualitative questions concern the structure, the process, and even the significance of such subject matter, careful, rigorous science may be necessary in order to overcome the prejudices and limitations of uncritical experience and assumptions, however well these may serve us in our everyday lives. After all, qualitative questions about the nature of phenomena such as "learning" and "intelligence," indeed of the very nature of "human beings" themselves, continue to be matters of conflicting claims and ongoing debate. Asking good qualitative questions and using careful, self-critical, methodical, and accountable procedures to answer them is crucial for science. Qualitative knowledge of human affairs and mental life has been a part of the human sciences since their institutionalization in the 19th century. However, the importance of research methods that produce qualitative knowledge in these disciplines has begun to become broadly accepted only in recent years. Careful procedures have been well established, justified, and made available. Important findings resulting from the use of these methods have demonstrated their value and utility, as well as their complementarity to established quantitative methods.

Although there is much to learn and to know about the design, data collection, and procedures in qualitative investigations, what is most perplexing to students and practitioners is qualitative *analysis*, which is so very different from quantitative analysis and has traditionally not been included in educational curricula. Few researchers or methodologists have had formal training and developed expertise in applying a variety of approaches to qualitative research, and few graduate institutions offer students an opportunity to learn a full spectrum of approaches to qualitative data analysis. In order to fill this gap and to facilitate a deeper understanding of a representative variety of available approaches, this book addresses the context and practice of researchers who have been immersed in distinctive, leading traditions of qualitative analysis.

An Adventure in Qualitative Research Methodology

This adventure began when we, five qualitative researchers widely separated by our geography, our training, our methodologies, and our areas of study, decided to undertake a unique challenge: analyses of the same written and interview data from our respective points of view. At the outset, none of us knew where this project would lead. Much like the beginning of any qualitative research project, we were only certain of our uncertainty. What subject matter would we analyze? How would we come into possession of an interview or other forms of qualitative data? How different and how similar would our methods of analysis turn out to be? Would our analyses lead to the similar insights or different findings? Might we be confronted with irreconcilable interpretations of the data and no means of resolution? What sense would each of us make of each other's work in comparison to our own? Would we be able to discern any fundamental unity among qualitative analytic approaches? What would we learn, individually and collectively, about our topic, about the analytic practices we use, about the various possibilities of qualitative analysis, about each other, and about ourselves? How might we and our understandings of our qualitative research methodology be changed in the course of this adventure?

We represent a spectrum of prominent, contemporary approaches to scientific knowledge. Because the methods of qualitative data analysis have built on and overlap with each other, we selected relatively distinct traditions with well-formulated procedures for this protocol analysis. *Phenomenology* (represented by Frederick Wertz) is a method originally formalized in philosophy that has also been employed across the humanities, social sciences, and service professions over the last century; since the 1960s, phenomenologists have used clearly defined methods for formulating meaning-oriented, descriptive knowledge in psychology. *Grounded theory* (Kathy Charmaz), which developed in sociology in the late 1960s with an emphasis on theory building, has contributed well-delineated procedures that have been widely utilized in diverse human sciences and professions. *Discourse analysis* (Linda McMullen) is one of a family of contemporary approaches that emphasizes human language as a socially contextual performance and that brings a socially critical lens to its study of science and human life. *Narrative research* (Ruthellen Josselson) draws upon the field of literary studies as well as interdisciplinary social and intellectual movements, ranging from psychoanalysis to feminism, and emphasizes the interpretive power of stories to disclose human meaning. *Intuitive inquiry* (Rosemarie Anderson) has joined the approaches to qualitative research more recently, emerging from the study of spiritual and transformative experiences, and contributing to the growing traditions of qualitative research by formally specifying methods that incorporate researchers' intuitive, emotional, and personal capacities, which have long been informally employed in scientific analyses and theorizing, in order to serve psychology's aspirations to foster personal and cultural transformation. These five approaches to qualitative analysis can be utilized across a broad spectrum of subject matters and with various kinds of data, including written descriptions, interviews, focus groups, and other human expressions. They can be combined with each other and used in a variety of research projects, including basic science, hermeneutics, heuristics, and ethnography; action, participatory, and emancipatory research; and clinical, evaluation, and case study research.

We are focusing on the analysis phase of qualitative research because the differences among various approaches can be best discerned there. Qualitative analyses are not the mere application of technical procedures; they are not simply additional tools for the researcher's toolbox. When properly practiced, such analyses require a unique qualitative stance and worldview. Therefore, our goal in this book is to provide a broad knowledge base that can serve as the foundation for understanding and employing the typical procedures used in our five specific approaches. In order to facilitate more in-depth understanding, which requires further reading, we provide references to the larger body of literature on qualitative methods and methodology, including the specific literatures of our five analytic approaches. We aim to provide readers with a concrete, detailed, and intimate experience as they enter the qualitative movement by following each of us through our analytic practices. We also hope to contribute original insights into how these different approaches relate to historically exemplary qualitative research and how they compare with each other, in order to promote a better understanding of their common features as well as their distinctive purposes and strengths. To these ends, each of us has confronted and delved into a broad spectrum of problems and challenges facing contemporary qualitative researchers, ranging from the philosophical underpinnings of our work to scientific issues of validity and ethical conundrums involved in the protection of human participants in highly personal research. We also place considerable emphasis on the role, style, and subjectivity of the individual researcher and offer reflexive examinations of our own personal presences in the process of analysis. Consequently, our adventure has not merely reiterated well-traveled paths. We have also made some exciting original advances into past, present, and future horizons of the qualitative movement.

All five of us have typically sought general knowledge through our research. The current project is unusual for us in that its main focus is the analysis using the data of only a single participant. We originally undertook this approach for demonstration purposes, in order to allow readers access to the nuts and bolts of our analytic practices with concrete material. However, in assuming the ethical responsibility involved in protecting the rights, preserving the well-being, and caring for the interests of our research participants, we entered into a relationship with the primary research participant and became attentive to her responses to this project. Although initially a subtext, this relationship inevitably became a significant part of our project that we share explicitly because of the general importance of the ethical and methodological issues it entails.

Norms regarding personal privacy are shifting in our culture, as reflected in the popularity of websites such as Facebook, which displays considerable personal information. Norms regarding the roles of research participants are also shifting in our science. The impact of research on participants and participants' experiences of research are provoking ethical and scientific debate. The boundaries between scientist and nonscientist have been shaken, problematized, and questioned. The model adapted from the physical sciences, in which the researcher is the subject and the participant is the object, has been viewed as inappropriate for the human sciences. Commentators, critics, and researchers themselves are increasingly calling on researchers to view participants as persons whose interests, methods of understanding, critical potential, and outcomes are acknowledged and valued within science. Scientists are also becoming increasingly sensitive to the political and ethical implications of the inequalities of power and privilege. Because the participant's role in research has become an important topic in contemporary research and has posed ambiguous and complex issues for research involving highly personal material, we explore and critically reflect on the variety and meanings of our research participant's responses to our analyses. We have found that even when researchers are seeking general knowledge and serving purposes other than those of the research participants, their analyses may have significant impact that calls for understanding and ethical responsibility on the part of scientists.

The Road Traveled

Our first difficulty was selecting an acceptable data set for this project. This decision was difficult because data do not just turn up on our doorstep out of nowhere. Each qualitative tradition and each individual researcher has ways of defining a research topic, critically engaging the literature on that topic, identifying significant research problems, designing an entire study, and collecting the data that will best serve the specific knowledge aims. Data analysis does not take place in a vacuum, or in a standard setting across approaches, but in the particular context of a research project. Therefore, adopting common material for analysis in this project involved some contrivance and artificiality. If we were conducting research in our natural contexts, we would design our studies in various ways and utilize different data. We discussed whether there were data that we could commonly use for demonstration and comparison purposes, and after a few weeks of dialogue, were able to overcome reservations and agree on common material for our analyses.

The primary data selected for this work are a stirring, in-depth written description and interview that emerged in a graduate class on qualitative research methods at Fordham University. The students in the class had decided to study "human resilience in the face of trauma" (what they called "misfortune"), and each student wrote a description of an example from their own personal lives, followed by interviews with each other. As primary data for the present project, we decided to use a written description and student-conducted interview with a young woman student whom we called "Teresa." Nineteen years old at the time of her "misfortune," Teresa was a student at a music conservatory, training to be an opera singer, when she developed cancer of the thyroid, which threatened her voice and career. As the cancer spread to her brain, she entered into a struggle for her life and lost much of what was of value to her. In a courageous effort to live as fully as possible, she profoundly altered and expanded her life.

We researchers were aware of the limitations of adopting these texts for our analyses. The interview was brief; the interviewer was a novice; only one participant's data would form the primary basis for analysis. Nevertheless, we accepted these limits because the richness of this material would enable us to demonstrate our analytic practices with sufficient authenticity to allow meaningful results and comparisons. In order to enable researchers to overcome the limits of a single participant's data set and to demonstrate their comparative analytic procedures, we chose a second written description and interview from the same class with another student whom we called "Gail." As a former Division I National Collegiate Athletic Association (NCAA) gymnast, Gail had suffered a traumatic injury in a fall from the uneven bars. Her data provided the researchers with an opportunity to work with more than one example of the subject matter if they so chose. Although we researchers do not ordinarily limit ourselves to one or two sets of data in our analyses, we were satisfied that these two examples would allow us to demonstrate our approaches for our present purposes.

This project developed in phases over 3 years. Each phase was followed by presentations at the Annual Convention of the American Psychological Association (APA), including symposia in the main program followed by formal discussion sessions in the Hospitality Suite of APA's Society for Humanistic Psychology. In the first phase, five of the coauthors analyzed the common data and presented accounts of their approaches, including their backgrounds, philosophies, and histories; their analytic procedures; and their findings in the analysis of Teresa's (and, in some cases, Gail's) descriptions and interviews at the APA convention in 2007. The researchers and those attending the presentations found the similarities and differences in these analyses to be fascinating, raising a host of previously unaddressed questions about qualitative research. Each researcher was surprised by the other analyses, which gave each of us a unique opportunity to explore and understand how the various approaches compare with, and relate to, each other. The task of the second phase was for each researcher to study the other four approaches and to compare them with specific references to his or her work and findings on the common data.

The Involvement of the Research Participant

Our comparisons of methods and findings provoked much thought and discussion at the APA convention in 2008. As we were musing over the discrepancies among the five analyses, one attendee suggested, "Have you asked Teresa [the participant] what *she* thinks of these analyses?" Although we had offered to share the results of our analyses with both research participants, we had not considered asking them for their responses. As qualitative researchers, we were accustomed to asking our participants to review and assess the accuracy of their interview transcripts as well as to delete any personal content that they did not want in print. Apart from these standard practices, the five of us researchers had not typically engaged our research participants in an extensive conversation about the results of our research. Aware that many qualitative researchers are involving participants in the various phases of the research, we decided to expand the scope of this project by inviting Teresa to respond to our analyses and to contribute a chapter to the present book as our sixth coauthor. Still a graduate student in psychology, she gladly accepted the invitation to join us as a collaborator and to write about her experiences participating in this research project, including her responses to our analyses.

After reading our material and in drafting her chapter, Teresa requested that we use her name, which would disclose her identity in our publication. We were concerned that she would thereby lose the protection of privacy that had been established by our rigorously upheld confidentiality. By inviting a research participant to read our analyses of her own words and respond to them, we anticipated a number of ethical challenges and complexities. We decided to address the ethical dilemmas of collaborative partnerships with research participants in our 2009 APA symposium and discussion. We teamed up with two researchers and ethicists, Professors Donna Mertens and Linda Silka, to explore the issues and options more deeply. In preparation, we (the original five) researchers discussed a range of ethical issues, centering on questions of anonymity, confidentiality, and the protection of privacy. We found ourselves facing a new set of concerns, such as the potential risks of making public our participant's medical history, which would then be available to future potential employers and insurers. We were concerned about the privacy not only of our participant but of others to whom she referred in her interview, such as her spouse, her parents, her voice teacher, and the physicians who had initially misdiagnosed her medical condition. We shared these concerns with the participant herself, who explored the issues we raised and steadfastly continued to request the use of her name. After lengthy and intense discussion, we arrived at a collective resolution. Given the unusual nature of this project, especially the participant's new role as a coauthor, we decided to continue to use the pseudonym of Teresa in the data, analyses, and comparisons contained in the present volume and to use her real name, Emily (Emalinda) McSpadden, as coauthor of the book and author of her chapter. Continuing to use the pseudonym *Teresa* pays respect to the important principle of confidentiality and marks the initial conditions under which the project and analyses were conducted. Using her real name acknowledges Emily McSpadden's particular role as a collaborator and coauthor of this volume. We hope readers understand how the unique conditions of this project have led us to this unusual arrangement.

The final phase of our work concerned our response to Emily's chapter, in which she expressed her responses to our analyses. We focused on and discussed some of the difficult ethical and scientific challenges posed by a collaborative partnership with a research participant and by the participant's responses to the analysis of her experience. In initially inviting our research participant to respond to our analyses, we deliberately did not direct or constrain her in any way and encouraged her to respond freely. Emily's responses were many and varied. She was grateful in some ways for how the researchers approached her story. She was at times taken aback, and yet also intrigued, by the methods used. She found some analyses to be in tune with her own self-understanding, and at times she felt embarrassed and disconcerted. She also objected to the apparent implications of some analyses, questioning their "accuracy." Our analyses sometimes confirmed and sometimes contradicted her view of herself. The researchers were all struck by the integrity, passion, and honesty with which Emily responded. They, too, had a variety of responses in turn, ranging from relief to fascination, to feeling misunderstood and underappreciated. These reactions posed a host of questions about the purpose of Emily's chapter, how it would be understood by readers, and about the power relationship between researchers and participant. Who has interpretive authority and on what basis?

The researchers had conflicting impulses as to how to proceed. Some felt strongly that Emily's responses should be presented as they were initially written. All agreed that Emily's responses were to be respected, protected, and presented here; the prospect of censoring our participant's responses to our analyses was abhorrent. And yet the researchers were concerned that, as a student and nonexpert in qualitative methods, Emily's responses might contain misunderstandings and consequently mislead readers about the analytic approaches. After all, Emily had not had the benefit of years of studying qualitative methods and the extensive process of collaboration and mutual correction that the researchers had with each other in writing their responses to each others' work. Might our inclusion of Emily's chapter inadvertently lead readers to bestow an interpretive privilege and authority on research participants that none of us five researchers endorses? None of us researchers believes that research participants are a final court of appeal in establishing the scientific value of procedures and the legitimacy of research findings. In comparing and responding to each others' analyses, at times we struggled to abstain from critique and to modify our statements in response to corrections by the other researchers, given their expertise. Should the participant's responses not be held to the same standards and process of revision? Who would have the final say in any disagreements that ensued?

In facing these ethical and scientific dilemmas, we chose a middle way—that of open, transparent, and respectful conversation. We thereby shed light on our differences of perspective, including those of researcher and research participant. We present Emily's initial, spontaneous responses to our analyses as originally written, and we later explicitly address the complex net of thorny issues raised by conflicting interpretations when participants are allowed to speak back to researchers in collaborative partnerships. This conversation between researchers and participant allowed us to better understand the complexities of power, privilege, ownership, interpretive authority, and validity in human scientific research.

The Organization and Uses of the Text

This text was written for student, novice, and seasoned professional qualitative researchers. The volume is organized in three parts. The first part tells the story of qualitative research in psychology, beginning with some of the greatest pioneering works and concluding with the contemporary movement and the typical organization of the qualitative research project. The second part and centerpiece of the volume presents Teresa's written description and subsequent interview about her struggle with cancer and accounts of each of the five approaches to qualitative analysis featuring the application to Teresa's story of traumatic loss. The third part of the volume addresses the contemporary problems of pluralism by providing a detailed comparison of the five approaches to analysis, the participant's response to the analyses, and an examination of such timely issues as research ethics, the meaning of the participant's responses to analysis, and specifications of the common fundaments and the distinctive features of five qualitative traditions.

The first chapter introduces the practice of qualitative research through an examination of noteworthy examples of its virtuoso practice in the history of psychology. After introducing the often unacknowledged wealth of seminal qualitative research in psychology, the work of master practitioners Sigmund Freud, William James, Abraham Maslow, and Lawrence Kohlberg reveals a goldmine of best practices. The methods and the knowledge developed by these pioneers, who address "the what" of psychopathology, dreams, religious experience, the healthy personality, human beings' best experiences, and the development of moral reasoning, serve as models and reference points throughout this volume. In this chapter we also discuss Gordon Allport's critical call for a formal methodology and practice norms for qualitative research, which anticipates the contemporary movement.

Chapter 2 focuses on the work of methodologists who have elevated qualitative analytic practice to praxis and have established various traditions of research by reflecting on their scientific basis and norms and formally specifying analytic practices to be used by researchers throughout the human sciences. Chapter 3 traces the recent appropriation and spread of growing knowledge and applications of qualitative analyses, including a focus on issues that most concern contemporary qualitative researchers and a summary of the problems and organization of the typical qualitative research project today.

Chapter 4 presents Teresa's verbatim written description and interview, providing readers with access to the raw data that the five researchers used in their analyses. The appendix includes the written description and interview offered by Gail, the elite gymnast who suffered and overcame a serious injury as a result of her athletic accident. Gail's texts, utilized in three of the five analyses that follow, also provide additional data for reference and use by readers, who can thereby apply the various analytic approaches detailed in this book to these data in their own, fuller way. Chapters 5–9 focus on the five analytic traditions and analyses of Teresa's texts (including some analyses of Gail's texts), in turn. Each chapter offers an overview of the history, philosophy, conceptual underpinnings, and procedures of the specified approach as well as its application to Teresa's texts.

Chapter 10 contains explicit comparisons of the five approaches to qualitative analysis, as viewed through the lenses of each of the five traditions. These comparisons bring to light the unique attractions, commonalities, distinctive features, strengths, and relevant applications of each approach. Chapter 11 includes Emily's responses to the analyses. The final chapter, Chapter 12, concludes with an examination of the main themes of the volume: ethics, the involvement of the participant in research, and methodological insights concerning the foundations of qualitative research and the distinctive features of its various traditions. Here we define the common fundaments of qualitative analysis that are shared by diverse practitioners, including the five traditions that are featured in this book and the virtuoso practitioners whose past works have had great impact. This generic foundation of qualitative analysis may be useful as a guide for researchers who do not affiliate with any single tradition. We also identify the options and unique advantages afforded by the five featured methodological traditions available among the multiple contemporary approaches to qualitative human science. The two raw data sets, multiple methods, and the involvement of the research participant herself, are elaborated in order to provide students and researchers with greater understanding of the achievements and challenges of the growing field of qualitative research.

This volume is intended to inform and provoke thought among qualitative researchers who study human experience. It also serves as an introduction to the "nuts and bolts" of qualitative research, addressing not merely the *why* and the *what*, but also the *how* of qualitative methods. We hope that our sharing of the history, movement, and contemporary applications of detailed analysis of lived experience (i.e., experience as it concretely and spontaneously takes place in actual human life)[1] is of interest to the full range of disciplines concerned with human existence. The psychological research and analytic methods featured in this text can be fruitfully extended by researchers working in such disciplines as anthropology, sociology, history, political sciences, and economics as well as in such interdisciplinary and professional fields as health, education, social service, business, counseling, and women's studies. This book is intended for independent investigators and students at graduate and advanced undergraduate levels in general courses on research methodology and in specific courses on qualitative research in human science disciplines. It can complement textbooks on quantitative methods and on qualitative methods. This book can also be used in courses on qualitative research methods in conjunction with readings from journal articles and other books that address such issues as data collection strategies and report writing. The inclusion of complete written and interview data sets from two participants allows readers to conduct their own original analyses, using the approaches detailed in this volume and others, in order to learn, explore, and compare variants of qualitative analysis.

Note

1. The term *lived experience*, frequently used by qualitative researchers, has been drawn from the continental tradition of the humanities and human sciences, as a translation of the German word *Erlebnis*. For a wonderfully informative exposition of the historical origins, meaning, usage, and complex concept of this term, see Gadamer (1960/1985, pp. 55–63). The word Erlebnis became common only in the 1870s as a derivation of the older word *Erleben*, which often appeared in the age of Goethe. The word Erlebnis began to be used in biographical writings in which it referred to *immediate* experience, in contrast to conceptual knowledge and interpretation, and connoted the weight and consequence and *temporal significance* of experience. The concept of *lived* experience, in contrast to the abstractions of experience in theory (e.g., "sensation") and measurement (e.g., "absolute threshold"), has included its inherent teleology, productivity, relationality, and above all, meaningfulness in the context of the person's larger life.

References

Denzin, N. K., & Lincoln, Y. S. (1994). Preface. In N. K. Denzin & Y. S. Lincoln (Eds.), *Handbook of qualitative research* (pp. ix–xii). Thousand Oaks, CA: Sage.
Gadamer, H.-G. (1985). *Truth and method.* New York: Crossroad Publishing. (Original work published 1960)

PART I

A STORY OF QUALITATIVE RESEARCH IN PSYCHOLOGY

CHAPTER 1

From Innovative Practices to the Call for Methodology

Q ualitative research methods were originally developed by individual investigators doing research through which new knowledge was acquired. Only later were these practices reflected upon, specified, spread through publication and education, and applied by other researchers. Research methodology is a rational articulation of performances by individual scientists. The qualitative research methodology that has guided the contemporary movement has not focused in detail on the research practices of psychologists prior to the emergence of qualitative methodologies. Contemporary investigators across all disciplines can draw valuable strategies, procedures, and principles from the practices of the qualitative researchers who produced landmark studies of the lived experience of individual persons. Grounded familiarity with a variety of best historical practices in qualitative research on human experience gives perspective and breadth to the understanding of the general methodologies that have followed them. Study of original practices that produced significant knowledge of lived experience can also provide new insights for the continuing development of methodologies for qualitative research.

In this chapter we first provide a historical overview of research that is well known for its important contributions to psychological knowledge but whose qualitative research methods have remained largely unexamined. They are an untapped resource for qualitative researchers in all disciplines and professions. With this road map, scholars and students of qualitative research methods can identify, revisit, study, and learn from the actual doing of qualitative research in successful works. We then explore in some detail the diverse qualitative research practices of four pioneers of research on human experience: Sigmund Freud, William James, Abraham Maslow, and Lawrence Kohlberg. The close study of their strategies provides contemporary researchers in many disciplines with methods ripe for appropriation and utilization in their own research. The variety of these ways of doing research will also foster a more concrete understanding of the methodologies that have more abstractly specified these practices. Finally in this chapter, we turn to Gordon Allport's critical review of these practice innovations and his call for a formal research methodology based on them. As part of an initiative across the social sciences in 1942, Allport argued that the establishment and utilization of qualitative research into subjective meaning requires the formal study of these methods and the legitimization of their scientific norms. This volume highlights the continuity in the historical development of qualitative research practices as well as the unity and complementarity of methods across diverse traditions, disciplines, and applications. Many of the ways of doing qualitative research found in the works discussed in this chapter are featured in the five methodological traditions introduced later in this volume, are employed in the five analyses of Teresa's narrative and interview, and can be used in a wide range of contemporary research.

Qualitative Research in the History of Psychology

Historians of psychology remind us that the first person to be called a "psychologist"—the founder of scientific psychology, Wilhelm Wundt—not only established the first experimental laboratory in 1879, marking the birth of this independent discipline, but also conducted qualitative research published in his 10-volume *Völkerpsychologie* (translated variously as "cultural psychology," "social psychology," and "folk psychology"; Wundt, 1900–1920, 1916). Recent scholarship has corrected longstanding misunderstandings of the legacies of Wundt's contributions, including his vision of psychology's disciplinary identity and research methods (Wong, 2009). Wundt argued for a close connection between psychology and philosophy. He defined psychology as a *Geisteswissenshaft* (human science), for which physics and physiology are auxiliary, and as an *interpretive* discipline that is foundational for the other mental sciences such as history and sociology. He viewed qualitative research as central to psychology and as a necessary complement to experimental psychology. Throughout his career, Wundt emphasized the importance of qualitative research on language, expressive movement, imagination, art, mythology, religion, and morality. In his autobiography, he characterized the investigations in the *Völkerpsychologie* (1900–1920) as his most satisfying life work (Wong, 2009).

Qualitative research methods used in psychology prior to World War II are still overlooked and sometimes derided within the field. Many who used such methods often did not report their procedures, and some acknowledged them only partially and apologetically. Methodologists in psychology have focused on quantitative methods in contrast to those in other disciplines, who have credited and featured the qualitative research practices of pioneers in their fields. When qualitative methods began to generate excitement and acceptance in late 20th-century psychology, much of the groundbreaking qualitative research in psychology was long past, and its methods have remained unstudied. Although their theories are still frequently cited, their research methods remain unknown. Consequently, the methods of the virtuoso practitioners in psychology have not received the attention and study they deserve.

Scholarship has begun to identify a treasure trove of research that involves the practice of qualitative methods in psychology. Giorgi (2009) traced the use of descriptive analyses in nonclinical areas of psychology in the work of Wilhelm Wundt, Alfred Benet, E. B. Titchener, the Würzberg school, the Gestalt school, John Watson, Wilhelm Stern, Jean Piaget, and Frederic Bartlett. The only psychologists to be awarded the Nobel prize, Herbert Simon and Daniel Kahneman, both used qualitative methods as a basis for their award-winning research (Ericsson & Simon, 1993; Kahneman, 2003). Giorgi discovered a virtually unknown and substantial manual of qualitative experimentation published by Titchener and also reviewed five rarely cited holistic schools of psychology at the time of the Weimar Republic: the *Gestalt* psychology in Berlin, Wilhelm Stern's personalistic psychology, Feliz Krüger's *Ganzheitpsychologie* (integral or holistic psychology) in Leipzig, David Katz's phenomenological school, and Edward Spranger's *Verstehenpsychologie* (psychology of understanding). None survived the Nazi period and World War II in Germany. Wertz (1983, 1987a, 1987b, 1993, 2001) has documented qualitative analytic procedures throughout the traditions of psychoanalytic, humanistic, and existential research.

Marecek, Fine, and Kidder (1997) have brought to light pervasive and influential qualitative research in social psychology (p. 632). They cite, in successive decades from the 1930s through 1970s, John Dollard's (1937) studies of race and class; Kurt Lewin's (1948) research on group processes; Muzafer and Carolyn Sherif's (Sherif & Sherif, 1953) study of intergroup conflict; Leon Festinger, Henry Riecken, and Stanley Schacter's (1956) study of cognitive dissonance; and Philip Zimbardo's (Zimbardo, Haney, Banks, & Jaffe, 1975) study of deindividuation. Irving Janis's (1972) discovery and investigation of "groupthink" is yet another example of qualitative research in social psychology. Marecek et al. (1997) note frequent ambivalence on the part of social psychologists who admit their employment of qualitative methods, for instance, in David Rosenhan's (1973) classic participant–observational research on being in a mental institution.

Detailed, systematic study of the qualitative methods used in the most fruitful investigations has barely begun. As noted, we consider the work of four exemplary practitioners: Sigmund Freud, William James, Abraham Maslow, and Lawrence Kohlberg. Unconstrained by any how-to manual or clear-cut procedural steps, they collected and analyzed data of human experience. In taking up significant research problems and tailoring methods to their human subject matter, these researchers offer models for practice that remain informative and valuable today. In describing their work, we make note of their telling but incomplete commentaries concerning their methods, which are more enacted than accounted for in their reports. In each of these presentations, we focus not only on research methods but also make references to the resulting knowledge and its presentation, for here rests the significance of the research. Although it is possible to understand and practice standard statistical methods with minimal regard to specific research problems and results, qualitative research methods are shaped by their subject matter and are best understood in light of the findings. The methods we explore in this chapter, together with findings and reporting strategies, provide relevant background for our later study of the well-established analytic approaches.

Sigmund Freud: Uncovering Meaning in Symptoms, Dreams, Errors, and Culture

Although Sigmund Freud, the founder of psychoanalysis, is best known for his theories and psychotherapy, he considered psychoanalysis first and foremost a new scientific research method (Freud, 1926/1978). In his new science, Freud used qualitative data and analytic procedures. He researched a range of topics, including psychopathology, dreams, errors, emotions, personality, creativity, group behavior, psychotherapy, religion, invention, literature, and art. Anticipating the breadth of contemporary qualitative data collection, Freud integrated naturalistic observations, descriptions of his own first-person experience, written anecdotes submitted by acquaintances and strangers, and interviews with others. He also used archival data such as letters, memoirs, autobiographies, biographies, inventions, art works, and literature. Addressing a spectrum of topics, Freud's research yielded concrete observations, comparative analyses, descriptive generalizations, broad and topical theories, and even (at times admittedly wild) speculations. Here we focus primarily on Freud's research on psychopathology with his own patients, though he himself recognized that the value of his research method extended far beyond clinical psychology. Freud ventured that the scientific value of his methods could be found in other areas of psychology and in other social sciences. Freud believed that psychoanalysis would make its most important contribution if investigators across all human sciences would "agree themselves to handle this new instrument of research [psychoanalysis] which is at their service. The use of analysis for the treatment of neurosis is only one of its applications; the future will perhaps show that it is not the most important one" (Freud, 1926, p. 97). Contemporary research—for instance, in literary studies, history, and critical theory—may bear out Freud's prophesy.

Freud began his professional practice as a physician by employing the standard treatments of the day with patients who suffered predominantly from hysteria. Initially Freud visited his patients' homes, sometimes daily, providing massage, electrotherapy, and hydrotherapy—physical treatments. Most decisive for the development of his research method was the *psychological* practice of hypnosis. Freud learned the procedure by studying with Liébeault, Bernheim, and Charcot, leading experts at inducing a somnambulistic trance in patients, who then became increasingly receptive to physicians' suggestions that their pathological symptoms would cease and that normal functioning would ensue. For instance, if a patient suffered from cheek pains and paralyzed legs, the physician would induce a hypnotic trance and suggest that the pains would vanish and that walking would resume normally. With noteworthy frequency, patients appeared to recover following treatment with hypnotic suggestion.

Freud employed hypnosis in an innovative manner, using suggestion not only to remove symptoms but also to encourage emotional expression or "catharsis" (Strachey, 1957). His first scientific breakthrough came from an even more original alteration of the use of hypnosis, which Strachey has characterized as Freud's "most important achievement . . . his invention of the first instrument for the scientific investigation of the human mind" (Strachey, 1957, p. xvi). Freud's practice of collecting life historical descriptions from medical patients under hypnosis yielded new insights, the scientific significance of which escaped neither Freud nor his senior colleague, Joseph Breuer (Breuer & Freud, 1895/1957). For instance, a patient whom they called "Anna O." sought Breuer's help in resolving her inability to drink water. This strange symptom, which forced Anna O. to subsist on fruit and melons for 6 weeks, proved amenable to hypnotic treatment. One evening under hypnosis, she grumbled in disgust about a disliked English maid-companion whose "horrid little dog" had drunk from Anna's glass. Wanting to be polite, Anna had said nothing at the time. Only later, under hypnosis, did she give energetic expression to the anger she had held back. After this cathartic session, she asked for something to drink and consumed a large quantity of water without any difficulty. The symptom never returned. For Freud, more important even than the effectiveness of this treatment was the insight that hysterical symptoms are psychogenic and related to the person's life historical experience.

Most important to Freud was the transformation of hypnotic procedures into a *method of investigating* these phenomena in order to discover their *meaning*. Having recognized the research potential of hypnosis in Breuer's earlier case of Anna O. (treated between 1880 and 1882), Freud began to regularly ask hypnotized patients to describe the life experiences in the course of which their hysterical symptoms first appeared. Freud collected hundreds of descriptions of life historical situations and mental processes in which symptoms originated. He compared them to each other and analyzed their commonalities. One of the commonalities Freud found among the observations he collected was what he called the patient's "strangulated affect." These patients all suffered disturbing experiences and negative emotions which, in a well-organized effort to maintain socially proper behavior, were not directly expressed and were suffered obscurely, both revealed and concealed, in their somatic symptoms. Freud's new methods of data collection and analysis formed the qualitative research foundation of a new kind of science of psychopathology that would guide therapy and theory and that would offer a model for the investigation of a wide spectrum of human experiences.

The procedures Freud developed for research did not come from a classroom, from a textbook, from Brucke's physiological laboratory, where he trained, or from the demonstrations of experts. They came from his patients, who increasingly demanded that he *listen to them*. Freud did indeed listen and observe. He also reflected, analyzed, and reported what he learned. He was as much the midwife of these new research procedures as their inventor. As Freud's practice of research evolved, he used hypnosis less frequently, coming to rely on what he called patients' "free associations." Freud made use of patients' spontaneous expressions in increasingly broad investigations of the origins and meanings of symptoms, dreams, errors, artistic and scientific productions, and a full spectrum of human activities. In this context, he realized the importance of understanding, of *interpretation*, in the analysis of psychological life (Strachey, 1957, p. xviii).

In Freud's case study of Emmy Von N. (Breuer & Freud, 1895/1957), we see the importance of a *trusting relationship* with the investigator, the earliest account of free association, the value of detailed and honest descriptions of experience, the role of the analyst as an accepting and respectful confidant, the role of the patient as truth teller and moral agent, and the necessary use of narrative on the part of both patient and researcher. Freud systematically asked Emmy to concentrate on each symptom and to express whatever came to mind in connection with it. In every case, with persistence, Emmy disclosed the life historical context and meaning of the symptom in her waking consciousness. Emmy herself then spontaneously began to adopt and to employ this method, leading Freud to comment on what Strachey (1957) believed was his first reference to "free association":

Even without questioning under hypnosis, [Emmy] can discover the cause of her ill-humor that day. Nor is her conversation . . . so aimless as it might appear. On the contrary, it contains a fairly complete reproduction of the memories and new impressions which have affected her since our last talk, and it often leads on, in quite an unexpected way, to pathogenic reminiscences of which she unburdens herself without being asked to. It is as though she had adopted my procedure and was making use of our conversation, apparently unconstrained . . . as a supplement to hypnosis. (Breuer & Freud, 1895/1957, p. 56)

Freud observed that a full emotional disclosure of life experience was more therapeutically effective in eliminating hysterical symptoms than was hypnotic suggestion. Anna O. had called this activity "chimney sweeping" and its consequence "the talking cure." For symptoms to be relieved, the patients had not only to tell the whole story of their symptoms' origins but to tell it with complete honesty, detail, and feeling. Anything less would result in a failing or incomplete cure. Pragmatic, therapeutic goals led Freud to innovatively transform traditional etiological research into what is called *hermeneutic* and *narrative* inquiry.

Perhaps more important than curative effects of this "talk" were the new forms of relationship with others, scientific data, interpretive insight, and general knowledge that this kind of analysis entailed. Freud's patients began to insist that he listen to their lengthy stories without interrupting them with hypnotic suggestions. "When, three days ago, [Emmy] had first complained about her fear of asylums, I had interrupted her after her first story, that the patients were tied onto chairs. I now saw that I had gained nothing by this interruption and that I cannot evade listening to her stories in every detail to the very end" (Breuer & Freud, 1895/1957, p. 61). Emmy even demanded to speak without Freud's asking any questions. "She then said in a definitely grumbling tone that I was not to keep on asking her where this and that came from, but to let her tell me what she had to say. I fell in with this . . ." (p. 69). In response to Freud's willingness to simply listen, Emmy went on to express the deepest life historical core of her disturbance. From that day on, she "treated me [Freud] with special distinction" (p. 63) and expressed her life experience of her own accord, without hypnosis, revealing the meaning of all her symptoms. Freud found that he could achieve understanding with all his patients on the basis of hearing an honest and detailed account of the experiential context in which the symptoms had emerged.

The "intimate connection between the story of the patient's suffering and the symptoms" (Breuer & Freud, 1895/1957, p. 160) required Freud not only to sensitively interpret their meanings but to adopt a narrative mode of knowing and reporting. Freud was willing to adopt such methods because they were demanded by the subject matter of this new science, which involved trauma, conflict, frustration, unfulfilled desire, the restraint of emotional expression, and the avoidance of facing difficult emotional situations. Freud explained:

I have not always practiced as a psychotherapist. Like other neurologists, I was trained to employ local diagnoses and electro-prognosis, and it still strikes me as strange that the case histories I write should read like short stories and that, as one might say, they lack the serious stamp of science. I must console myself with the reflection that the nature of the subject matter is evidently responsible for this, rather than any preference of my own. The fact is that local diagnosis and electrical reactions lead nowhere in the study of hysteria, whereas a detailed description of mental processes such as we are accustomed to find in the works of imaginative writers enables me . . . to obtain at least some kind of insight into the course of that affliction. (Breuer & Freud, 1895/1957, pp. 160–161)

What Freud called "the fundamental rule" of psychoanalytic therapy was also an original and crucial research tool that yielded a huge body of data. Patients were instructed to express everything they experienced in Freud's presence, holding nothing back, no matter how seemingly irrelevant or disagreeable—the two conditions that limited complete disclosure.

So say whatever goes through your mind (regardless of its importance, apparent relevance, etc.). Act as though you were sitting at the window of a railway train and describe to someone behind you the changing views you see outside. Finally, never forget that you have promised absolute honesty, and never leave anything unsaid because for any reason it is unpleasant to say it. (Freud, 1913/1963, p. 147)

Such open expression required, on the part of the analyst, a nonjudgmental attitude of "evenly hovering attention" to all the details of the patient's speech. The analyst was to be nondirective, to remain silent and to listen, to speak only about signs of inhibition that might be limiting the patient's observation and description of his or her life experience. Eventually, the analyst gained greater understanding of these inhibitions—the patient's "resistance," rooted in past experiences with significant others ("transference"). In response to the analyst's interpretation of the patient's speech, patients became increasingly expressive, and the interpretations of the psychological processes became more revelatory and refined. By alternately collecting data and interpreting their meaning, Freud improved his understanding of each individual person. By continually comparing each case with others and analyzing their similarities and differences, Freud produced a general body of knowledge.

Freud considered his greatest work *The Interpretation of Dreams*, in which he presented the procedure he invented for investigating the meaning of dreams. Freud reported numerous analyses and interpretations of his own and others' dreams, accounts of the general psychological processes he inferred on the part of dreamers, and a general theory of dreaming (Freud, 1900/1965). At the heart of this work are Freud's careful techniques of observation, data collection, interpretation of meaning, and comparative analysis. He began with the descriptive report of the actual dream, in as much detail as possible. In order to investigate its meaning, Freud meticulously differentiated each of the elements of the dream. Then, in connection with each manifest dream content, he instructed the dreamer to adopt an open attitude and report all thoughts, feelings, memories, and so on, that occurred. In view of these laboriously collected data, understood in the relevant life context of the dreamer, Freud interpreted the dream with reference to significant experiential patterns of which the dream was a part. In order to arrive at a general knowledge of dreaming, Freud methodically compared the analyses of a large number of individual dreams by dreamers of varied ages and life circumstances. In comparing analyses of children's dreams with each other and with those of adults, Freud was able to relate many dreams to the dreamers' wishes that were unfulfilled during the previous day. Freud found that a "wish-fulfilling aim," quite obvious in many children's dreams, was often not immediately evident in adults' dreams but could be discerned by employing an extended contextual analysis of adult dreamers' past experiences and the lack of emotional satisfaction he observed in them.

Freud found that the investigation of human experience required meticulous investigations of living persons who could provide fresh data through observations, verbal reports, and interviews. Such investigations were not sufficient and required supplementation by archival data of many sorts, including personal letters, memoirs, autobiographies, inventions, artistic and literary creations, as well as cultural and symbolic products such as jokes, language, religious rituals and doctrines, and social institutions. Freud drew upon all of these sources in his analyses and argued, against the American medical establishment, that rigorous research of human experience requires a broad interdisciplinary education and training. In *The Question of Lay Analysis*, Freud (1926/1978) insisted that the special demands of human subject matter require background knowledge quite different from that of natural science and medicine. He concluded that medical training not only is useless but is the opposite of what is needed; it develops skills and knowledge that are detrimental and inappropriate in psychoanalysis. Freud asserted that when natural scientists and physicians ridicule genuinely psychological methods and knowledge as unscientific, they are failing to recognize the obligations that derive from mental life; they "therefore fall into the layman's lack of respect for psychological research" (Freud, 1926/1978, p. 73). Freud held that the knowledge and skills required by the psychological scientist are acquired in the study of humanities and other social sciences, including the history of civilization, sociology, religion, mythology, and the study of art and literature (Freud, 1926/1978). In this way, Freud anticipated the rich cross-disciplinary breadth required by qualitative research in psychology.

Although Freud did not provide a systematic research methodology for human science, his research strategies anticipate this later work and are consistent with current best practices. Freud recognized that knowledge of the subject matter precedes knowledge of the science itself. In one of his last papers, he acknowledged that research involves two persons, analysand and analyst, and that he had not focused on the latter. "The dynamic determinants of this process [of the analysand becoming conscious] are so interesting that the other portion of the work, the task performed by the analyst, has been pushed to the background" (Freud, 1937, p. 258). Freud noted the importance, for instance, of learning more about the procedures though which the analyst "works over observations" in the process of interpretation. Many of the procedures Freud used in this work, as described above, have been highlighted by later qualitative methodologists. The diversity of data collected by Freud, including first-person descriptions, interview conversations, behavioral observations, documents, artistic products, language, social practices, and cultural phenomena, anticipated current qualitative research practices and methodologies. Freud emphasized the importance of a trusting, nonjudgmental relationship with research participants to overcome habitual social prohibitions and to elicit the full, honest, detailed, emotional expression of lived experience. He meticulously differentiated parts of experiential reports and collected more extensive data about related experiences in individuals' lives. Freud took his primary task to be the data-based interpretation of meaning, and he gained insight by focusing on the purposes and contexts of experiences within a person's larger life story. Freud shared his interpretations with those whose lives he interpreted, and he used their extended responses to confirm or reshape his understandings, alternately collecting data and offering insight in an ongoing conversation. He continually compared analyses of the same and different persons in order to form more general knowledge. Finally, Freud insisted on the distinctiveness and unity of the human science disciplines in contrast to the physical sciences.

William James:
Analyzing the Forms of Spiritual Experience

William James was educated as a physician, though he never practiced medicine. He began his career as a physiologist. Although James is considered the father of American psychology and is held in high regard as one of its most brilliant and influential pioneers, his works are seldom studied in psychology. *The Varieties of Religious Experience* well exemplifies James's psychological research and remains a showcase of practices in the qualitative research of human experience. James wrote this book after he moved from the Department of Psychology to the Department of Philosophy at Harvard. Though over 100 years old, James's investigation is a classic and continues to be used by scholars in all the humanities and cultural sciences that are concerned with human spirituality.

The goal of James's research was to answer a qualitative psychological question: What is the nature, the constitution, of religious experience? (1902/1982, p. 9). Like Freud, James's research practice was guided by careful reflections on the disciplinary distinctiveness of experiential study and on the demands that human subject matter makes on research. James emphasized the need to focus on the "existential conditions" (p. 9) of these experiences, that is, to abstain from viewing his subject matter from the standpoints of theology (supernatural beliefs), neurobiology (physical conditions), and psychopathology (deficiency in relation to norms). Instead, religious experience was to be understood by "the significance for life of religion, taken 'on the whole'" (p. 485). The scientific study of this subject matter, James emphasized, requires research that does not repudiate, as does physical science, the *personal point of view*. Instead, psychology must respect the meanings that subjective experience has for individuals. James's articulation of meaning verges on the poetic as he insists that the psychologist attend to

> the terror and beauty of phenomena, the "promise" of the dawn and of the rainbow, the "voice" of the thunder, the "gentleness" of the summer rain, the "sublimity" of the stars, and not the physical laws which these things follow. . . . [A]s soon as we deal with private and personal phenomena as such, we deal with realities in the completest sense of the term . . . the world of experience. (p. 498)

James was defining what is now called the *qualitative research stance.*

At the start of his research, James conceptually delineated his subject matter in a way that was at once highly specific regarding inclusion and exclusion criteria and yet open with regard to conclusions. He distinguished *religious experience*, what we today call "spirituality," from individuals' involvement in religious institutions, including their organized rituals and dogmatic beliefs, and he restricted his study to the former. James deliberately abstained from adopting rigid definitions and previously established conceptualizations of religious experience in order "not [to] fall immediately into a one-sided view of our topic" (1902/1982, p. 26). Believing that abstract conceptions are "more misleading than enlightening" (pp. 26–27), James sought to gain an "intimate acquaintance with particulars" with regard to "*the feelings, acts, experiences of individual men* [humans] *in their solitude, so far as they apprehend themselves to stand in relations to whatever they may consider the divine*" (p. 31, italics in original). James's research practice involved an open, unprejudiced attention to concrete human life.

James's method was to collect hundreds of examples of religious living that were as widely ranging and variable as possible. "To understand a thing rightly we need to . . . have acquaintance with the whole range of its variations" (1902/1982, p. 22). The plan of his inquiry was to utilize data that best expressed his subject matter in the ordinary lives of those who experienced it most fully, namely:

> subjective phenomena recorded in literature produced by articulate and fully self-conscious men [humans], in works of piety and autobiography. . . . [T]he documents that will concern us most will be those of the men [humans] who were most accomplished in the religious life, and the best able to give an intelligible account of their ideas and motives. . . . The *documents humains* which we shall find most instructive need not then be sought for in the haunts of special erudition—they lie along the beaten highway.

These ordinary humans who had lived through his research phenomenon and expressed their experience, James believed, would yield knowledge "close to the essence of the matter" (p. 3). James engaged in intimate contact with actual instances of his subject matter from the start of his data collection to the final presentation of his research. "In my belief that a large acquaintance with particulars often makes us wiser than the possession of abstract formulas, however deep, I have loaded the lectures with concrete examples" (p. xxxv). James's research method involved conceptualization not derived from preconceptions but emerging from an encounter with singular realities.

James observed that religious and nonreligious experiences are seamlessly blended in the lives of those who experience the former most abundantly. Therefore, collecting examples of distinctly religious experience in order to conceptually differentiate its qualities from other experiences is very difficult. Because of this difficulty James selected his data from reports of the most extreme examples of religious experience, for instance, those that led to radical transformations, such as the conversion of an atheist to a formal religion; those who gave up habits of alcohol, smoking, and violence under the influence of a religious revelation; mystics whose revelations and insights had great personal and social consequence; saints who habitually chose charity, poverty, and physical deprivation; and martyrs who undertook hardship, suffered torture, and even embraced death in their acts of faith. James stated what appears to be a profound principle of qualitative method: "It always leads to a better understanding of a thing's significance to consider its exaggerations and perversions" (James, 1902/1982, p. 22). To achieve sufficient variety and extremity of real-life examples, James used archival data from letters, observations, journals, autobiographies, and biographies that contained descriptions of religious experiences ranging from West to East, from theistic to atheistic, and spanning Jewish, Christian, Islamic, Hindu, Buddhist, Emersonian transcendentalist, and even psychopathological and drug-induced religious experiences. The dramatic and often aberrant character of James's material tends to obscure his insightful methodological rationale for choosing extremity over normality in his sampling.

In the most extreme examples of martyrs' imperturbability, for instance, James was able to grasp the reversal of ordinary human values and the sense of well-being that may paradoxically encompass suffering in religious experience. Mundane bodily safety and comfort take on an altered meaning in connection with experiences of the heavenly. James's research vividly supported his insights with abundant and extensive quotations directly from his data. James cited Blanche Gamond's description of her religious persecution under Louis XIV:

> Six women, each with a bunch of willow rods as thick as the hand can hold . . . tied me to a beam in the kitchen. They drew the cord tight with all their strength and asked me, "Does this hurt you?," and they discharged their fury on me, exclaiming as they struck me, "Now pray to your God." But at this moment I received the greatest consolation . . . since I had the honor of being whipped in the name of Christ. . . . Why can I not write down the inconceivable influences, consolations, and peace I felt interiorly? . . . They were so great that I was ravished, for there where afflictions abound grace is given superabundantly. In vain the women cried, "We must double our blows; she does not feel them, for she neither speaks nor cries." And how should I have cried, since I was swooning with happiness within. (James, 1902/1982, pp. 288–289)

With mountains of data before him, James's method of analysis is detailed, comparative, thematic, and generalizing. He focused on, identified, and descriptively elaborated such typical experiential patterns and themes of religious life as "the reality of the unseen," "healthy religion," "unhealthy religion," conversion, the lifestyle of saintliness, the value of religious experience, and many others. In attempting to grasp higher levels of generality, James compared widely varying experiences and discerned the common characteristics that qualitatively distinguish various types of religious experience as well as the even more general characteristics of all human experiences. In order to achieve conceptual precision at the highest level of generality, James compared religious experiences to nonreligious experiences that included similar behaviors and environmental conditions. For instance, he found a peculiar kind of happiness on the part of Christian saints as they ministered to the sick that was not present in the moral resignation characteristic of work on the part of stoics. James's comparative analysis identified the essential qualitative characteristics of religious experience "to get at its typical *differentia*" (James, 1902/1982, p. 48). As an outcome of his comparative analyses, James consolidated the insight that in the fluidity of real-world lived experience, religiosity and stoicism may pass from one to the other, may blend with each other, and may manifest in intermediate stages (pp. 46–47). However, on the basis of extreme, relatively pure examples of each, James was able to sharply delineate qualitative knowledge of their differences. Particularly in the face of the same objective conditions of sickness and death, the happy, easeful, even rapturous approach of the saint was understood in sharp contrast with the moralist's tense muscles, uneasy breath, and strained effort to achieve a worldly goal.

Discerning the essence through variations, James outlined and detailed the most general characteristics of religious experience in the cognitive, behavioral, and affective lives of individuals of both genders and various cultures, ages, and walks of life. In these findings, James aimed at what is most general: "I am expressly trying to reduce religion to its lowest admissible terms, to that minimum, free from individual variations, which all religions contain as their nucleus, and on which it may be hoped that all religious persons may agree" (James, 1902/1982, p. 503). James found the following invariants in religious beliefs: (1) The visible world is part of a more spiritual world from which it draws its significance; (2) union or harmony with that higher universe is our true end; and (3) communion with the spirit thereof produces real effects, psychological and material, in the phenomenal world. He found the following invariants in religious emotional and social experience: (4) a new zest, as if a gift to life, taking the form of either lyrical enchantment or earnestness and heroism; and (5) An assurance of safety, a temper of peace, and a preponderance of loving affections in relation to others. James concluded that the faith state may hold a very minimum of intellectual content; it may involve "a mere vague enthusiasm, half spiritual, half vital, a courage, and a feeling that great and wondrous feelings are in the air" (p. 505). James found the fruits of religious experience in the charity, devotion, trust, patience, and bravery of saints, illustrated by St. Francis and St. Ignatius exchanging their clothes with beggars, by saints kissing lepers, and by brawling alcoholics turning a cheek to abusive others after religious conversion. The saint loves enemies, cares for the sick, and endures pain and suffering with a light and uplifting attitude in spiritual experience. In the face of failure, loss, sickness and death, the ordinary believer quietly receives consolation from faith.

James was aware that his investigation involved a new attitude and method, a new kind of science that contrasts with the natural sciences. He assumed that the limits of the latter would come into greater relief in the future. "The rigorously impersonal view of science might one day appear as having been a temporarily useful eccentricity rather than a definitively triumphant position which the sectarian scientist at present so confidently announces it to be" (James, 1902/1982, p. 501). James's research on spiritual experience acquired a kind of knowledge that functions evocatively and that verges on wisdom. It enriches those who share it and opens one's heart and mind to understanding the experience as it is lived by oneself and by others. This knowledge involves a rigorous investigation of the psychological reality under study that is analytical, systematic, and above all thoroughly empirical. For James, this kind of research alone enables science to unflinchingly confront the subject matter of the human person.

James's research practices, like Freud's, anticipate later qualitative methodologies. James emphasized the importance of focusing on subjective experience, the "personal," "existential" point of view, in contrast to theistic dogma, on the one hand, and materialistic facts, on the other. He insisted on holism—taking experiences in the whole of life. He placed aside abstract conceptualizations of the subject matter and instead worked with highly detailed, concrete examples of his subject matter offered by ordinary people who had genuinely lived through and articulately expressed the experiences under investigation. James noted the methodological value of extreme real-life examples of his subject matter, and he deliberately sought out many cultural and historical variations. His analytic work involved continual comparison of differences, through which he found both highly general characteristics of the experiences under study as well as typical variations. James used and advocated dramatic, evocative language in conveying his findings, viewing this kind of discourse as appropriate for knowledge of personal subjective experience. His hope that the legitimacy of this new kind of personal science would become more respected and practiced has been realized in the work of later qualitative methodologists and researchers.

Abraham Maslow:
Identifying Qualities of the Healthy Personality

Abraham Maslow was trained as an experimental psychologist studying primate dominance and sexuality in the laboratory of Harry Harlow. He was the cofounder, with Anthony Sutich, of humanistic psychology and of transpersonal psychology. Maslow became dissatisfied by the psychology of the first half of the 20th century because its dominant paradigms—the experimental study of animals and the clinical study of psychopathology—failed to provide knowledge of human beings at their best. He later studied with Alfred Adler and adopted mentors in Max Wertheimer and Ruth Benedict—both pioneers in qualitative research. Unlike Wundt, Freud, and James, who explicitly insisted on the scientific nature of qualitative methods, Maslow viewed them as deficient in an academic field dominated by behaviorism. Maslow did not consider his research "science." His well-known study of *self-actualization* (a term he borrowed from Kurt Goldstein [1934/1995], the Gestalt neurologist who formulated the concept in his qualitative study of brain-injured soldiers after World War I) "was not planned as ordinary research." Maslow's study was undertaken as a private quest, as personal learning in order to satisfy his own curiosity, a way of solving "personal moral, ethical, and scientific problems" (Maslow, 1954/1987, p. 199). Maslow did not initially intend to publish his groundbreaking study, but its unexpected enlightenment and exciting implications for general psychology demanded that "some sort of report should be made to others in spite of its methodological shortcomings" (p. 199).

Although Maslow was ambivalent about the scientific nature of his study, he believed that the importance of the subject matter—the healthy personality—and the impossibility of approaching it through traditional research methods justified his unusual approach. "I consider the problem of psychological health to be so pressing, that any suggestions, any bits of data, however moot, are endowed with great heuristic value. . . . [I]f we wait for conventionally reliable data, we should have to wait forever" (Maslow, 1954/1987, p. 199). Maslow reported having to overcome his fear of mistakes in this uncharted territory, to plunge in, to do his best, to learn from his blunders, and eventually to correct the shortcomings of his investigation, lest he refuse to work on the problem at all. Given the importance of his topic for psychology, Maslow presented his report "with due apologies to those who insist on conventional reliability, validity, sampling, and the like" (p. 125).

Maslow began this informal personal investigation by taking careful observational notes on the behaviors of Max Wertheimer and Ruth Benedict, whom he considered "wonderful human beings." As he expanded his pool of research participants, Maslow utilized mainstream research tools (diagnostic assessment) and measurement instruments (tests of personality and psychopathology) in order to eliminate individuals with mental disorders from his research sample. However, he believed that the positive delineation of "psychological health" required qualitative procedures. Maslow developed a technique he called "iteration," a cyclical practice in which conceptual definition and empirical investigation alternate, each inform the other, and gradually yield a more precise and adequate definition of his subject matter, "psychological health."

Maslow's analysis began with nontechnical, personal, and cultural formulations of the features of psychological health, and from these he assembled what he called a "folk definition." He first collated extant expressions about psychological health in everyday speech (the "lexicographical stage") and carefully synthesized them, still remaining within ordinary semantics. After modifying this definition in order to eliminate logical and factual inconsistencies and to achieve greater internal consistency, Maslow formulated a "corrected folk definition." On this basis, he selected and compared two groups of participants—one that seemed to manifest the characteristics designated in the corrected folk definition and the other that did not manifest these qualities of healthy personality. After collecting data from these two groups using "clinical methods" (psychological tests and in-depth interviewing), Maslow conducted a comparative analysis of participants that yielded a sharper, "clinical definition." The negative criterion in this definition was the absence of neurosis, psychopathic personality, psychosis, or strong tendencies in this direction. The positive criterion, though difficult to describe and not yet fully articulated, was the utilization of talents, capacities, and potentialities, such that the person has developed, or is developing, the full stature of which she or he is capable. At this stage of his research, Maslow conceptualized self-actualized individuals as being relaxed; as having gratified their basic emotional needs for safety, belongingness, love, respect, and self-esteem; as engaged in fulfilling their cognitive needs for knowledge and understanding; and as having developed their philosophical, religious, and axiological bearings. This more empirically informed clinical definition led Maslow, in selecting individuals for further study, to retain some, to drop others, and to add new participants to the "healthy personality" group. Maslow did acknowledge the general applicability and scientificity of this method as a legitimate way of clarifying a psychological construct. "In this way, an originally vague and unscientific folk concept can become more and more exact . . . [and] therefore more scientific" (Maslow, 1954/1987, p. 127).

Maslow used multiple data sources because he, like James, aimed to discriminate what is common among diverse concrete examples of his subject matter. He identified healthy personalities among friends and personal acquaintances. He also carefully studied texts describing the lives of such public and historical figures as Albert Einstein, Eleanor Roosevelt, and Lao Tsu, the founder of Taoism. Further observations, testing, interviews, and readings provided the data for Maslow's comparative analyses. Maslow's sampling was not random but quite purposeful and critical. He initially intended to include college students and even fictional characters from literary works in his sample of healthy personalities. However, as Maslow's understanding of "self-actualization" evolved through the series of tentative definitions, participant selections, comparative analyses, and increasingly refined definitions, college students appeared to fall short of his emerging criteria, as did fictional characters, so he excluded them from further research. Although Maslow was clear about the general characteristics of his procedure—"the spiral-like process of self correction"—he did not make any of his raw data available, nor did he (1) specify the procedures of analyzing the data collected on individual persons, (2) detail the procedures of comparison within and between his research groups, (3) report how many series of iteration took place, nor (4) provide abundant examples of how each series of data collection and analysis achieved more refined concepts and empirical groupings of individuals. Maslow did indicate, as an illustration of the increasing adequacy of his knowledge, that the original folk definition tended to define the healthy personality in overly idealized, even perfectionistic terms, "so unrealistically demanding that no living human being could possibly fit the definition" (Maslow, 1954/1987, p. 202). The evidence-based nature of this study, including both data and analysis of particular persons in the "healthy personality" group, required and provided a definition of the healthy personality that included foibles, mistakes, foolishness, and imperfections of various sorts.

Like James, who found it difficult to define the religious experience, Maslow evidently struggled to classify individuals as "self-actualized." He characterized participants as "fairly sure," "highly probably," "partial," and "developing in that direction," and reported the number of persons in each group. It is interesting to note that as Maslow's study continued longitudinally, the number of self-actualized contemporaries increased from three, who were "fairly sure" in Maslow's first edition (1954), to seven, who were "fairly sure" in the third edition (1954/1987), but the reported qualities of the healthy personality did not change. Maslow finally included nine contemporaries who were interviewed, nine historical and public figures, and five "partial cases," who fell short of the full criteria but nevertheless were helpful in the study.

In conducting this basic theoretical research about personality, Maslow borrowed methods from clinical psychology. He often characterized his method as "clinical," by which he meant that his procedures were flexible, were adapted to each individual research participant, and aimed at understanding each person's spontaneous life in great concrete detail. Practical and ethical problems required compromise, making it difficult for Maslow to acquire complete data commensurate with the deepest and most extensive clinical studies, which he held as a methodological ideal. For instance, the older participants, when informed of the nature of this research, became self-conscious, froze up, or often terminated participation. Consequently, Maslow observed and studied some individuals "indirectly, almost surreptitiously," including them in his study without formal interviews. Because participants' names could not be divulged, the usual public availability and repeatability of investigation were not possible. However, Maslow attempted to adhere to the ideal of public verification of his knowledge claims by including public and historical figures in his study.

Maslow likened the understanding that he developed on the basis of this data collection to "the slow development of a global and holistic impression of the sort that we form of friends and acquaintances" (1954/1987, p. 128). It was not possible to set up situations as one would an experiment or to do testing with some participants. Maslow took advantage of fortuitous opportunities that presented themselves in everyday life, where he spontaneously invited persons to participate in his research and interviewed them to whatever extent circumstances allowed. Consequently, standardization was not possible, and the data were often incomplete. Using a procedure he called "holistic analysis," Maslow formed an overall comprehensive conceptualiza-tion of the healthy personality by integrating various insights into the data from his participants. Maslow expressed his findings in a composite portrait of the psychology of "self-actualization" by describing the interrelated themes that characterize the lives of these most healthy persons.

Maslow's findings, in spite of the great care and rigor he employed in this unusual empirical method, must have struck him as unfamiliar given the models of psychological knowledge he encountered in contemporary educa-tion, training, and professional journals. Consequently, Maslow appears to have had doubts about the scientific validity of his findings. In his first pub-lication, after lamenting the small number of participants, the incomplete-ness of the data, and the impossibility of quantitative analysis, he says, "only composite impressions can be offered for whatever they may be worth (and of course they are worth much less than controlled objective observation, since the investigator is never quite certain about what is a description and what is a projection)" (1954/1987, p. 203). It is interesting to note that this last paren-thetical phrase in Maslow's methods section is removed in the third edition (1954/1987) of his classic text. One can only wonder whether his confidence in the scientific legitimacy of his findings increased over time.

Maslow's findings, which he considered *observational* despite his reser-vations, are rich and provocative. Drawn from and descriptive of his data, Maslow's knowledge claims amount to an empirically grounded, general, dimensional conceptualization of the psychological processes in the life of a healthy person, which he illustrated by means of the empirical details of his cases. The characteristics Maslow brought to light and clarified include the following:

- ♦ Efficient perception of and comfortable relations with reality
- ♦ An open and accepting attitude regarding self
- ♦ A spontaneous style
- ♦ Problem-centered and self-transcendent cognition
- ♦ Comfort in and enjoyment of solitude
- ♦ Autonomous self-direction
- ♦ A fresh appreciation of novel and ordinary experiences of work, others, and nature
- ♦ Frequent peak or "mystical" experiences
- ♦ A sense of kinship with humanity
- ♦ Humility, respect for, and a tendency to learn from a variety of other people different from oneself
- ♦ A democratic political stance

♦ Deep and close, though perhaps few, interpersonal relationships

♦ Strong ethical standards

♦ A high intrinsic value orientation

♦ A thoughtful (nonhostile) sense of humor

♦ Pervasive creativity

♦ An ability to resist social pressure

♦ Acknowledgment of fallibility

♦ An individually based value system

♦ The resolution of typical dichotomies of personality

Regarding this interesting final characteristic, Maslow detailed the balance, the "both–and" rather than "either–or" integration, of often polarized psychological characteristics, such as intellectual–emotional, selfish–unselfish, spiritual–sensual, sexual–loving, work–play, animalistic–refined, kind–ruthless, acceptant–rebellious, serious–humorous, introverted–extroverted, intense–casual, conventional–unconventional, mystic–realistic, Dionysian–Apollonian, masculine–feminine, and childlike–mature.

Maslow was evidently satisfied enough with his method, based on his confidence in the resulting composite portrait of psychological health, that he undertook a second qualitative research project in order to investigate special, euphoric moments he called "peak experiences," which he discovered occurring with the greatest frequency in the healthiest persons. Maslow gathered written descriptions from 190 college students and conducted interviews with over 80 participants detailing "the most wonderful experience or experiences of your life. . . . Tell me how you felt . . . the ways the world looked different" (Maslow, 1968, p. 71). In addition, Maslow analyzed 50 unsolicited letters written to him in response to previous publications as well as archival texts in the areas of mysticism, religion, art, creativity, and love. He constructed another composite portrait of "peak experiences" from the partial aspects given by these many and various participants and data sources, for no one participant or verbal report included all the features of peak experiences. Maslow's empirical data included such instances and activities as a new mother gazing lovingly at her baby, a biologist looking into a microscope, writing poetry, flying a plane, meditating, communing with nature, sexual orgasm, intellectual insight, painting, and athletic fulfillment.

Maslow found and described in detail the following cognitive characteristics of peak experiences, and again he expressed them in a single composite. The object of the peak moment is experienced (1) as a whole, detached from usefulness or instrumental values; (2) as exclusively, fully, and caringly attended to; (3) as wondrously independent of the perceiver; (4) with a heightened intraobject richness; (5) as ego transcending; (6) as intrinsically valuable; (7) with time–space disorientation; (8) as good and desirable; (9) as absolute, not relative; (10) effortlessly; (11) passively and receptively; (12) as forming a unity with the participant; (13) with wonder, awe, reverence, and humility; (14) as a resolution of contradictions; (15) with godlike acceptance; (16) ideographically and without classification; and (17) without fear, anxiety, prohibition, or restraint. In these experiences, the world becomes more unified, persons become more themselves, and conduct is more easeful and effortless. These experiences are characterized by spontaneity, efficiency, freedom from conflict, and virtuosity: "To put it simply, [the person] becomes more whole and unified, more unique and idiosyncratic, more alive and spontaneous (leaving fears and doubts behind), more ego-transcending and self forgetful" (Maslow, 1959, p. 61). Maslow went on to report that, in such "peak experiences," ordinary persons and even psychopathological individuals temporarily experience the world the way self-actualizing individuals more consistently do. He drew the conclusion that "self-actualization" should be conceived less statistically, less as a rare, all-or-none achievement and rather on a continuum that exists in every person's life. Self-actualizing persons have peak experiences more frequently, but the potential for peak experiences is shared by all. Maslow also analyzed the consequences of these experiences, including their possible dangers (e.g., passivity, invalid illusion, self-absorption, irresponsibility, excessive tolerance, overaestheticism) as well as their potential for personal transformation and identity formation when they are part of healthy, psychological growth process.

Maslow's research was rejected for publication by the *Psychological Review*, *American Psychologist*, and *Psychiatry* (Hoffman, 1999, p. 206, as cited in Coon, 2006, p. 266). However, as the newly elected president of APA Division 8 (the Society for Personality and Social Psychology) in 1956, Maslow delivered his findings as a keynote address and eventually published his report in 1959 in the *Journal of Genetic Psychology*, entitled, "Cognition of Being in the Peak Experiences." Maslow (1959) wrote that "this is then a chapter in the Positive or Ortho-Psychology of the future, in that it deals with fully functioning and healthy human beings" (p. 45). It is interesting that in the 1959 publication, Maslow does not report his method. The method described above was reported in an edited and somewhat expanded report of this research as a chapter in his book (Maslow, 1968), *Toward a Psychology of Being*.

Although Maslow had no doubt about the intrinsic scientific value of his research, he did not view it as ordinary science ("normal science," in Kuhn's [1962] sense) because there had been no widespread disciplinary legitimization of the procedures he had used. Its incongruity with his training and his difficulties publishing this work must have intensified Maslow's insecurity. Although he was evidently not in a position to detail and argue for the scientificity of his research, he felt badly stung by the rejection of this work by scientific venues. After his article on peak experiences was turned down,

Maslow never again submitted his work to mainstream journals (Coon, 2006). Throughout these projects, Maslow's research was aimed at revealing what is uniquely human in a holistic, rigorous way. His research was carefully and critically conducted, made extensive use of empirical data, provided systematically organized conceptualizations beyond common sense, transparently reported the methods used, and presented an opportunity for critique and challenges of both procedures and findings based on subsequent scholarship and research.

Maslow's research practices included some novel features and others that Freud and James have made familiar. Maslow's research topic arose from a highly personal quest and served his vision of a better future for humanity. His science was also a quest for enlightenment and wisdom. Maslow used mainstream quantitative research tools, such as personality measurements, to rigorously identify his participants and to guide his behavioral observations and interview data collection. He adapted his methods to his individual participants with ethical sensitivity to their responses, given the highly personal and private nature of the lived experiences he was studying. Maslow developed a cyclic, iterative procedure in which he began with common folk understandings of his subject matter, and through successive cycles of data collection and analysis, achieved a conceptual clarity that surpassed prior knowledge with a new scientific precision. He stressed the corrigibility of this kind of knowledge along with a confidence in the self-corrective process through which it undergoes improvement. Like Freud and James, Maslow constantly compared the experiences of various participants, and his general knowledge of the healthy personality and the peak experience was formulated in holistic, composite portraits that conceptually articulated numerous, interrelated constituents.

Lawrence Kohlberg: Discovering Types of Moral Reasoning in Human Development

Lawrence Kohlberg was a leader of the cognitive revolution that, together with the humanistic movement, displaced behaviorism as the dominant trend in psychology, reintroduced mental life as a subject matter, and contributed to legitimizing qualitative research methods. In his outstanding doctoral dissertation, Kohlberg (1958/1994) studied the development of moral reasoning— the chief adaptation of humankind—in order to address problems in the ways that common sense and psychological theories treated the topic. Kohlberg's investigation was, in part, a response to the qualitative study of moral thinking by Piaget (1932), who had used observational and interview methods with his own three children. Kohlberg's dissertation research, which used what is now called "mixed methods" (an integration of qualitative and quantitative methods), has shaped the psychology of moral development. This advance in psychology was made possible by the interdisciplinary milieu at the University of Chicago, whose anthropologists and sociologists exposed Kohlberg to the rich methodological tradition of qualitative research in those disciplines. Kohlberg forged his procedures from Max Weber's seminal work on the Protestant work ethic and received help in his qualitative analysis from dissertation committee member Anselm Straus, who later co-invented the grounded theory method. "I owe much to the understanding and stimulation I have received from Mr. Anselm Strauss. Among the many forms this has taken, I may mention the unusual help he gave in going over the raw data with me in a remarkably insightful and suggestive way" (Kohlberg, 1958/1994, p. 3).

Kohlberg's primary research participants were 72 Chicago-area boys, ages 10, 13, and 16 years, from upper-middle-class and lower- to lower-middle-class families; half were socially popular and half were socially isolated. These participants were supplemented by groups of 24 delinquents, 24 6-year-olds, and 50 boys and girls (13 years old) living outside of Boston. Each child was presented with 10 hypothetical situations in which obedience to authorities or rules/laws conflicted with the serving of human needs. Modeled on Piaget's (1932) procedure, participants were presented with these hypothetical moral dilemmas and were asked probing questions about their thinking and choices. Kohlberg collected the children's verbal responses in 2-hour, tape-recorded, open-ended interviews with each participant. The best known of these situations is the "Heinz dilemma," in which a man named Heinz steals an unfairly priced drug that he cannot afford in order to save the life of his ill spouse. In another hypothetical dilemma, for instance:

> Joe's father promised he could go to camp if he earned the $50 for it, and then changed his mind and asked Joe to give him the money he had earned. Joe lied and said he only earned $10 and went to camp using the other $40 he had made. Before he went, he told his younger brother Alex about lying to their father. Should Alex tell their father? (Kohlberg, 1963/2008, p. 9)

Kohlberg also conducted focus groups composed of three participants, where he instructed participants to discuss their different views of the 10 situations and to attempt to come to an agreement on the moral resolutions.

After completing the transcription of all recordings, Kohlberg used the ideal-type analysis developed by Weber (1904/1949) to empirically identify the various kinds of moral thinking. Weber had been aware of the potential for this method to contribute to developmental analyses, as he himself had traced the development of "Protestantism" into "capitalism." To Kohlberg, this seemed to be "an almost necessary technique" for selecting, summarizing, and interpreting age trends, because the conceptualization of developmental stages amounts to the analytic delineation of a genetic series of types of psychological life. Ideal typological methods enabled Kohlberg to understand and coherently interpret consistent, complex relations among constituents of moral reasoning, as well as distinct qualitative cognitive structures, from this great mass of verbal data. "It [the qualitative analytic procedure] involves the simultaneous willingness to select out and stress empirical consistencies which can be coherently interpreted and the willingness to revise and reform principles of observation and interpretation as new empirical patterns seem to emerge" (Kohlberg, 1958/1994, p. 88). This procedure enabled Kohlberg to detect generally important dimensions of the subject matter, to define them, and to trace their developmental trajectories by comparing examples of thinking among children of various ages with increasing integration of each newly discovered constituent of moral thinking. Kohlberg's aim was to articulate stages/types that were not purely theoretical constructions that externally characterized humans, but rather were psychological structures that described how individuals think and the values they actually hold, in line with the empirical data.

Kohlberg analyzed the data by carefully considering each action choice mentioned by the children, their way of thinking about the conflict, and their reasoning about what makes each choice "good" or "bad." In analyzing the data, Kohlberg noticed a number of striking responses that clustered together across a number of individuals (of various classes and ages), expressive not of social conventions but of internal reasoning patterns and principles. For instance, the working-class 10-year-old Danny replied to Alex's (Joe's brother) dilemma, "In one way it would be right to tell on his brother or his father might get mad at him and spank him. In another way it would be right to keep quiet or his brother might beat him up" (Kohlberg, 1963/2008, p. 9). Kohlberg saw in these and other choice considerations offered by Danny a way of thinking in which punishment plays the key role in which action is considered "wrong." Kohlberg found forms of moral thinking organized by this principle of *concrete power and punishment* in many other cases as well, especially among children ages 6–7. There was a limited number of organizing principles evident in various patterns of thinking, and these formed the preliminary "types." By comparing the concrete illustrations of these principles, as given by the children in response to the moral dilemmas posed, the internal coherence of each type and the differences between its important features and those of other types became clearer and were revised in order to improve the findings. Once basic types were established, each child's interview was then analyzed in its entirety to further support and revise the features of the types to more accurately reflect the interview items that most closely approximated them.

With 4-, 5-, and 7-year-old children, Kohlberg explored stories in which disobedience to an order and the breaking of rules was followed by reward or punishment. For instance, in one story a boy was ordered to watch a baby on a couch while his mother left the house. As soon as the mother left, the boy ran out into the yard and played. The research participant was asked to complete the story and was then told that when the mother came home, she gave the disobedient boy some candy, or in another version of the story, she sent an obedient boy to his room. Four-year-olds defined the boy's action as good or bad according to the reward or punishment rather than according to whether they boy followed the adult command, whereas the older children showed conflict. Some 7-year-olds, who said it was wrong of the mother to reward the disobedient boy, defined right and wrong according to the mother's previous order. They expressed being concerned about the "injustice" of rewarding the boy who disobeyed the order and punishing the boy who followed the rule. These older children did not base the meaning of "good" and "bad" on the action's consequent rewards and punishments. Instead, they construed the meanings of "right" and "wrong," as well as the meaning of the rewards and punishments themselves (i.e., fair or unfair), according to the principle of following orders and rules—considerations that were absent in the thinking of younger children (Kohlberg, 1963/2008, p. 14).

From this kind of analysis, Kohlberg (1958/1994) found three major stages/types, each divided into two subtypes. In formulating these six types of reasoning, Kohlberg used three criteria: they must express morality, have genetic implications, and be relevant to various moral theories. These types were not derived merely from abstract, a priori thinking on his part but from consistencies in the data. Not all data had equal value to Kohlberg in his qualitative analysis. Kohlberg reported that he was best able to identify distinct types in participants who were more consistent, understandable, and engaged in their thinking. The children with the most frequent manifestations of a particular type also tended to be ones whose thinking provided the most extreme examples, which thereby illustrated the organizing "principle" most clearly. Like James, Kohlberg found these extreme, prototypical instances of moral reasoning to be of greatest methodological value, even if not necessarily frequent, in identifying types that could be applied to all participants. Rare cases were especially informative for explaining development in general. Kohlberg likened this strategy to the method Freud had used in identifying highly general principles of psychopathology by scrutinizing the now statistically rare hysterical type. "The most illuminating and 'quotable' responses are usually the most unusual or idiosyncratic. A principle of thinking that we believe common to the type is caught in one response to one question in one child, in another for another" (Kohlberg, 1958/1994, p. 102). Thereby recurrent patterns were systematically interpreted and classified.

In the interviews with children 10–16 years old, Kohlberg found six very different general types of moral reasoning that form a developmental sequence:

- ♦ Level I: Premoral
  - • Type 1: Punishment and obedience orientation, external consequence based
  - • Type 2: Naïve instrumental hedonism, need based
- ♦ Level II: Conventional role—conformity
  - • Type 3: Good-boy morality of maintaining good relations, approval of others, stereotyped virtue
  - • Type 4: Authority, rule, law, and society maintaining morality
- ♦ Level III: Morality of self-accepted moral principles
  - • Type 5: Morality of contract and democratically accepted law
  - • Type 6: Morality of individual principles of conscience

Once these stages/types were established, Kohlberg returned to all data and placed each statement of moral thinking into one of the types. Every thought content expressing a moral judgment in the data was assigned to a type. Participants had a range of 43–117 total expressions that were coded. In meticulously analyzing these data, Kohlberg identified 30 general aspects or dimensions of moral reasoning, some that had been previously reported and emphasized by Piaget and other theorists. These included, for instance, conception of rights, orientation toward punitive justice, considerations of intentions versus consequences of action, motives justifying action, and reciprocity. These general dimensions were found to have a distinctive meaning for each of the six types of moral thinking. Each of these types was viewed as being coherently structured by characteristic patterns of motivation and cognition, which Kohlberg was able to delineate. The six types of moral reasoning were taken to represent successive emergent restructures of the meanings of "right" and "wrong."

The 50–150 moral ideas or statements in each child's interview could be individually placed in the classification system constructed of the six levels and 30 dimensions, which formed a grid of 180 cells. Individual participants were not restricted to one level of moral reasoning within and across the moral dilemmas. The percentage of each participant's statements falling into each of the six types of moral thinking was assessed, and participants were classified according to their modal response. For instance, 15 of the 72 boys were found to be thinking modally on the first level, meaning that at least 45% of their moral statements were Level I.

Perhaps Kohlberg's most difficult problem was empirically supporting his conclusion that the types of thinking form a developmental sequence. Guttman's (1950) technique was used to quantitatively analyze consistent age trends of types, thereby triangulating evidence of developmental sequence. A correlation matrix verified the sequential nature of the types by showing decreasing correlations among types that are presumably more develop-mentally remote from each other. Quantitative findings also indicated that earlier types of moral reasoning decreased from ages 10–16 years, and more advanced types increased with age. However, Kohlberg realized that the superior evidence of a developmental sequence is qualitative. "More strongly than the quantitative data, we believe that the qualitative data and interpretations contained in our stage descriptions makes the notion of developmental trans-formations in moral thought more plausible and meaningful" (Kohlberg, 1963/2008, p. 19). In other words, these "types" progressively encompass each other in an orderly sequence, wherein the meanings of right and wrong in one stage are included in, as well as surpassed, in an orderly sequence of sub-sequent types, with more complex ways of thinking integrating the simpler ones. The above described 7-year-olds, in their considerations of the mother's reward of the disobedient child, understood that rewards and punishments have reference to the goodness and badness of behavior, but their view went beyond this and also included another criterion—whether the child followed the order—and this additional concern led to an evaluation of whether the rewards and punishments were themselves just. Therefore, these types form a sequence of less to more complex wholes, and that which is new takes priority over and encompasses older considerations. Hence, the structure and value of these experiences show qualitative evidence of their hierarchical organi-zation and sequential complexity. The qualitative differences indicate that development is not merely the reflection of greater knowledge or greater con-formity to culture.

Kohlberg struggled mightily with the means to present his complex, extensive findings and to draw out their many theoretical implications. He referred to these types in lengthy discussions within chapters of the text (over 200 pages), which addressed each of the three overall stages and discussed the theoretical implications of his findings. Abundant quotations are provided in order to illustrate the way in which each type of thinking approaches general moral issues such as punishments, discipline, rights, duty, laws, respect for authority, responsibility, conscience, virtue, and justice.

Kohlberg's research was published in *Vita Humana* in 1963 as a short arti-cle, which was republished in *Human Development* in 2008. Very little descrip-tion of his method of analysis was included. Kohlberg's dissertation, which contains the full exposition of his qualitative method, was published only in 1994, well after his work had shaped the field. Kohlberg's work led to a volu-minous subsequent research and, even with criticisms and controversies, is featured in psychology textbooks and remains a fundamental reference point in the psychology of morality. Despite the tremendous attention this classic research has been given, there has been very little, if any, attention given to its complex and highly refined qualitative methods. Most psychologists are familiar with Kohlberg's theory but remain unfamiliar with Weber's "ideal type" methods and are unaware of how Kolhberg adapted them for research in developmental psychology.

Kohlberg's practices include the deliberate selection of participants of diverse ages, socioeconomic levels, degrees of socialization, and (to some extent) gender. Using carefully designed hypothetical situations, Kohlberg invited his participants to live through the experiences he studied in the immediacy of the research situation. He collected data by tape recording interactive Socratic conversations with individuals and focus groups, which provided access to his phenomenon in real-life social situations. Kohlberg offers an explicit account of his handling and analysis of data. He thoroughly differentiated his voluminous data and analyzed every action choice in comparison with others, looking for patterns within and among subjects' performances. Kohlberg discovered that not all data were of equal value for qualitative insights. Prototypical patterns and their principles were best discerned not in average, modal responses but rather in the data of unusual participants who were most consistent, understandable, and engaged. Paradoxically, rare and idiosyncratic thinking offered the greatest methodological value in the achievement of general understandings. In this iterative process of comparing the most extreme examples of moral reasoning, Kohlberg revised conceptualizations as new patterns emerged. These comparisons revealed, at midlevel generality, a relatively small number of typical structures, each unified by intelligible principles. Once these were clear, Kohlberg returned to the data and found one of these patterns in each of his participant's statements. Through qualitative analysis, Kohlberg delineated a developmental series of complex psychological structures, each composed of multiple constituents whose meaning followed from the holistically pervasive principle. Kohlberg used qualitative and quantitative analyses to independently confirm developmental relationships among qualitative types. He carefully documented each step of his research and illustrated the findings regarding development through typical forms of moral reasoning in presentations with real-life examples and direct quotations from his participants.

Gordon Allport's Call for Methodology: The Social Science Research Council's Initiative

In the 1930's, increasing attention turned to the widespread and growing use of qualitative research across the social sciences. The Committee on Appraisal of Research, part of the Social Science Research Council, called for a critical review of research that had used "personal documents," defined as "account(s) of individual experience which reveal the individual's actions as a human agent and as a participant in social life" (Blumer, as cited in Allport, 1942, p. 21). These "documents" included such texts as autobiographies, interviews and other recordings, diaries, letters, expressive and projective creations, and questionnaires. In 1940, the committee asked Gordon Allport of Harvard University to recommend a scholar to conduct the review in psychology, and Allport himself volunteered. Allport's 1942 monograph, now out of print for more than four decades, inventoried and evaluated all research in psychology that utilized such first-person data. Allport studied the various types of personal documents used, the data collection and analytic methods, and the value of such documents with the help of his graduate assistant, Jerome Bruner, who later became a leader of the narrative approach to qualitative methods. In the monograph, Allport voiced a passionate, critical-minded, and courageous claim of the highest scientific legitimacy for qualitative research. This monograph remains today a thorough and compelling argument for qualitative research methods.

One of Allport's conclusions was that although personal documents have tremendous potential in generating psychological knowledge, such methods were too often conducted in uncritical ways. Although in the 1920s some psychologists had begun to focus on the methodological issues involved in such research—reliability, validity, classification, and prediction—there remained few clear accounts of how highly personal material was selected, organized, and analyzed. Consequently, the researchers had little understanding of the methodological norms and standards of quality that would assure sound science. Allport contrasted the increasing use of first-person documents in clinical psychology with the regrettable lack of sophisticated methodological discussions of the procedures involved. He called for a new journal devoted entirely to the case study, one that would not simply present findings but that would focus on the procedures used and their underlying principles. Allport was impressed by the variety of topics these methods could address, their value in acquiring new empirical knowledge, their guidance in the development of theories, their practical utility, and their contributions to interdisciplinary studies. Allport reported on such psychological topics, practical uses, inductive theorizing, interdisciplinary investigations, forms of scientific reporting, and the relationship to quantitative research (e.g., questionnaire and test construction). He insisted on the importance of both "ideographic" (individual, case study) and "nomothetic" (population frequency and aggregate analyses) knowledge in psychology and showed that the analysis of personal documents is indispensible for both.

One virtue of the use of personal documents, according to Allport, is to prevent science from becoming artificial by providing a "touchstone of reality" (1942, p. 184). He asserted that this kind of research is necessary for knowledge of subjective meaning, which is indispensable in psychology. Allport argued that the close analysis of personal documents is not limited, as is often thought, to the mere generation of hypotheses that would require verification by quantitative methods, or to the mere illustration of principles that would be established by behavioral observation and measurement. He considered qualitative methods to be valuable in their own right and superior to other methods in the investigation of meaning and many important human phenomena, such as love, perception of beauty, religious faith, experience of pain, ambition, fear, jealousy, frustration, memory, fantasy, and friendship. He concluded that this kind of research is capable of its own forms of generalization and validation. One of Allport's interesting points is that, in the use of personal documents, validity may rightfully exceed reliability. He thereby called into question the traditional methodological canon that validity presupposes reliability. Instead of mandating consistency as a precondition of true knowledge, Allport advocated using many different perspectives in research on personal experience and argued that multiple different knowledge claims may achieve greater truth. Allport insisted that these methods are scientific and meet the crucial criteria of understanding, prediction, control, and generalization when properly employed.

Allport enumerated the criticisms of qualitative methods and demonstrated the irrelevance, triviality, misconceptions, and downright falseness of many common complaints. He did not downplay the difficulty of the methodological problems involved in using personal documents. However, he argued that all research methods have problems and that the difficulties in using personal documents could be addressed and resolved no less successfully than could the problems of quantitative and experimental methods.

Allport concluded that "bold and radical" innovation doing research with personal documents should be encouraged and undertaken in psychology. Alternative and new ways of organizing documents, analyzing data, validating knowledge claims, predicting and interpreting, and writing reports should be encouraged and undertaken. Clear accounts of the methods used and sophisticated methodological critique should be undertaken to establish the unique scientific norms appropriate for these methods. "Strong countermeasures are indicated against theorists who damn the personal document with faint praise, saying that its sole merit lies in its capacity to yield hunches or to suggest hypotheses . . . . They fail to express more than a small part of the value of personal documents for social science" (Allport, 1942, p. 191).

In this strong, visionary monograph, Allport anticipated the events that were to come in the second half of the 20th century. In the decades of the 1950s through the 1970s, various new traditions of research methodology were established. Each of these involved the formal development of practices that were employed in the work of Freud, James, Maslow, and Kohlberg, as well as in the work of many other researchers who lacked formal training, conducted their investigations in relative isolation, and did not assert the general applicability of the methods even though they successfully answered important research questions about human experience. Only in the 1970s did extensive scholarship on the basic principles and procedures of qualitative research develop on a broad scale. New traditions were established by individuals who experimented boldly and radically, as Allport had recommended, who carefully thought about the research methods they practiced, who offered compelling scientific rationales for their approaches, who described rigorous procedures that could be taught and carried out on a wide scale, and who established the use of qualitative methods in educational institutions, professional organizations, journals, and book publications. Only in the last few decades have these various qualitative methodological traditions gained widening attention and use. The recent proliferation of journals, textbooks, graduate courses, and professional organizations has been called "the qualitative revolution" in the social sciences (Denzin & Lincoln, 1994, p. ix) and has become a major historical "force" in psychology (Ponterotto, 2002). In the next chapter, we turn to the work of those scholars who delineated and made more available qualitative methods akin to those featured in this chapter.

References

Allport, G. W. (1942). *The use of personal documents in psychological science* (prepared for the Committee on the Appraisal of Research; Bulletin #49). New York: Social Science Research Council.

Breuer, J., & Freud, S. (1957). *Studies on hysteria.* New York: Basic Books. (Original work published 1895)

Coon, D. J. (2006). Abraham H. Maslow: Reconnaissance for eupsychia. In D. A. Dewsbury, L. T. Benjamin, & M. Wertheimer (Eds.), *Portraits of pioneers in psychology* (Vol. VI, pp. 255–272). New York: Psychology Press.

Denzin, N. K., & Lincoln, Y. S. (1994). *Handbook of qualitative research.* Thousand Oaks, CA: Sage.

Dollard, J. (1937). *Caste and class in a Southern town.* Garden City, NY: Doubleday Books.

Ericsson K. A., & Simon, H. A. (1993). *Protocol analysis: Verbal reports as data.* Cambridge, MA: MIT Press.

Festinger, L., Riecken, H., & Schachter, S. (1956). *When prophesy fails.* Minneapolis: University of Minnesota Press.

Freud, S. (1959). Psycho-analysis. In J. Strachey (Ed. and Trans.), *The standard edition of the complete works of Sigmund Freud* (Vol. 20, pp. 259–270). London: Hogarth Press. (Original work published 1926)

Freud, S. (1963). *Therapy and technique.* New York: Collier Books. (Original work published 1913)

Freud, S. (1964). Constructions in psychoanalysis. In J. Strachey (Ed. and Trans.), *The standard edition of the complete works of Sigmund Freud* (Vol. 23, pp. 255–269). London: Hogarth Press. (Original work published 1937)

Freud, S. (1965). *The interpretation of dreams.* New York: Basic Books. (Original work published 1900)

Freud, S. (1978). *The question of lay analysis.* New York: Norton. (Original work published 1926)

Giorgi, A. (2009). *The descriptive phenomenological method in psychology: A modified Husserlian approach.* Pittsburgh: Duquesne University Press.

Goldstein, K. (1995). *The organism: A holistic approach to biology derived from pathological data in man.* New York: Zone Books. (Original work published 1934)

Guttman, L. (1950). The basis for scalogram analysis. In S. A. Stouffer, L. Guttman, E. A. Suchman, P. F. Lazerfeld, S. A. Star, & J. A. Clausen (Eds.), *Measurement and prediction* (pp. 60–90). Princeton, NJ: Princeton University Press.

James, W. (1982). *The varieties of religious experience.* New York: Penguin Books. (Original work published 1902)

Janis, I. L. (1972). *Victims of groupthink.* Boston: Houghton Mifflin.

Kahneman, D. (2003). Experiences of collaborative research. *American Psychologist, 58*(9), 723–730.

Kohlberg, L. (1963). The development of children's orientation toward a moral order: Sequence in the development of moral thought. *Vita Humana, 6,* 11–33. (Reprinted in 2008, *Human Development, 51,* 8–20.)

Kohlberg, L. (1994). *Moral development: A compendium* (Vol. 3, B. Puka, Ed.). New York: Garland. (Reprint of Kohlberg, L. [1958]. *The development of moral thinking and choice in the years 10 through 16.* Unpublished doctoral dissertation, University of Chicago, Chicago, IL.)

Kuhn, T. (1962). *The structure of scientific revolutions.* Chicago: University of Chicago Press.

Lewin, K. (1948). *Resolving social conflict: Selected papers on group dynamics.* New York: Harper & Row.

Marecek, J., Fine, M., & Kidder, L. (1997). Working between worlds: Qualitative methods and social psychology. *Journal of Social Issues, 53*(4), 631–644.

Maslow, A. H. (1959). Cognition of being in the peak experiences. *Journal of Genetic Psychology, 94,* 43–66.

Maslow, A. H. (1968). *Toward a psychology of being.* New York: Van Nostrand Reinhold.

Maslow, A. H. (1987). *Motivation and personality.* New York: HarperCollins. (Original work published 1954)

Piaget, J. (1932). *The moral judgment of the child.* Glencoe, IL: Free Press.

Ponterotto, J. (2002) Qualitative research methods: The fifth force in psychology. *Counseling Psychologist, 30*(3), 394–406.

Rosenhan, D. (1973). On being sane in insane places. *Science, 179,* 250–258.

Sherif, M., & Sherif, C. W. (1953). *Groups in harmony and tension: An integration of studies on intergroup relations.* New York: Harper & Brothers.

Strachey, J. (1957). Editor's introductions. In J. Breuer & S. Freud, *Studies on hysteria* (pp. ix–xxviii). New York: Basic Books.

Weber, M. (1949). *Methodology of the social sciences* (E. A. Shils & H. A. Finch, Trans.). Glencoe, IL: Free Press. (Original work published 1904)

Wertz, F. J. (1983). Some components of descriptive psychological reflection. *Human Studies, 6*(1), 35–51.

Wertz, F. J. (1987a). Common methodological fundaments of the analytic procedures in phenomenological and psychoanalytic research. *Psychoanalysis and Contemporary Thought, 9*(4), 563–603.

Wertz, F. J. (1987b). Meaning and research methodology: Psychoanalysis as a human science. *Methods: A Journal for Human Science, 1*(2), 91–135.

Wertz, F. J. (1993). The phenomenology of Sigmund Freud. *Journal of Phenomenological Psychology, 24*(2), 101–129.

Wertz, F. J. (2001). Humanistic psychology and the qualitative research tradition. In K. J. Schneider, J. F. T. Bugental, & J. F. Pierson (Eds.), *The handbook of humanistic psychology: Leading edges in theory, research and practice* (pp. 231–246). Thousand Oaks, CA: Sage.

Wong, W. (2009). Retracing the footsteps of Wilhelm Wundt: Explorations in the disciplinary frontiers of psychology and in *Völkerpsychologie. History of Psychology, 12*(4), 229–265.

Wundt, W. (1900–1920). *Völkerpsychologie* (Vols. 1–10). Leipzig, Germany: Engelmann.

Wundt, W. (1916). *Elements of folk psychology: Outlines of a psychological history of the development of mankind* (E. L. Schaub, Trans.). New York: Macmillan.

Zimbardo, P., Haney, C., Banks, W. C., & Jaffe, D. (1975). The psychology of imprisonment: Privation, power, and pathology. In D. Rosenhan & P. London (Eds.), *Theory and research in abnormal psychology* (pp. 271–287). New York: Holt, Rinehart & Winston.

CHAPTER 2

The Establishment
of Methodological Traditions

I n the second half of the 20th century, a series of explicitly methodological works in psychology specified formal procedures for qualitative analysis. Many of these procedures were used by practitioners but had not
been systematically articulated and made available for general use. Starting
in the 1970s, the five approaches featured in this volume developed relatively
independently, later becoming part of a broad movement. In the milieu of
current methodological pluralism, they continue in relative independence of
each other and are also sometimes used jointly. The presence of these methods, when encountered in journals, textbooks, professional conferences, and
educational venues, raises a host of questions about their relations to each
other. How are these analytic methods similar? How are they different? Do
they share any common fundamentals? What distinctive capabilities does
each offer? Can they be compatibly combined with each other? Here we trace
the emergence of general methods in the second half of the 20th century
through the personal and professional contexts of those who established the
traditions. In the next chapter, we focus on the multifaceted movement they
engendered, the problems of contemporary methodological pluralism, and
the common issues that qualitative researchers are encountering as these traditions infuse virtually every area of psychology.

Critical Incident Technique: James Flanagan

To our knowledge, James Flanagan's (1954) critical incident technique (CIT)
was the first qualitative research method that offered psychological research-

ers a clearly formulated set of specific procedures concerning research purpose, design, data collection, analysis, and report. Although this technique is not one of the approaches featured in this volume, it is historically important and remains useful due to its extraordinary flexibility and particular strength in the area of data constitution, which nicely complements our subsequent focus on procedures of analysis. Flanagan's work has gone largely unacknowledged by scholars in the contemporary movement, perhaps because Flanagan was uncritical of the positivistic philosophy underlying psychological research. However, Flanagan's contributions to research method are fundamentally pragmatic and modular to the extent that the components of his method (e.g., his very useful procedures of data collection) can be employed with other approaches, including the explicitly nonpositivistic approaches to qualitative analysis that we focus on next. Like all good scientific methods, Flanagan's CIT arose out of significant research problems, on the one hand, and a genuine respect for the realities of the subject matter, on the other hand.

Flanagan developed the CIT in the Aviation Psychology Program of the United States Army Air Forces (USAAF) in World War II. His task was to formulate procedures for the selection and classification of air crews, especially the identification of successful and unsuccessful pilot trainees. Questionnaires filled out by flight instructors about candidates who had been dismissed from flight training schools had previously provided only brief, stereotyped and clichéd reasons for their failure—empty phrases like "insufficient progress," "unsuitable temperament," or "poor judgment" (Flanagan, 1954, p. 328). Rather than asking the instructors to convey their general knowledge about the characteristics of successful and unsuccessful pilot trainees, Flanagan solicited instructors' observations of specific *critical incidents* in which they observed success and failure in trainees learning to fly. The most important feature of the CIT, and its greatest virtue as a qualitative method, is the concreteness of its data. In subsequent research on "disorientation while flying," Flanagan asked pilots themselves to provide first-person descriptions of actual incidents in which they experienced disorientation and vertigo—what they saw, heard, felt, and did in such situations. The analysis of these incidents led to recommendations of changes in the cockpit and instrument panel to prevent vertigo while flying.

In order to be "critical," an incident must occur in a situation where the purpose and effects of a human activity are clear. For instance, Flanagan collected recorded interviews with pilots who described particular successful and unsuccessful incidents of taking off, flying on instruments, landing, and using controls. Descriptions of such critical incidents were also collected and analyzed to study the failure in bombing missions in 1943–1944 and to study combat leadership in 1944. This new method, which contrasts sharply with the testing of hypotheses (even based on expert hunches), surpassed brief questionnaires by allowing investigators to analyze reports of actual effective and ineffective behaviors in their natural contexts—a touchstone of reality. For instance, several thousand soldiers were asked to describe incidents in which an officer's action was "especially helpful" or "inadequate" in accomplishing a mission (Flanagan, 1954, p. 328). Flanagan and his team developed procedures to analyze such protocols in order to yield knowledge of effective combat leadership, the "critical requirements for leadership."

The procedures for this qualitative method were written up in a USAAF document in 1946. The CIT has two purposes: to solve practical problems and to develop broad psychological principles. Flanagan provided a set of procedures for formulating questions, collecting data, and analyzing and synthesizing such observations. He acknowledged that this method was not new, for many great writers—as keen observers of human life—have made such observations of significant incidents, described them carefully, and gained insight based on them. Flanagan's original achievement was the systematic development of such practices for scientific psychological research using detailed memories, reporting, and inductive analysis.

After the war, Flanagan and other researchers in the USAAF Aviation Psychology Program established the American Institute for Research, a nonprofit scientific and educational organization, with the aim of further developing the CIT method. The first published application was on job analysis—what makes the difference between success and failure in the performance of hourly wage earners (Miller & Flanagan, 1950). In this study, researchers collected data from 2,500 interviews in which plant foremen described situations of satisfactory and unsatisfactory performance of workers. Other early studies focused on attitude and aptitude (Flanagan, 1954). In dissertations, students at the University of Pittsburgh researched human activities in various occupations such as dentistry. Descriptions of critical incidents by dental patients, dentists, and dental school instructors were used in elaborating the principles of good dentistry practice and effective dentistry instruction along with a battery of selection tests used by the University of Pittsburgh School of Dentistry. The CIT was also used to analyze best practices in education. Psychology instruction was studied using critical incidents described by students and faculty, and interesting differences were discovered in their partly divergent points of view. The CIT was also extended beyond applications to practical problems as a method used to generate basic qualitative knowledge of psychological phenomena in various subfields. In studies of personality, for instance, the phenomenon of "emotional immaturity" was analyzed and a classification system with diagnostic criteria was developed from data provided by psychologists, psychiatrists, social workers, and nurses.

In his seminal 1954 publication, Flanagan elaborated the typical procedures in each of the five phases of a CIT study: (1) aim of research, (2) design and participant instructions, (3) data collection, (4) analysis (summary and description), and (5) interpretation and reporting. In the CIT, there is no one rigid rule for data collection. The CIT is a flexible set of principles that can be modified for various research problems and situations. The crucial principle of selecting and collecting incidents is their relevance to the research topic and problem. Flanagan stressed the importance of critical incidents that contain "extreme behavior" (1954, p. 138)—either especially effective or ineffective—as the most useful for research, echoing the insight of James and Kohlberg that applies equally to the research of Freud and Maslow. The selection of observers is also important: They must have direct access to the research phenomenon. Data can be gathered following observation or memory. Flanagan enumerated procedures for explaining studies and formulating questions to participants. He emphasized the importance of choosing the right words in the instructions given to research participants, words that are readily understood by participants and that clearly specify the activities or topic under investigation. Descriptions can be obtained by individuals or groups and can be written, given verbally, or solicited in a conversation with the researcher. Data analysis proceeds inductively by identifying the common elements of various incidents. Additional incidents are analyzed until no new knowledge is acquired. Identification of practical implications follow from the inductively established findings. Flanagan discussed the frame of reference of the researcher, the formation of analytic categories, the structural organization of the subject matter, the naming of meanings, the generalization of results, the interpretation of findings, and the writing of a research report. The CIT can be used in applied areas such as measuring instrument development, job description, training program design, procedures of selection and classification, and psychotherapy and counseling practice (e.g., to establish areas and means of change). The CIT is not limited to practical problems but can be used in clarifying basic psychological constructs and in discerning psychological principles of motivation, leadership, attitudes, and personality by utilizing accounts of actual situations involving the psychological phenomenon under investigation. The main virtue of this method is the establishment of knowledge that surpasses any based on opinions, hunches, estimates, and assumptions.

The CIT has been used extensively in industrial organizational psychology. Although its use declined in the late 1950s, interest rose again in the 1980s with the increase in recognition of the value of qualitative research (Norman, Redfern, Tomalin, & Oliver, 1992). It has been used in virtually all areas of applied psychology and in many other basic areas as well as by those involved in health care (e.g., nursing), business, and education. It has potential application across the full spectrum of social sciences and even the humanities. In one noteworthy, though not well-known application, the CIT has been *the* method used in the development of ethical principles and standards for psychologists. In research leading to the first ethical principles for psychologists in 1948, approximately 7,500 members of the APA were instructed to describe actual situations in which a psychologist made a decision having ethical implications and to indicate the ethical issues involved. The analysis of more than 1,000 such incidents submitted by APA members was the basis of the first ethical code for psychologists (Adkins, 1952). The critical incident method has been employed in successive revisions and in the completion of the current APA Ethics Code (American Psychological Association, 2002), and critical incidents of ethical violations continue to be collected today on the website of the American Psychological Association.

Phenomenological Psychology: Amedeo Giorgi

The research methods that were developed for psychology by Amedeo Giorgi have their origin in the transdisciplinary movement of phenomenology. With roots in ancient Greek thought and the humanistic tradition, phenomenology was initially developed as a philosophical method for investigating consciousness by Edmund Husserl (1859–1938) at the turn of the century (Husserl, 1900–1901/1970, 1913/1962). Following his teacher Franz Brentano (1874/1973), Husserl held that by virtue of their capacity for consciousness, humans are fundamentally different from material nature and therefore require methods other than those developed by the physical sciences to be scientifically investigated. Husserl aimed to develop methods appropriate for the study of conscious experience that would enable science to overcome the limitations of objectivism, that is, the universal application of the materialistic concepts and methods of the natural sciences. His work in epistemology and the philosophy of science branched into other areas of philosophy and the human sciences, influencing generations of diverse scholars. It should be noted that the term *phenomenology* is not always used in reference to the tradition begun by Husserl in European philosophy. In psychology, the word has been used more broadly to characterize any work in research, theory, or practice that emphasizes first-person experience. The term is also used in psychiatry to denote descriptive knowledge of the symptoms of mental disorders. In this volume, the term is used to refer only to the approach to knowledge developed and strongly influenced by Husserl and those who followed him.

Husserl meticulously investigated consciousness in both everyday life and science, articulating methods appropriate for its study and working to clarify the foundations of philosophy and the sciences. In keeping with Brentano, Husserl emphasized the *intentionality* of consciousness, the self-transcending way that consciousness relates to other objects, including ordinary things like blackbirds, imaginary creations like novels, scientific theories, and mathematical formulae. Husserl's work gave rise to phenomenology, a 20th-century movement that continues to grow in the field of philosophy and throughout the full spectrum of the humanities, human sciences, and fine arts study.

Perhaps most impressive about Husserl's work is the range of scholarship he inspired in the many intellectual currents that extended the phenomenological tradition. Embree (2010) estimates that there are currently over 180 local phenomenological organizations and 3,500 self-identified phenomenologists in over 50 countries, working in more than three dozen disciplines.

Taking seriously the maxim that science begins with the unprejudiced description, Husserl (1900–1901/1970) expressed the fundamental orientation of phenomenology in his inspired call, "*Zu den Sachen selbst*" (to the things themselves), meaning that knowledge must be grounded in contact with the unique characteristics of its subject matter. Husserl wrote extensively on the foundations of scientific knowledge and of psychology in particular. He clarified the essential characteristics of human lived experiences and the reflective methods proper to its investigation, thereby clarifying the foundations of psychological science. Further contributions to psychology have been made by such followers as Martin Heidegger, Jean-Paul Sartre, Maurice Merleau-Ponty, Alfred Schutz, Aron Gurwitsch, Paul Ricoeur, and Emanuel Levinas as they moved phenomenology in existential, hermeneutic, social constructionist, and narrative directions. The earliest discipline outside philosophy to adopt phenomenology was psychiatry, beginning with the work of Karl Jaspers and extending through the 20th century with, for instance, Ludwig Binswanger, Medard Boss, Eugene Minkowski, Erwin Straus, J. H. van den Berg, and Ronald Laing, who had considerable influence in America.

Amedeo Giorgi has played the leading role in adapting and systematizing the use of phenomenological methods for empirically based psychological research. As an undergraduate at St. Joseph's College in Philadelphia, Giorgi switched his major from English to psychology after reading William James. Beginning his graduate study in experimental psychophysics at Fordham University in 1953, Giorgi avidly read history and systems texts while assisting Prof. Rev. Richard Zegers, S.J., in research and running his mentor's lab. Adopting the department's commitment to foundational disciplinary research, Giorgi conducted his master's research on monocular movement parallax thresholds and his dissertation on critical flicker frequency. Giorgi learned in psychophysics that relatively few subjects (two subjects in his master's thesis and three in his doctoral dissertation research) could generate masses of data that would produce highly general scientific results if analyzed meticulously. However, during his graduate study Giorgi developed growing doubts about the relevance of experimental methods for psychology.

After graduation, Giorgi accepted a position at Dunlap and Associates and was responsible for operational research on the Hawk missile system. Although he learned to adapt his methodological ideals to the practical problems of human factors, he remained critical of experimental methods for addressing human problems. In 1960, while Giorgi was teaching at Manhattan College, former classmate Ed Hogan informed him of his colleague

Adrian Van Kaam, a priest who had worked in the Dutch underground during World War II and who made the same criticisms of psychology that Giorgi had voiced. Giorgi met Van Kaam and learned of the European phenomenological research in nonclinical, experimental, and physiological areas by, for instance, Buytendijk, Graumann, and Linschoten. Giorgi enrolled in courses at the New School with Aron Gurwitsch, Rollo May, and Paul Tillich before joining the faculty of Duquesne University in 1962, when Van Kaam started a new doctoral program in phenomenological psychology. As the research methods specialist, Giorgi developed a course on the Phenomenological Foundations of Psychology, which was the basis for his first book, *Psychology as a Human Science.* In this work, Giorgi (1970) documented the historically persistent criticisms of psychology, such as its difficulties with defining its subject matter, its theoretical fragmentation, and the inability to bridge the gap between pure and applied areas. He argued that the common origin of these continuing problems in psychology is the erroneous adoption of the *natural science approach* to its subject matter. Giorgi claimed that the discipline of psychology must be understood not only with attention to its subject matter and methods, but also with regard to what he called its "approach," by which he meant its implicit assumptions and underlying philosophy. He called for a critical assessment of the naturalistic assumptions that had dominated psychology throughout its history and for a radical reorientation to a *human science approach,* which would allow the inclusion of research methods specifically designed to investigate human subject matter.

Charged with developing phenomenological research methods, Giorgi traveled throughout Western Europe and Scandinavia in the 1960s and found that the phenomenological psychologists offered brilliant philosophical and theoretical critiques of psychology but provided no positive alternative model for research methodology. At Duquesne, as Giorgi studied phenomenological philosophy with the help of faculty in the Philosophy Department, he explored and developed empirical, data-based research methods with doctoral students in psychology. One of Giorgi's first students, Paul Colaizzi (1967), replicated experiments in serial learning and collected first-person descriptions of participants' experience in experimental situations, analyzing the "fundamental psychological structure" of the perception of nonsense syllables. With students, Giorgi began flexibly crafting modes of qualitative data collection and descriptive analyses in response to the demands of various research problems and a wide range of human phenomena.

In 1970, Giorgi introduced a course on phenomenological research methods and offered a weekly seminar in which he, with dissertation students and their mentors, designed research methods on the full range of psychological topics. Some of Giorgi's students replicated traditional hypothesis-testing experiments supplemented with phenomenological analyses, and others researched situations in the lifeworld that served as analogues to experimental situations, such as McConville's (1974) study of "perception of the horizontal" on a golf course. In what has been referred to as the Duquesne Circle, Giorgi developed expertise on research methodology in diverse areas of psychology. Rolf Von Eckartsberg, William Fischer, Anthony Barton, Edward Murray, Constance Fischer, Frank Buckley, David Smith, Charles Maes, Richard Knowles, Paul Colaizzi, and Paul Richer contributed empirical research and theory across the full spectrum of traditional and new psychological subject matter. Doctoral research played a key role in the adaptation of phenomenologically based methods to the full range of psychological phenomena, including some that had not previously been approached by quantitative psychology, such as "the natural athlete" (Alapack, 1972), "transcendental, yoga, and Ignatian meditation" (Barnes, 1980), and "the psychology of courage" (Asarian, 1981). Typically, researchers collected descriptions of situations as experienced by human beings (e.g., through writing, interview, and audiotaped speech).

Giorgi adapted methods originally developed by phenomenological philosophers, such as the intentional analyses of meaning and the analysis of the essences of phenomena, for empirically based psychological research. These practices and the know-how that he developed in modifying them for psychology formed the basis for his methodological writings and the Duquesne academic curriculum in research methods. In methodological writings, Giorgi articulated and justified the key procedures involved in descriptive psychological research. Representative research and methodological advances of the Duquesne Circle were published in a four-volume series: *Duquesne Studies in Phenomenological Psychology* (Giorgi, Von Eckartsberg, & Fischer, 1971; Giorgi, Fischer, & Murray, 1975; Giorgi, Smith, & Knowles, 1979; Giorgi, Barton, & Maes, 1983). Giorgi has continued to develop his methodological work at the University of Quebec at Montreal and at the Saybook Institute. Full expositions, with careful attention to the relationship of philosophy and psychology, are found in Giorgi's (1985) *Phenomenology and Psychological Research* and his (2009) *The Descriptive Phenomenological Method in Psychology: A Modified Husserlian Approach.*

Because mainstream venues such as the *Journal of Experimental Psychology* would not publish descriptive research, Giorgi founded the *Journal of Phenomenological Psychology* in 1970. The phenomenological approach and the journal, in particular, led the publication of qualitative research in psychology. Investigating the emergence of qualitative research in psychology prior to 1980, Rennie, Watson, and Monteiro (2002) found that the term *phenomenological* (and *existential phenomenological psychology*) yielded a total of 126 hits in psychology journals, in comparison with *qualitative research, grounded theory,* and *discourse analysis,* which had no hits in psychology journals and combined for a total of nine hits in venues of other disciplines. Of journals publishing articles that used the search terms, the *Journal of Phenomenological Psychology* has included the most hits consistently over the last three decades (195 hits).

In an effort to reduce the isolation of phenomenological psychologists and to increase their impact with like-minded professionals, Giorgi formed professional alliances with others who shared the vision of a uniquely *human science*, including philosophical psychologists, humanistic psychologists, and qualitative researchers employing various approaches and methods across the full range of human science and service professions. For instance, Giorgi played a leading role in founding such professional organizations as the interdisciplinary International Human Science Research Association in 1981, which has met annually in North America, Japan, Scandinavia, Western Europe, and South Africa. Shunned in his original home in the APA Division of Experimental Psychology, Giorgi brought phenomenological psychology into the APA's Society of Theoretical and Philosophical Psychology and Society of Humanistic Psychology. As an executive board member and president of both APA divisions, Giorgi introduced phenomenological philosophy and qualitative research methods to North American psychologists and supported the broad qualitative research movement.

Grounded Theory: Barney Glaser and Anselm Strauss

The concrete origins of grounded theory clearly reside in sociologists Barney G. Glaser and Anselm L. Strauss's (1967) cutting-edge book *The Discovery of Grounded Theory*. The authors introduced grounded theory as a systematic, inductive, iterative, and comparative method of data analysis for the purpose of sociological theory construction. Glaser and Strauss's book spoke to the disciplinary debates of the 1960s. By that time, the development of sophisticated quantitative methods had undermined and marginalized an earlier robust tradition of qualitative research in sociology. Quantitative researchers had become skeptical about the value of qualitative research, which they saw as subjective, impressionistic, and anecdotal, rather than objective, systematic, and generalizable. Quantitative researchers had assumed control of departments, journals, and research funding. Simultaneously, qualitative research in sociology had increasingly become the purview of a few major scholars and their students, and theorizing had become the prerogative of elite armchair theorists who constructed theories without conducting empirical research. Glaser and Strauss wrote the *Discovery* book for sociologists to challenge and counter these trends. Neither Glaser nor Strauss foresaw that grounded theory would be adopted by multiple disciplines and professions.

Glaser and Strauss's book provided a powerful rationale for the logic and legitimacy of qualitative research and its potential for creating new theories and for democratizing theory construction. They argued that grounded theory answered criticisms of qualitative research because of its rigor, explicit strategies, and development of generalizations. Quantitative researchers of the day may not have been persuaded by Glaser and Strauss's arguments but aspiring qualitative researchers were. *The Discovery of Grounded Theory* played a vital role in igniting the "qualitative revolution" (Denzin & Lincoln, 1994, p. ix) that grew during the last decades of the 20th century and spread throughout the social sciences and professions (Charmaz, 2000, 2006).

The Discovery of Grounded Theory was the first major attempt to codify and systematize implicit methodological strategies for analyzing qualitative data and moving the analysis into explicit theoretical statements. Although less acknowledged than theory construction, Glaser and Strauss (1967) also developed grounded theory to analyze and explain social and social psychological processes. Some University of Chicago ethnographers and life history scholars had studied these processes and had long invoked similar analytic strategies that Glaser and Strauss explicated and named in the *Discovery* book. These sociologists had not, however, written about their analytic strategies, and likely most of them invoked implicit principles for data analysis. Before the publication of Glaser and Strauss's book, sociologists had learned qualitative research through a combination of mentoring and immersion in field research.

The intellectual foundations of grounded theory are subtle but somewhat contradictory. Although Glaser and Strauss constructed new analytic methods, each drew upon and extended the intellectual heritage represented in their respective doctoral training departments. Columbia University, Barney Glaser's alma mater, stood at the forefront of conventional 1950s sociology when he entered the doctoral program. At that time, sociologists at Columbia aimed to make sociology a "scientific" discipline based on a unitary vision of scientific method that embraced mid-20th-century assumptions of empiricism, objectivity, and quantification. The doctoral program in sociology at Columbia University emphasized (1) rigorous quantitative inquiry; (2) structural–functional theorizing, which focused on the structure and functioning of society and its institutions; and (3) the development of testable theories that explained specific social phenomena.

Glaser studied with Paul Lazarsfeld, who systematized quantitative inquiry, and Robert K. Merton (1957), who proposed constructing middle-range theories. By this term, Merton meant theories that would explain the structure and functioning of particular social institutions and answer empirical questions. Merton's proposal attempted to redirect sociological theorizing away from its midcentury emphasis on speculative macro theories, which explained the structure of society by creating abstract analyses of social action and social systems (Parsons, 1937, 1951). A classic example of Merton's turn toward middle-range theorizing can be found in his theoretical explanation of deviant behavior as resulting from an imbalance between individual aspirations and the structure of available opportunities (Merton, 1938).

The logic of quantitative research influenced Glaser's approach to grounded theory. His strong quantitative training surfaced in his treatment of grounded theory as a form of variable analysis and in the language of coding and sampling that he adopted to categorize grounded theory strategies. He (Glaser & Strauss, 1967; Glaser, 1978) borrowed quantitative terms to describe key grounded theory strategies, which has resulted in some confusion about the method. In grounded theory, for example, *coding* became inductive and open-ended rather than preconceived and deductive, as in quantitative research.

Lazarsfeld's influence is particularly evident in Glaser's goal to systematize qualitative analysis. Similarly, Glaser's (Glaser, 1978; Glaser & Strauss, 1967) emphasis on developing middle-range theories hearkened back to Merton's (1957) call for middle-range theories addressing measurable empirical problems. Glaser extended Merton's goal of constructing specific middle-range theories by arguing that researchers could generate these theories through inductive qualitative analysis. Threads of the structural–functionalism that informed Merton's work can be identified throughout Glaser's writings.

Perhaps the most profound early influence on Glaser was Anselm Strauss. In the festschrift for Strauss, Glaser thanked him by saying, "... you have taught me that the 'sociological word' is seldom received from on high: It is discovered in the data" (1991, p. 16). Glaser, a native San Franciscan, had returned to Northern California after finishing his doctoral studies. He met Strauss, who was at the University of California, San Francisco, and joined him, as did Jeanne Quint (Benoliel), in studying the social organization of dying. Quint did considerable fieldwork for the project and wrote *The Nurse and the Dying Patient* (1967), which became a classic study in nursing and changed the way nurses dealt with dying patients. Glaser (1991) credits Strauss for teaching him how to work autonomously and to engage the data with honesty. Their collaboration gave Glaser the freedom to develop his ideas and his methodology.

The path of Glaser's career may have led him away from Columbia, but its influence framed his approach to grounded theory. The influences of Strauss's doctoral training in sociology at the University of Chicago and his Chicago colleagues, in contrast, were simultaneously more apparent and continuous throughout his career. Strauss studied with scholars and researchers who were associated with the "Chicago school" of sociology. Chicago school sociologists had long engaged in field research and viewed the city as a natural setting in which to pursue it. Many of its proponents subscribed to its pragmatist philosophical underpinnings as articulated by John Dewey (1920, 1922, 1925; Dewey & Bentley, 1949) and George Herbert Mead (1932, 1934), although neither the sociology department at Chicago nor the Chicago school was as monolithic as typically portrayed. Those Chicago school sociologists who were influenced by pragmatism adopted its sociological derivative: symbolic interactionism. This theoretical perspective views self, situation, and society as social constructions that people accomplish through their actions and interactions. Symbolic interactionism is predicated on the use of language and symbols. Both pragmatists and symbolic interactionists (1) view humans as active agents who can interpret and act upon their situations; (2) take language and interpretation into account; (3) treat events as open-ended and emergent; (4) study individual and collective action; and (5) acknowledge the significance of temporality. Symbolic interactionism also challenged dominant 1960s social scientific assumptions about a single scientific method, a unitary external reality, objectivity and reliability, and the superiority of quantification over qualitative inquiry.

The notion of an agentic actor, with its assumptions of choice and action, distinguished Chicago school sociologists from other social scientists who espoused various forms of determinism. George Herbert Mead (1934) theorized that language is pivotal for the development of self and the conduct of social life. In Mead's view, subjective meanings emerge from experience, are given form through language, and change as experience changes. Thus, interpretation and action entail dynamic, reciprocal relationships. In this view, people interpret what is happening and, through their actions, fit diverse forms of conduct together. The implications of Mead's social psychology for method foster the value of gaining an empathic understanding of how research participants define their situations.

The seeds of Strauss's Chicago roots took form during his undergraduate career as a biology major at the University of Virginia, where he chanced to take a sociology course from Chicagoan Floyd House. Strauss became fascinated by works of coauthors W. I. Thomas and Florian Znanicki (1918) and John Dewey (1920), whose ideas formed the foundation for his theoretical perspective. With House's encouragement, Strauss went on to the University of Chicago, where Robert E. Park and Ernest W. Burgess's (see Park, Burgess, & MacKenzie, 1925/1967) studies sparked his lifelong interests in the city and in qualitative research. The influence of Everett C. Hughes's (1958) studies of work is evident in Strauss's coauthored grounded theory studies of patients' and families' work in pain management (Fagerhaugh & Strauss, 1977) and in caregiving (Corbin & Strauss, 1988). From Herbert Blumer (1969), Strauss developed his symbolic interactionist sensibilities and learned about Mead's theory of the development of self. Most social psychologists have focused on Mead's contributions to studying the self, but Strauss also built on Mead's conceptions of temporality, which can be traced back to Henri Bergson's (1922/1965) insights about duration.

Strauss's (1993) theory of action drew on both Mead and Dewey and their conceptions of action and process. Strauss may seem like a direct descendent of Mead, yet the influence of Dewey consistently reemerges from his earliest works to his last statement in *Continual Permutations of Action* (1993). His theoretical essays are replete with sensitizing concepts from which researchers can begin inquiry. Sensitizing concepts consist of general concepts such as self, identity, performance, work, and definition of the situation for initiating, but not determining, research. In *Mirrors and Masks* (1969/1959), for example, Strauss drew on Dewey and Bentley (1949) to illuminate relationships between naming and knowing. For Strauss, to name is to know—to identify a type, to locate an object, event, individual, or group in relation to others (Charmaz, 2008). Naming marks boundaries and suggests one's relationship to what is named. Thus, naming a phenomenon and evaluating it are blurred. Both are embedded in experience, and renaming this phenomenon means changing one's relationship to it. So too, constructivist grounded theory, a 21st-century revision of Glaser and Strauss's classic statement, marks new meanings of the method and changes our relationship to it.

The ideas of the first Chicago school drew Strauss to Chicago, where he later played a major role in establishing what became known as the second Chicago school (Fine, 1995). Strauss was part of a lifelong community of scholars linked by ties to Chicago School sociology that he extended through his international networks. Peers as well as protégés deeply engaged him throughout his career. Strauss collaborated on writing projects such as his early textbook on social psychology with Alfred Lindesmith (Lindesmith & Strauss, 1949) and remained involved in team research throughout his life.

Grounded theory continues to be closely associated with Glaser and Strauss, in part because each has written major texts explicating the method and, in part, because they each took grounded theory in different directions. The constructivist version of grounded theory offers another direction that takes into account methodological developments of the past 40 years. Constructivist grounded theory joins the fluidity and open-endedness of Anselm Strauss's early approach to social psychology with the specific strategies for analyzing data that Barney Glaser developed.

Discourse Analysis:
Jonathan Potter and Margaret Wetherell

The theory and practice of discourse analysis, as applied to questions and issues that concern social scientists, have been influenced by the writings of many people. Philosophical contributions on language by scholars such as Ludwig Wittgenstein, John Austin, Roland Barthes, Michel Foucault, and Jacques Derrida, and theoretical critiques of traditional psychological concepts such as cognition, self, and emotion advanced by Kenneth Gergen, John Shotter, Rom Harré, among others, have provided a rich source of ideas for the development of new ways of thinking about language and how people use it and of new analytic tools for empirical research.

Notwithstanding the importance of the rich scholarship on which the development of discourse analysis, as applied to social psychology, rests, two psychologists are clearly at the forefront of theoretical, methodological, and empirical work in this area: Jonathan Potter and Margaret Wetherell. Although both trained in mainstream psychology in the 1970s, each was influenced by ideas and developments outside of the dominant (American) psychology of the day. Potter studied at the University of York with Michael Mulkay and was influenced by writings in philosophy, literary theory, and the sociology of science, while Wetherell did her doctoral work at the University of Bristol, where a distinctly different (European) approach to the discipline was being formed by scholars such as Henri Tajfel, Howard Giles, and John Turner, and where Michael Billig's work on intergroup relations and on fascists was generating considerable excitement (Potter & Wetherell, 2006a).

Disenchantment with the narrow way in which central concepts in social psychology were theorized and the near-exclusive use of experimental designs and questionnaires in mainstream psychology fueled Potter's and Wetherell's engagements in new ways of thinking about and doing psychology. It was while they were lecturers in the Psychology Department at The University of St. Andrews in Scotland—a department whose faculty specialized in neuroscience and animal behavior and appreciated in-depth descriptive work—that they wrote what would be one of their most influential texts: *Discourse and Social Psychology: Beyond Attitudes and Behaviour* (Potter & Wetherell, 2006a). Published in 1987, the book's theoretical foundations included a focus on the performative aspects of language as developed in Austin's speech act theory; on Harold Garfinkel's view of ethnomethodology (the study of ordinary people's methods); and on Ferdinand de Saussure's work on semiotics (the science of signs). With this foundation, Potter and Wetherell reworked traditional notions in social psychology—such as attitudes, accountability, self, and categories—along discursive lines. For example, rather than taking attitudes as something fixed and inside the person, Potter and Wetherell emphasized the function (or, in contemporary terms, the action or action orientation) and construction of "attitudinal" statements—that is, how such statements are produced and what they achieve.

In addition to reworking some central concepts in social psychology, Potter and Wetherell further developed Gilbert and Mulkay's (1984) notion of an interpretative repertoire as "the recurrently used system of terms used for characterizing and evaluating actions, events and other phenomena" (Potter & Wetherell, 1987, p. 149)—a notion that has been used extensively since—and set out a model for how to conduct discourse analysis. In their chapter on methodology they stressed, among other points, that (1) "participants' discourse or social texts are approached in *their own right* and not as a secondary route to things 'beyond' the text like attitudes, events or cognitive processes" (p. 160); (2) research questions are focused primarily on construction and function; (3) data from a variety of sources and contexts should be analyzed; (4) interviews must be understood as "conversational encounters" (p. 165), which require that the researcher's and the participant's contributions be analyzed; (5) analysis involves a search for pattern, that is, for variability, and a concern with function and consequence (p. 168); (6) extracts from transcripts or documents are not illustrations of the data, but are instances of the data analysis itself; and (7) discourse analysts have an obligation to apply their research.

The publication of *Discourse and Social Psychology: Beyond Attitudes and Behaviour* has contributed to a rethinking of psychological concepts in non-objectivist terms. It has also fueled a great deal of discursive research, sparked further articulation of discursive methodologies and of methods of data collection, generation, and analysis, and generally enhanced the legitimacy of qualitative research in the social sciences (although its greatest impact remains outside of American psychology) (Potter & Wetherell, 2006b). A few notable examples of such ensuing contributions include (1) Wetherell and Potter's (1992) work on commonplace patterns of explanation and argumentation used by white New Zealanders to sustain racism and exploitation of the Maori minority; (2) Edwards and Potter's reformulation of attribution from the privileging of the real-world stimulus and the cognition of the actor to a focus on the activity of the actor—that is, how people produce particular versions of causality (e.g., Edwards & Potter, 1992); (3) Edwards's (1999) reconsideration of emotion as displays and discursive categories that are used to achieve particular effects, as something that is jointly managed and constructed, rather than as a physiological and cognitive experience; (4) Potter and Hepburn's (2005) critique of the research interview as the preferred method of data generation and their call for the expanded use of so-called naturalistic sources of data; and (5) Wood and Kroger's (2000) detailed specification of resources and strategies that can be employed in doing discursive analysis.

Potter's and Wetherell's contributions to discourse analysis and discursive psychology continue to be groundbreaking, although their paths have diverged. In the late 1980s Potter took a post in the Department of Social Sciences at Loughborough University, where he has pursued interests in reconstructing constructionism (Potter, 1996), in the relation between discourse and cognition, particularly the role that cognitive states should play in the analysis of interaction (Molder & Potter, 2005), and in the application of discourse analysis to a variety of interactions, including family mealtimes and calls to child protection helplines. In his empirical work, he has embraced more fully the conversation analytic perspective and is developing a discursive psychological approach to audio and video records of natural interaction (see *potter.socialpsychology.org*).

In the mid-1980s Margaret Wetherell joined the faculty of social sciences at the Open University, and from 2003 to 2008 was Director of the UK Economic and Social Research Council Identities and Social Action Programme.

Her current theoretical work focuses on the possible lines of engagement between psychoanalysis and discourse theory as a new way of thinking about and analyzing subjectivity and the psychosocial domain, while her empirical work on identity has focused on ethnicity, racism, and gender (Wetherell, 2009a, 2009b), in particular, on masculinities and men's identities, and has extended to an analysis of the discursive practices that constitute democratic deliberation and citizen participation (Davies, Wetherell, & Barnett, 2006). With an emphasis on social action, Wetherell's work provides a model for the application of discourse analysis.

In addition to Potter's and Wetherell's significant influence on ways of thinking about and doing social psychology, their work has contributed to a climate in which new journals such as *Discourse and Society, Feminism and Psychology*, and *Theory and Psychology* have flourished, and in which the traditional boundaries between psychology and disciplines such as sociology, literary theory, anthropology, and philosophy are dissolving (Potter & Wetherell, 2006a).

Narrative Psychology:
Jerome Bruner, Ted Sarbin, and Don Polkinghorne

There is no single figure to whom one could attribute the narrative research tradition in psychology. Certainly, it can be traced to Freud, Piaget, Allport, and Erikson, all of whom were working with narratives, although they would not have defined themselves as developing narrative research. Many contemporary narrative researchers situate their work as emanating from ideas propounded by psychologists Jerome Bruner, Ted Sarbin, or Don Polkinghorne but resist the idea that there is a definable "method" through which narratives can be elicited or analyzed. Rather, narrativists ground their mode of inquiry on works by such writers as the Russian philosophical anthropologist Bakhtin or the French philosopher Ricoeur. They see their work as rooted in the hermeneutic tradition, tracing their epistemological heritage to Dilthey, Husserl, and Heidegger. Many draw on ethnographic approaches, particularly the work of anthropologist Clifford Geertz. Feminist scholars in a number of disciplines have turned to and developed narrative modes of inquiry in order to investigate "voice," a concept elaborated by Carol Gilligan (1982) who, with her colleagues and students at Harvard, developed a "listening guide" to voices of experience as expressed in narrations (Brown & Gilligan, 1992). Narrative research has been particularly appealing to life history researchers because people compose stories to understand their lives. Narrative inquiry borders and draws on scholarship and methodology from anthropology, history, and literary theory. In contemporary days, Dan McAdams and Jefferson Singer have furthered narrative research in psychology by developing the idea that personality and identity are constructed narratively. Psychologists Ruthellen Josselson and Amia Lieblich coedited six volumes of a series called *The Narrative Study of Lives* published by Sage, and, with Dan McAdams, five more volumes published by the American Psychological Association (2003). See the reference list in Chapter 8 for the specific reference entries cited here. Since 1998, Michael Bamberg has edited a journal called *Narrative Inquiry.* In these volumes, the most prominent narrative researchers in psychology have published their work, including Bert Cohler, Michelle Fine, Mark Freeman, Ken and Mary Gergen, Gary Gregg, Suzanne Ouellette, William McKinley Runyan, and others.

Born in 1915, Jerome Bruner was a student of Gordon Allport at Harvard and later taught at Harvard, at Oxford University, and at the New School. A major figure in the history of psychology, Bruner led several "revolutions" in the field. His first revolution, the "New Look" in psychology in the 1940s, explored perception from a functional orientation, taking into account how needs, motivations, and expectations (or "mental sets") influence perception. Bruner understood that perception is a form of information processing that involves interpretation and selection and argued that psychology must concern itself with how people interpret the world, as well as how they respond to perceptual stimuli. Later, influenced by the work of Vygotsky, Luria, and Piaget, he championed the "Cognitive Revolution" in the 1960s and developed cognitive and constructivist psychological approaches in psychology. His book, *A Study of Thinking* (1956), written with Jacqueline Goodnow and George Austin, is often viewed as the herald of the cognitive sciences. Bruner was drawn to linguistic philosophy for insight into human language capacities and to cultural anthropology for insight into how thinking is culturally bound. He was most interested in the distinctly human forms of gaining, storing, and integrating knowledge, and his work had profound effects on education. When he became disillusioned with the more concrete and piecemeal direction that the cognitive revolution was taking, he began writing the foundational works for the "narrative turn" in psychology in the 1990s. In this phase, he reemphasized the fundamental cultural and environmental aspects to human cognitive response and used the concept of narrative as an organizing principle. At the end of his career, he taught at the New York University Law School, where he attempted to integrate narrative theory with legal processes. Throughout his long and highly productive career, Bruner focused his interests on perception, language, communication, and culture, all leading eventually to an integration of these phenomena into what he called the "narrative paradigm."

Reacting against what Gordon Allport had labeled "methodolatry," Bruner remained dedicated to the larger questions: questions about the nature of mind, about how people create meaning and construct their reality, and how people are affected by culture and history. All these, he believed, needed to be addressed through a consideration of the stories people tell about their experiences. Bruner believed that people have an "innate" predisposition to narrative organization of their experiences, whereas cultures offer forms of telling and interpreting that make narratives comprehensible both to the self and to others (Bruner, 1990).

Bruner's early work in cognitive psychology focused on language and other representations of human thought. Bruner took many of his ideas from literary theory and taught that narratives take place over time and deal with particular events. He recognized that stories are fundamental building blocks of human experience and argued that stories represent some kind of brain processing of the events that the individual has experienced and made meaning of, rather than reflections of some uninterpreted reality. Life stories link story and life as we create stories of our lives and live our stories.

Perhaps most important, Bruner distinguished the narrative mode of knowing from the paradigmatic one. Whereas paradigmatic knowing is based upon classification and categorization, narrative modes of thought (Bruner, 1986) aim to create interpreted descriptions of the rich and multilayered meanings of historical and personal events. The search is for truths that are unique in their particularity, grounded in firsthand experience, in order to extend and enhance conceptualization. Narratives, then, are viewed as the building blocks of the construction of reality and meaning. "It is our narrative gift that gives us the power to make sense of things when they don't" (Bruner, 2002, p. 28).

Bruner continually linked narrative and culture. Cultures create the realm of stories that are deemed acceptable, defining a tension between the expected life and what is humanly possible. Sharing common stories creates a community and promotes cultural cohesion. In his reflections on law and literature, Bruner elaborated his belief that interpretation, through narrative, is central to being human; it is how we bring meaning and order to life.

Ted Sarbin was a professor of psychology and criminology at the University of California, Santa Cruz, and also a professor of psychology at Berkeley. He was strongly influenced by the American philosopher Stephen Pepper and the social theorist George Herbert Mead. In 1986, he edited *Narrative Psychology: The Storied Nature of Human Conduct*, in which he argued for the transformation of psychology. His thesis was that the metaphor of the machine underlay much of psychology. In opposition, he proposed narrative as a "root metaphor" for psychology. "In giving accounts of ourselves or of others, we are guided by narrative plots. Whether for formal biographies or autobiographies, for psychotherapy, for self-disclosure, or for entertainment, we do much more than catalog a series of events. Rather, we render the events into a story" (Sarbin, 1986, p. 23). This book contained chapters by a number of psychologists who were developing techniques for investigating the ways that people narrate life events.

A few years later *Narrative Knowing and the Human Sciences,* by Donald Pol-kinghorne (1988), called psychology's attention to the work of Paul Ricoeur, a French philosopher whose immense body of work detailed the centrality of narrative for meaning making. With ideas converging with those of Bruner and Sarbin, Polkinghorne wrote, "We achieve our personal identities and self concept through the use of the narrative configuration, and make our exis-tence into a whole by understanding it as an expression of a single unfolding and developing story" (Polkinghorne, 1988, p. 150). Polkinghorne empha-sized the dynamic aspect of the self-as-a-story. Because we are in the middle of the plots of our lives, we have no clear idea about how they will evolve and end. We have to revise our stories constantly, reshuffle the memories of the past and perform new selection of events and characters, in accordance with new current experiences or life development, and with the changing expecta-tions regarding our future.

Since the 1990s, work in narrative research has burgeoned, resting on the foundations detailed above, as researchers use narrative analysis to understand how various people—including those marginalized by hypothetico–deductive psychological research—construct their lives. Inductive in its essence, narra-tive research requires work from a reflexive stance; it focuses on holistic aspects of participants' biographies and utilizes the capacity to meld observation and theory in meaningful ways. Narrative work is conducted within a postmodern frame in which knowledge is constructed rather than discovered; as such, it is assumed to be localized and perspectival, occurring within intersubjective relationships to both participants and readers. "Method," then, becomes not a set of techniques and procedures, but ways of thinking about inquiry, modes of exploring questions, and creative approaches to offering one's constructed findings to the scholarly community. This inquiry occurs without certitude. We face the uneasiness and complexity of the work in the absence of well-trodden paths to "truth."

Intuitive Inquiry: Rosemarie Anderson

Intuitive inquiry applies elements of European hermeneutics to qualitative data analysis. Following the hermeneutical traditions established by the writ-ings of Fredrick Schleiermacher (1768–1834) and Hans-Georg Gadamer (1900–2002), hermeneutics has had wide application in the interpretation of sacred and literary texts in religion, philosophy, and literature and, more recently, in the interpretation of textual data in qualitative research. Although the practices of hermeneutics vary considerably, interpretation is generally understood as self-reflective, iterative, and ongoing, with the interpreter mindful that his or her pre-understandings influence interpretation and that new insights influence how a text is understood as a whole. Acknowledging that interpretation inevitably arises within a cultural context with implicit values and symbols, hermeneuticians often employ human imagination and aesthetic sensibilities in interpretive acts. Intuitive inquiry stands within and expands this tradition to qualitative research.

Psychologist Rosemarie Anderson developed intuitive inquiry in the mid-1990s, incorporating scholarly and aesthetic elements embedded in her personal and professional life. Anderson was born in 1947, the first child of Scandinavian parents who held strong political opinions on the radical left and a deep appreciation for the arts, especially music and theater. As a teen and young adult, she was a gymnast specializing in floor exercises and dance. The Anderson family home was within metropolitan New York City, and frequent visits to the Metropolitan Museum of Art, Guggenheim Art Museum, Lincoln Center, and the Broadway theater district forged her early education.

Anderson's undergraduate and graduate psychology training was strongly influenced by the learning theories of Clark Hull and B. F. Skinner, experimental methods, and statistical analyses. During her doctoral training in experimental social psychology at the University of Nebraska–Lincoln in the early 1970s, the psychology department was well known for innovations in theory and experimental research. In her own research and analyses, Anderson came to understand quantitative multivariate analysis as a complex form of pattern recognition that required intuitive insights to "unlock" patterns embedded in statistical arrays, an understanding that was formative for her in subsequent research and influenced her development of intuitive inquiry almost 30 years later.

After graduate school, Anderson continued to conduct research in experimental social psychology at Wake Forest University but, over time, became increasingly disquieted with the limitations of experimental methods as applied to research in psychology. In the context of the influx of spiritual traditions from the East that infused American culture in the 1970s, her spiritual life was also quickening. Anderson resigned her position at Wake Forest and accepted a position with the University of Maryland's Asian Division, teaching psychology courses at U.S. military bases in Japan, South Korea, and Australia. Fortunately for her, Asia in the late 1970s was still the Orient, far from Europe or the Americas, ideologically and culturally. The cultures and art of Asia and the monasteries she visited while still in her early 30s left a strong spiritual and aesthetic impression that asked her to look anew at her personal and professional life direction.

Upon returning to the United States in 1979, Anderson accepted a research position at Florida Mental Health in Tampa, a position that required a 1-year commitment. Her spiritual interests still emerging and seeking to integrate her interests in psychology and spirituality, Anderson decided to pursue a theological education to explore life's great existential questions within her own spiritual tradition. She attended the Graduate Theological

Union in Berkeley, California, and completed a Masters of Divinity degree at the Pacific School of Religion in 1983. Under the tutelage of many fine teachers, Anderson was classically educated in ancient Hebrew, New Testament Greek, Biblical hermeneutics, and philosophy. This formal training in philosophy and especially hermeneutics gave her the intellectual background to develop intuitive inquiry some 20 years later.

At the completion of seminary training, Anderson rejoined the University of Maryland but this time to teach in the European Division. After teaching in Italy for a few months, she accepted a position as a university dean to oversee the University of Maryland's undergraduate and graduate programs in Germany.

When Anderson was ordained a priest in the Protestant Episcopal Church in 1987, she returned to the United States to serve as a parish priest in San Diego, California, and a university chaplain in Santa Cruz, California. As a parish priest and chaplain, Anderson began to apply her knowledge of Biblical hermeneutics to sermon preparation. As Biblical hermeneutics requires, each week she studied the scripture chosen in terms of what it might have meant to the audience to whom it was originally addressed, including the text's historical context, genre, and the possible purposes of the author(s). Thereafter, she interpreted meanings embedded in the text as relevant to the congregation's hopes and needs in the delivered sermon.

In 1991, Anderson began to teach as adjunct faculty at the Institute of Transpersonal Psychology (ITP) and, in a year's time, accepted a position on ITP's core faculty, a position that encouraged Anderson to combine her interests in psychological research and spirituality. Abraham Maslow (1971), one of the founders of transpersonal psychology, described the new field as dedicated to the study of the "farther reaches of human nature." With historical roots in the political and social movements of the 1960s in the United States, transpersonal psychology explores a full spectrum of human experience, including topics often neglected in mainstream psychological research, such as peak experiences, alternative states of consciousness, and experiences of nonduality.

Anderson's professorial colleagues at ITP represented spiritual traditions worldwide, inviting her into new dialogues about psychospiritual development, perennial philosophy, and research methods appropriate to the study of transpersonal phenomena. William Braud also joined the ITP Core Faculty in 1992. Soon, both Anderson and Braud recognized that the experimental methods of their graduate training were ill suited to a full exploration of transpersonal and spiritual phenomena. Subsequently, in 1995, a set of unexpected circumstances led them to coteach quantitative and qualitative research methods together. This course became a "laboratory" in which to expand and extend established quantitative and qualitative research methods to meet the needs of transpersonal topics. Anderson and Braud's ongoing conversations and interactions with doctoral students and colleagues led them to coauthor *Transpersonal Research Methods for the Social Sciences*, a book that has set a standard for transpersonal research since its publication in 1998.

In the mid-1990s, Anderson also began to develop intuitive inquiry by integrating her appreciation of the intuitive nature of human understanding and European hermeneutics. Aware that research analyses often required intuitive insight to deepen interpretation, she began to formulate structured processes to prompt intuitive insights in qualitative research. Encouraged by the writings of Michael Polanyi, Carl Jung, and Clark Moustakas and by research on intuition and its relationship to right- and left- brain processes, Anderson developed intuitive inquiry as a qualitative approach to research and began to invite her doctoral students to "test" the approach in their dissertation research. In the early 2000s, she gave intuitive inquiry the structure of a hermeneutical circle, an iterative process that enfolds pre-understandings and intuition into data collection, analysis and interpretation, and presentations of findings. Integrating intuitive ways within a hermeneutical structure proved fruitful, resulting in a structured but flexible approach to qualitative research that could be used by researchers who do not necessarily consider themselves intuitive. At this point in the development of intuitive inquiry, Anderson looks forward to the variants on intuitive inquiry that other researchers will improvise and propose.

From Qualitative Practice to Methodological Traditions

The genius of systematizers is in their clear discernment and explicit delineation of general research practices that embody fundamental principles of good scientific method. Their work has gone beyond that of isolated virtuoso practitioners by specifying qualitative methods and principles of practice to be learned and employed by researchers on a large scale. In the methodologies described in this chapter, we find many procedures that were used by isolated practitioners prior to the establishment of qualitative traditions. In some cases, underlying principles were identified by lone qualitative pioneers prior to their being systematized for broad usage. For instance, Freud made use of extreme examples of dreams, neuroses, and parapraxes that presented themselves spontaneously to him. Maslow deliberately undertook the collection of extreme examples of healthy personality and, like Freud, made use of them without ever recognizing or commenting on the general value of that practice. James, too, made extensive use of extreme cases, and he explicitly drew attention to the practice and its great value, but he justified it on the basis of the specific demands of spirituality as a subject matter and did not suggest it as a general principle of qualitative methodology. Kohlberg did not set out to collect extreme examples of moral reasoning, but he gravitated to them and made special use of them in order to sort out what was most significant in his voluminous sea of data. Kohlberg reflected on the practice, commented on its general value, and even called attention to its utilization by Freud. However, he did not offer the research community a general set of procedures that would make this good practice available to researchers on a large scale. Only after Flanagan raised the collection of extreme examples to methodological status in a general system of practice has its application spread and born fruit in human science.

Similarly in the case of Giorgi, the phenomenological procedures of intentional analysis of meaning and eidetic analysis of the essence of phenomena had been practiced by many. Not only did Freud, James (who explicitly used the word *essence*), Maslow, and Kohlberg employ these practices, but researchers throughout psychoanalytic and existential research used such methods without explicitly raising them to methodological status (Wertz, 1983, 1987a, 1987b, 1993). Psychologists and human scientists of all stripes have focused on the essential meaning of their phenomena. Giorgi's generative contribution was to specify general, practical procedures for collecting and analyzing lived experiences that could be employed across the spectrum of human subject matter by an unlimited movement of researchers.

Glaser and Straus explored the procedures for developing theories that are in close touch with concrete reality, and presumably Straus even conveyed these practices in mentor relationships to students such as Kohlberg, before they articulated the underlying principles of the method for more general use. It is quite likely that these practices have been employed by many theorists, who have done so informally and sometimes haphazardly. Glaser and Strauss provided the research community with an explicit understanding of the principles underlying theory development and practices through which it could be carried out on a broad scale.

Potter's and Wetherell's contributions to the development of procedures for the analysis of naturally occurring language (talk), which is unquestionably of the most profound significance for the human sciences, were based in underlying principles and justifications whose genesis lay in diverse disciplinary traditions. It was, however, their elaboration and articulation of analytic concepts and strategies, along with a critique of traditional social psychology, that contributed to a broad movement of discursive research in psychology and other human sciences and to further development and specification of how to analyze human talk.

When Freud recognized that his research reports sometimes sounded more like stories than scientific reports, he was astonished. To his credit, he recognized that this characteristic of his work was not driven by personal proclivity but demanded by his subject matter, and he did view his practice as scientific. Bruner's contributions to narrative psychology, late in his career, extended the work he had done in the early 1940s as Allport's (1942) assistant when he originally studied the importance of premethodological work with personal documents in psychology. But only by virtue of the work of methodologists such as Bruner, Sarbin, and Polkinghorne have the principles and general practices of narrative research become available to the broad research community and begun to produce volumes of human science research.

Intuition has been practiced to the benefit of scientific research throughout history. Freud and James were certainly masters of intuitive insight, and Maslow's study of healthy personality was deeply rooted in personal concerns related to a mysterious historical vision of the healing transformation of humanity. However, these practices and aspirations were described in detail and elevated to methodological legitimacy in the work of Anderson.

Human science researchers who are interested in qualitative inquiry now have available to them not only a varied and rich array of theoretical and conceptual principles, but a complementary and diverse set of analytic concepts, strategies, and practices. We now turn to the broad movement in the human sciences and to the contemporary issues and questions engendered by the explication and dissemination of these research methods.

References

Adkins, D. C. (1952). Proceedings of the sixteenth annual business meeting of the American Psychological Association, Inc., Washington, DC. *American Psychologist, 7,* 645–670.

Alapack, R. J. (1972). *The phenomenology of the natural athlete.* Unpublished doctoral dissertation, Duquesne University, Pittsburgh, PA.

Allport, G. W. (1942). *The use of personal documents in psychological science* (Prepared for the Committee on the Appraisal of Research; Bulletin #49). New York: Social Science Research Council.

American Psychological Association Ethics Committee. (2002). Report of the Ethics Committee, 2001. *American Psychologist, 57,* 650–657.

Anderson, R., & Braud, W. (1998). *Transpersonal research methods for the social sciences.* Thousand Oaks, CA: Sage.

Asarian, R. D. (1981). *The psychology of courage: A human scientific investigation.* Unpublished doctoral dissertation, Duquesne University, Pittsburgh, PA.

Barnes, R. M. (1980). *A study of the psychological structures of transcendental, yoga, and Ignatian meditation* Unpublished doctoral dissertation, Duquesne University, Pittsburgh, PA.

Benoliel, J. Q. (1967). *The nurse and the dying patient.* New York: Macmillan.

Bergson, H. (1965). *Duration and simultaneity, with reference to Einstein's theory.* Indianapolis, IN: Bobbs-Merrill. (Original work published 1922)

Blumer, H. (1969). *Symbolic interactionism.* Englewood Cliffs, NJ: Prentice-Hall.

Brentano, F. (1973). *Psychology from an empirical standpoint* (A. C. Rancurello, D. B. Terrell, & L. L. McAlister, Trans.). New York: Humanities Press. (Original work published 1874)

Brown, L. M., & Gilligan, C. (1992). *Meeting at the crossroads: Women's psychology and girls' development.* Cambridge, MA: Harvard University Press.

Bruner, J. S. (1986). *Actual minds, possible worlds.* Cambridge, MA: Harvard University Press.

Bruner, J. S. (1990). *Acts of meaning.* Cambridge, MA: Harvard University Press.

Bruner, J. S. (2002). *Making stories: Law, literature, life.* Cambridge, MA: Harvard University Press.

Bruner, J. S., Goodnow, J. J., & Austin, G. A. (1956). *A study of thinking.* New York: Wiley.

Charmaz, K. (2000). Constructivist and objectivist grounded theory. In N. K. Denzin & Y. Lincoln (Eds.), *Handbook of qualitative research* (2nd ed., pp. 509–535). Thousand Oaks, CA: Sage.

Charmaz, K. (2006). *Constructing grounded theory: A practical guide through qualitative analysis.* London: Sage.

Charmaz, K. (2008). The legacy of Anselm Strauss for constructivist grounded theory. In N. K. Denzin (Ed.), *Studies in symbolic interaction* (pp. 127–141). Bingley, UK: Emerald Publishing Group.

Colaizzi, P. F. (1967). An analysis of the learner's perception of the learning material at various stages of the learning process. *Review of Existential Psychology and Psychiatry, 7,* 95–105.

Corbin, J. M., & Strauss, A. (1988). *Unending care and work.* San Francisco: Jossey-Bass.

Davies, C., Wetherell, M., & Barnett, E. (2006). *Citizens at the centre: Deliberative participation in healthcare decisions.* Bristol, UK: Policy Press.

Denzin, N. K., & Lincoln, Y. S. (1994). *Handbook of qualitative research.* Thousand Oaks, CA: Sage.

Dewey, J. (1920). *Reconstruction in philosophy.* New York: Henry Holt.

Dewey, J. (1922). *Human nature and conduct.* New York: Henry Holt.

Dewey, J. (1925). *Experience and nature.* Chicago: Open Court.

Dewey, J., & Bentley, A. F. (1949). *Knowing and the known.* Boston: Beacon Press.

Edwards, D. (1999). Emotion discourse. *Culture and Psychology, 5,* 271–291.

Edwards, D., & Potter, J. (1992). *Discursive psychology.* London: Sage.

Embree, L. (2010). Interdisciplinarity within phenomenology. *Indo-Pacific Journal of Phenomenology, 10*(1), 1–7.

Fagerhaugh, S. Y., & Strauss, A. (1977). *The politics of pain management: Staff–patient interaction.* Reading, MA: Addison-Wesley.

Fine, G. A. (Ed.). (1995). *A second Chicago School?: The development of a postwar American sociology,* Chicago: University of Chicago Press.

Flanagan, J. C. (1954). The critical incident technique. *Psychological Bulletin, 51*(4), 327–358.

Gilbert, G. N., & Mulkay, M. (1984). *Opening Pandora's box: A sociological analysis of scientists' discourse.* Cambridge, UK: Cambridge University Press.

Gilligan, C. (1982). *In a different voice.* Cambridge, MA: Harvard University Press.

Giorgi, A. (1970). *Psychology as a human science.* New York: Harper.

Giorgi, A. (1985). *Phenomenology and psychological research.* Pittsburgh, PA: Duquesne University Press.

Giorgi, A. (2009). *The descriptive phenomenological method in psychology: A modified Husserlian approach.* Pittsburgh, PA: Duquesne University Press.

Giorgi, A., Barton, A., & Maes, C. (Vol. Eds.). (1983). *Duquesne studies in phenomenological psychology: Volume IV.* Pittsburgh, PA: Duquesne University Press.

Giorgi, A., Fischer, C. T., & Murray, E. L. (Vol. Eds.). (1975). *Duquesne studies in phenomenological psychology: Volume II.* Pittsburgh, PA: Duquesne University Press.

Giorgi, A., Smith, D., & Knowles, R. (Vol. Eds.). (1979). *Duquesne studies in phenomenological psychology: Volume III.* Pittsburgh, PA: Duquesne University Press.

Giorgi, A., Von Eckartsberg, R., & Fischer, W. F. (Vol. Eds.). (1971). *Duquesne studies in phenomenological psychology: Volume I.* Pittsburgh, PA: Duquesne University Press.

Glaser, B. G. (1978). *Theoretical sensitivity: Advances in the methodology of grounded theory.* Mill Valley, CA: Sociology Press.

Glaser, B. G. (1991). In honor of Anselm Strauss: Collaboration. In D.R. Maines (Ed.), *Social organization and social process: Essays in honor of Anselm Strauss* (pp. 11–16). Hawthorne, NY: Walter de Gruyter.

Glaser, B. G., & Strauss, A. L. (1967). *The discovery of grounded theory.* Chicago: Aldine.

Hughes, E. C. (1958). *Men and their work.* Glencoe, IL: Free Press.

Husserl, E. (1962). *Ideas: General introduction to pure phenomenology* (W. R. B. Gibson, Trans.). New York: Collier Books. (Original work published 1913)

Husserl, E. (1970). *Logical investigations.* (L. Findlay, Trans.). London: Routledge & Kegan Paul. (Originally published in 1900–1901)

Josselson, R., Leiblich, A., & McAdams, D. (Eds.). (2003). *Up close and personal: The teaching and learning of narrative research.* Washington, DC: American Psychological Association.

Leech, N. L., & Onwuegbuzie, A. J. (2008). Qualitative data analysis: A compendium of techniques and a framework for selection for school psychology research and beyond. *School Psychology Quarterly, 23*(4), 587–604.

Lindesmith, A., & Strauss, A. L. (1949). *Social psychology.* New York: Dryden.

Maslow, A. H. (1971). *The farther reaches of human nature.* New York: Viking.

McConville, M. (1974). *Perception of the horizontal dimension of space: A phenomenological study.* Unpublished doctoral dissertation, Duquesne University, Pittsburgh, PA.

Mead, G. H. (1932). *Philosophy of the present.* LaSalle, IL: Open Court Press.

Mead, G. H. (1934). *Mind, self and society.* Chicago: University of Chicago Press.

Merton, R. K. (1938). Social structure and anomie. *American Sociological Review, 3,* 672–682.

Merton, R. K. (1957). *Social theory and social structure.* Glencoe, IL: Free Press.

Miller, R. B., & Flanagan, J. C. (1950). The performance record: An objective merit-rating procedure for industry. *American Psychologist, 5,* 331–332.

Molder, H., & Potter, J. (2005). *Conversation and cognition.* Cambridge, UK: Cambridge University Press.

Norman, I. J., Redfern, S. J., Tomalin, D. A., & Oliver, S. (1992). Developing Flanagan's critical incident technique to elicit indicators of high and low quality nursing care from patients and their nurses. *Journal of Advanced Nursing, 17,* 590–600.

Park, R. E., Burgess, E. W., & McKenzie, R. D. (1967). *The city.* Chicago: University of Chicago Press. (Original work published 1925)

Parsons, T. (1937). *The structure of social action.* Glencoe, IL: Free Press.

Parsons, T. (1951). *The social system.* Glencoe, IL: Free Press.

Polkinghorne, D. E. (1988). *Narrative knowing and the human sciences.* Albany, NY: State University of New York Press.

Potter, J. (1996). *Representing reality: Discourse, rhetoric and social construction.* London: Sage.

Potter, J., & Hepburn, A. (2005). Qualitative interviews in psychology: Problems and possibilities. *Qualitative Research in Psychology, 2,* 281–307.

Potter, J., & Wetherell, M. (1987). *Discourse and social psychology: Beyond attitudes and behaviour.* London: Sage.

Potter, J., & Wetherell, M. (2006a). Preface to Chinese edition of *Discourse and Social Psychology.* Beijing: China: Renmin University Press.

Potter, J., & Wetherell, M. (2006b). Postscript to Chinese edition of *Discourse and Social Psychology.* Beijing: China: Renmin University Press.

Quint, J. C. (1967). *The nurse and the dying patient.* New York: Macmillan.

Rennie, D. L., Watson, K. D., & Monteiro, A. M. (2002). The rise of qualitative research in psychology. *Canadian Psychology, 43*(3), 179–189.

Sarbin, T. R. (Ed.). (1986). *Narrative psychology: The storied nature of human conduct.* New York: Praeger.

Stoppard, J. M. (2003). Navigating the hazards of orthodoxy: Introducing a graduate course on qualitative methods into the psychology curriculum. *Canadian Psychology, 43*(3), 143–153.

Strauss, A. L. (1961). *Images of the American city.* New York: Free Press.

Strauss, A. L. (1969). *Mirrors and masks.* Mill Valley, CA: Sociology Press. (Original work published 1959)

Strauss, A. L. (1993). *Continual permutations of action.* New York: Aldine de Gruyter.

Thomas, W. I., & Znaniecki, F. (1918). *The Polish peasant in Poland and America.* New York: Knopf.

Wertz, F. J. (1983). Some components of descriptive psychological reflection. *Human Studies, 6*(1), 35–51.

Wertz, F.J. (1987a). Common methodological fundaments of the analytic procedures in phenomenological and psychoanalytic research. *Psychoanalysis and Contemporary Thought, 9*(4), 563–603.

Wertz, F.J. (1987b). Meaning and research methodology: Psychoanalysis as a human science. *Methods: A Journal for Human Science, 1*(2), 91–135.

Wertz, F. J. (1993). The phenomenology of Sigmund Freud. *Journal of Phenomenological Psychology, 24*(2), 101–129.

Wetherell, M. (Ed.). (2009a). *Identity in the 21st century: New trends in changing times.* Basingstoke, UK: Palgrave.

Wetherell, M. (Ed.). (2009b). *Theorizing identities and social action.* Basingstoke, UK: Palgrave.

Wetherell, M., & Potter, J. (1992). *Mapping the language of racism: Discourse and the legitimization of exploitation.* New York: Columbia University Press.

Wood, L. A., & Kroger, R. O. (2000). *Doing discourse analysis: Methods for studying action in talk and text.* Thousand Oaks, CA: Sage.

CHAPTER 3

Contemporary Movement,
Methodological Pluralism, and Challenges

S
o far our story of qualitative research methods has focused on innova-
tors of methods and founders of established traditions. In the last two
decades, qualitative research has become a *movement*, spreading through
almost every area of psychology to encompass researchers, faculty, and students of many stripes. The excitement is evident in accounts characterizing
this movement as a "revolution" (Denzin & Lincoln, 1994, 2000, pp. 923–
936), a "force" (Ponterotto, 2002), a "tectonic change" (O'Neill, 2002), and
a "paradigm shift" (O'Neill, 2002; Ponterotto, 2005). Psychology has been a
latecomer to this movement, which transformed other social sciences earlier
and with greater impact. A qualitative–quantitative debate has taken place
largely outside but also inside psychology, voicing historical criticisms of
research methodology with unprecedented philosophical, political, ethical,
and scientific concerns. As qualitative research appears in new journals dedicated to it, in more mainstream journals, in established and new scientific
and professional forums, in new course curricula, and in advanced student
research, psychologists are becoming more comfortable with methodological
pluralism and are learning how to integrate multiple methods. Journal editors, established researchers, methodologists, educators, funding agencies,
practitioners, and students at all levels are becoming increasingly familiar
with the values, skills, and criteria for qualitative research. In this chapter we
discuss these recent historical developments, the issues that have been under
discussion in the qualitative movement today, and the typical problems and
organizational components of the contemporary qualitative research project.
We conclude with a summary of the contributions of the qualitative movement to psychology.

Institutionalization of Qualitative Methods as Normal Science

The qualitative movement in psychology has gained widespread attention only within the last 20 years. Psychologists have been conspicuously few in *The Handbook of Qualitative Research*, edited by Denzin and Lincoln (2000), which is now in its third edition. Marecek, Fine, and Kidder (1997) reported that a flowering of qualitative research—which had already occurred in the United Kingdom, Continental Europe, Australia, New Zealand, and Canada—has finally gotten underway in the United States. The American Psychological Association Books published *Qualitative Research in Psychology: Expanding Perspectives in Methodology and Design*, edited by Camic, Rhodes, and Yardley in 2003. Along with methodological volumes, there are currently many volumes containing exemplary empirical studies in psychology (e.g., Fischer, 2005).

Journals

Rennie, Watson, and Monteiro (2002) documented the terms *qualitative research, grounded theory, discourse analysis, empirical phenomenological,* and *phenomenological psychological* in *PsycINFO* and *Dissertation Abstracts*. One interesting finding is that before the 1980s, the search term *qualitative research* yielded no hits. Whereas before the 1980s, only terms containing *phenomenology* were present, a sharp rise in the other terms, including *qualitative research,* took place in the 1990s. Krahn, Holn, and Kime (1995) noted that APA President Frank Farley's 1993 prediction of a movement away from quantitative research methods has been born out. They found only 30 qualitative articles in mainstream psychology journals from 1993 through 1997, followed by a dramatic increase. Poulin (2007) noted a paucity of available educational opportunities in qualitative methods in psychology during the early 1990s that is still being addressed. Kidd (2002, citing Azar, 1999) reported a growing but not ubiquitous interest and a call for more qualitative articles among mainstream journal editors. Shank and Villella (2004) detected a similar shift in journals through the 1990s.

Qualitative research has become a common term, expressed with great interest, in American universities. For instance, the Qualitative Research Committee in the graduate school of St. Louis University, in order to promote qualitative research across the disciplines, has established a clearinghouse of relevant materials (*www.slu.edu/organizations/qrc*), including a list of web links to organizations and conferences (*www.slu.edu/organizations/qrc/QRCweblinks. html*) and a list of journals "friendly" to the publication of qualitative research (*www.slu.edu/organizations/qrc/QRjournals.html*). This incomplete and growing list currently contains over 135 journals, many of which are interdisciplinary and 10 of which contain *psychology* in the title. According to Krahn et al. (1995), this diverse, heterogeneous movement has been unified by its data-based emphasis on context, meaning, holism, and process with common roots in the phenomenological paradigm and the *Verstehen* (understanding) continental traditions.

Professional Organizations and Conferences

Over this last 40-year period, professional organizations and conferences in psychology have become increasingly hospitable to qualitative researchers, studies, and methodological works. The Society for Humanistic Psychology (APA Division 32) and the Society for Theoretical and Philosophical Psychology (APA Division 24) of the American Psychological Association have led the way. The former has had a Human Science Research interest group primarily focused specifically on qualitative research. The Society for Humanistic Psychology has dedicated symposia, paper sessions and poster sessions in its annual convention program and at least one issue per year of *The Humanistic Psychologist* to qualitative research methodology. Both societies have encouraged the career development of qualitative psychologists at all levels with regular bestowals of awards ranging from the Sidney Jourard Award for Outstanding Student Paper, given by The Society for Humanistic Psychology to the Theodore Sarbin Award for distinguished scholarship, by The Society for Theoretical and Philosophical Psychology.

In 2008, qualitative researchers led by Ken Gergen, Ruthellen Josselson, and Mark Freeman petitioned the APA with 863 verified signatures of members for a new division, the Society for Qualitative Inquiry, which did not succeed in gaining enough votes in the Council of Representatives to become a division. Nevertheless, this effort received major support from the Society for Counseling Psychology (17), the Society for Theoretical and Philosophical Psychology (24), the Society for Humanistic Psychology (32), the Society for the Psychology of Women (35), Psychoanalysis (39), and the Society for the Psychological Study of Lesbian, Gay, Bisexual, and Transgendered Issues (44) and significant support from the Society for Industrial and Organizational Psychology (14), Psychotherapy (29), Psychology of Religion (36), Health Psychology (38), the Society for Family Psychology (43), the Society for the Study of Ethnic Minority Issues (45), Media Psychology (46), the Society for Group Psychology and Group Psychotherapy (49), and the Society for the Study of Men and Masculinity (51). By now the group has increased its membership to over 1,200, and APA Division 5—Evaluation, Measurement, and Statistics— has, with genuine enthusiasm and a highly supportive executive board discussed inviting the group to join and form a larger division on research methods. This inclusion of the qualitative psychologists in APA Division 5 would more than double the membership and would broaden the focus to equally involve quantitative and qualitative research methods. The expanded organization would have a more inclusive name, such as the Division of Research Methods and Practices. The qualitative group would form a subdivision (called the Society for Qualitative Inquiry in Psychology [SQUIP]) with its own journal and program time at APA annual conventions. The SQUIP has undertaken plans to launch a journal, form a website, organize a listserv, and generate membership guidelines. Other initiatives under discussion include a task force to promote the teaching of qualitative research in undergraduate and graduate curricula, an initiative to ensure that APA journals are open to publishing qualitative research, and a summer educational program for qualitative inquiry.

The British Psychological Society has a Qualitative Methods in Psychology Section with over 1,000 members. Aiming to raise the profile of qualitative methods and offer opportunities for collaboration and networking, the section has an annual conference, a bulletin, a discussion board, and a Facebook group.

Many of the professional organizations and conferences that have attracted, supported and inspired qualitative researchers in psychology have been multidisciplinary. For instance, the International Human Science Research Conference (IHSRC) has been dedicated explicitly to the promotion and utilization of qualitative research methods in the human sciences since 1982. At the time this group formed, no other conferences allowed, let alone encouraged, the presentation of research that used exclusively qualitative methods. Quantitative methods were accepted for presentation as long as they were combined with qualitative ones. This organization traces its origin to phenomenology seminars and conferences at the University of Michigan in the late 1970s. It has held meetings in 10 countries and has been hosted by seven different disciplines in annual meetings over the last 28 years (Giorgi, 2010). The International Association for Qualitative Inquiry has held an annual International Congress of Qualitative Research since 2005 at the University if Illinois. Last year there were more than 900 attendees from more than 55 nations who presented over 800 papers in 120 sessions. Other annual or biannual conference organizations include the Interdisciplinary Coalition for North American Phenomenologists; Qualitative Research on Mental Health; The International Institute for Qualitative Methodology at the University of Alberta; the Center for Interdisciplinary Research on Narrative at St. Thomas University, which organizes and cosponsors biannual Narrative Matters conferences; and the Association for Qualitative Research in Australia.

The Spread of Qualitative Research through Subfields

Publications on qualitative research in specific areas of psychology have appeared in recent decades in social psychology (Marecek et al., 1997), industrial-organizational psychology (Cassell & Symon, 2006), educational psychology (Shank & Villella, 2004), school psychology (Leech & Onwueg-buzie, 2008; Michell, 2004), health psychology (Dickson-Swift, James, Kippen, & Liamputtong, 2007; Russell-Mayhew, 2007; Yardley, 2000), coun-seling psychology (Hoyt & Bhati, 2007), clinical child psychology (Krahn et al., 1995), cultural and multicultural psychology (Ratner, 2008; Kral & Burkhardt, 2002; Ponterotto, 2002), evaluation (Mark, 2001), sport psychol-ogy (Weinberg & Gould, 2007), professional psychology (Goldman, 1993), and health care systems (Hodges, Hernandez, Pinto, & Uzzell, 2007). Special issues of leading journals have been devoted to qualitative research in social and community psychology (e.g., the *Journal of Community and Applied Social Psychology* [Henwood & Parker, 1994] and the *American Journal of Community Psychology* [Banyard & Miller, 1998]), counseling psychology (the *Journal of Counseling Psychology* [Havercamp, Morrow, & Ponterotto, 2005; Polkinghorne, 1994]), and evaluation research (*American Journal of Evaluation* [Mark, 2001]). This trend has led rehabilitation psychologists to view their subfield as being "behind the curve" (Chwalisz, Shah, & Hand, 2008), indicating their recog-nition of a trend that is setting new general standards that demand advance-ment in specialty areas.

Qualitative approaches are becoming increasingly mainstream and rec-ognized as what Kuhn (1962) called *normal science*. However, rather than being "normal" in the traditional sense, in which science adopts a set para-digm involving standardized methods that are employed without questioning their assumptions or making modification in response to anomalies, qualita-tive research is occurring in a movement whose very character is pluralistic, self-questioning, continually changing, and adaptive to anomalies, as we have seen in the innovations of Anderson's intuitive inquiry. It is as if Allport's (1942) call for "bold experimentation" in research with personal documents continues to echo in this movement more than 50 years later. From semi-nal leaders to undergraduate students, whether collecting data or in class-rooms, critical questioning at basic levels, fresh thinking, and innovations of all sorts are welcome and taking place. With no single approach to research dominating psychology, the choice of method(s) can no longer be taken for granted and must be critically undertaken in light of alternatives with differ-ent assumptions.

Key Issues in Qualitative Research

Philosophy and Human Science

One of the most exciting and challenging dimensions of the qualitative movement is its common consensus that philosophy matters and is relevant to empirical research with humans. Many qualitative researchers, from Wundt and James to the founders of the five approaches featured in this book, have held that the attempt on the part of scientists to break absolutely with phi-losophy was impossible and naïve, because all research makes basic philo-sophical assumptions about existence (ontology), knowledge (epistemology), value (axiology), and the good (ethics). Although these perennial and dif-ficult issues have been thoughtfully addressed in diverse cultures and histori-cal periods, many psychologists and social scientists—even those who write about research methodology—have had little formal philosophical educa-tion. Qualitative researchers have struggled to understand and to become more reflective about and more responsible for the philosophical underpin-nings and implications of research. An important part of conducting qualita-tive research is literacy concerning the philosophical assumptions underlying research.

A strong tradition in philosophy justifies the importance and even prior-ity of qualitative research based on the characteristics of the human being. In order to introduce this line of thinking as it has developed in the context of modern science, we turn to the philosophy of Wilhelm Dilthey, who compel-lingly insisted on the priority of qualitative research in human science. Dilthey is well known for addressing the distinction between *Naturwissenschaften* (nat-ural science) and *Geisteswissenschaften* (human science) and for his striking advocacy for the method of *Verstehen* (understanding) in the human sciences: "We explain nature, but we understand psychic life" (1894/1977, p. 27).

Dilthey (1894/1977) acknowledged that the method of "theory-deducted hypothesis-inductive test" has had tremendous success in the physical sciences because their subject matter is external to experience and its parts are inde-pendent of each other. Because the nature and functional relations of physical variables are beyond immediate subjective experience, they must be inferred by hypotheses and verified by quantitative tests. Dilthey argued, however, that this way of knowing physical nature is neither required nor appropriate in psychology and the human sciences because their subject matter is given in experience and because the constituents of human experience are internally related to each other by virtue of their *meaning*, which is their distinctive and most important characteristic. Dilthey argued that in psychology, as a human science, description must play a far more profound role than it does in natu-ral science. It provides an "unbiased and unmutilated" view of psychological life in its full, complex reality. *Interpretive* analysis is required to distinguish parts of mental life and to grasp their meaningful interrelations within the context of the whole. The structural unity of psychological life, which must be taken into consideration by all human science disciplines, according to Dilthey, entails such special characteristics as teleological development, the role of learning and temporal context, the centrality of motivation and feel-ings, reciprocal and efficacious relations with the external world, and the irreducibility of such basic constituents as cognition, feeling, and behavior to each other and to material reality. Based on these ontological characteristics, especially *meaningfulness*, Dilthey concluded that the primary method for the study of lived experience is description, interpretation, and understanding—qualitative procedures—and only secondarily, and on the basis of these methods, would the human sciences construct theories, deduce hypotheses, and test them using measurements and quantitative analyses. Dilthey's epistemology reversed the received methodological hierarchy in the human sciences by making interpretive methods the gold standard and hypothetical methods a supplementary procedure.

Consistent with Dilthey's ontology and epistemology, continental philosophy has developed through the 20th century on the basis of the conviction that physical and psychological realities are different kinds and therefore require different ways of knowing. Following this philosophical position, many qualitative methodologists assert that their methods have priority in the human sciences, in which inferential methods are relegated to a subordinate role, in contrast to mainstream researchers in psychology whose methodological hierarchy privileges hypothesis testing by quantitative analysis. This difference in philosophical positions has led to a fierce debate between qualitative and quantitative researchers.

The Qualitative–Quantitative Debate

Since the late 1970s, as qualitative methods were being proposed and promoted, there has been considerable discussion about the relative value and role of qualitative versus quantitative methods in social science. The qualitative–quantitative debate took place mostly outside of psychology in applied areas such as education, public health, and evaluation, which are interdisciplinary, but it has also erupted in marginal and mainstream venues in psychology (Rabinowitz & Weseen, 1997). On both sides of the quantitative–qualitative debate, some argued for their own approach to the complete exclusion of the other. Others argued that each research method has its place. To some, the origin of this debate was in differing philosophical assumptions and systems underlying the different human science research methodologies, which were therefore viewed as irreconcilably opposed. Others have insisted that different methods are rightfully driven by different research problems, questions, and aims, in which case no one method is intrinsically superior in human science, and multiple methods are legitimate for multiple purposes. Within this pluralistic context considerable work has occurred on how to integrate or "mix" qualitative and quantitative methods. Some have strongly argued that research benefits from integrating qualitative and quantitative methods in the same research project, for instance, in community psychology (Griffin & Phoenix, 1994) and educational psychology (Yin, 2006).

One virtue of this debate was to call psychologists' attention to questions about epistemology and the philosophy of science as well as to articulate multiple ways of knowing that could enrich the discipline. Profound differences in the definition of "science" have come to light, and these broad disciplinary debates continue. Following scholars in other fields (Smith & Heshusius, 1986), a growing number of psychologists consider the debate unnecessarily "contentious and fractious" (Greene, 2007) and have advocated multiple methods and mixed methods (the combination of qualitative and quantitative in single studies) as well as multiple and mixed philosophies (Griffin & Phoenix, 1994; Michell, 2004; Powell, Mihalas, Onwuegbuzie, Suldo, & Daley, 2008; Yin, 2006). Although effort is being made to integrate multiple methods at the level of practice and principle, purists from various camps continue to assert their positions. Although these issues appear unlikely to be resolved in the near future, we view the debate as healthy and generative. Knowledge of philosophy and of both qualitative and quantitative traditions and procedures is certainly a prerequisite for addressing and resolving the issues concerning the role, value, and compatibility of newly emerging and established methods.

The Generative Tensions of Pluralism

The contemporary literature about qualitative research includes lively attention to the implications for multiple research methodologies in such varied philosophical orientations as positivism, neopositivism, phenomenology, existentialism, hermeneutics, pragmatism, constructionism, structuralism, poststructuralism, and postmodernism. These philosophical orientations have grown out of, and in response to, each other. Although there may appear to be sharp differences among these orientations, deeper and more careful thought may discover unexpected commonalities and compatibilities. The relationship of philosophy to empirical research is no simple matter. It has often been noted that Freud's work, for instance, implicitly utilized very different philosophies, such as positivism, naturalism, phenomenology, and hermeneutics. Although many have assumed that philosophical consistency is a virtue and that apparent philosophical contradictions within a researcher's methods are a defect, it has also been argued that freely drawing on opposed philosophical traditions is a virtue and that human science is enriched by creative, even if impure, combinations such as Freud's work involved (Ricoeur, 1970). Kohlberg's work was theoretically guided by a neo-Kantian structuralist philosophy along with a mixed methodology, including Weber's *Verstehen* (understanding) approach and mainstream positivism using quantitative procedures, and yet it produced excellent knowledge with fruitful impact on psychology, despite these philosophical incongruities.

The philosophical problems surrounding qualitative research remain unresolved and pose exciting challenges and opportunities for advancing human science as researchers become more philosophically sophisticated and better understand multiple methodological approaches. Currently, there remain questions and debates about the nature of "description," "interpretation," "explanation," "theory," and how they are related to each other. Fascinating discussion is taking place about the meanings and relationships between realism and idealism, objectivism and perspectivism, foundationalism and relativism, language and reality, modernism and postmodernism.

As important as philosophical issues are, qualitative researchers are often called to contribute practical solutions to human problems. The human sciences have a strong empirical orientation, and research is often driven by practical problems. These aspects of human science research make it refreshingly nonideological and creatively responsive to the concrete demands of its subject matters. Innovative and fruitful methods can develop without much attention to complex philosophical issues and debates. One of the most important lessons of the works of Freud, James, Maslow, Kohlberg, and the human science pioneers is that breakthroughs are made by working closely with empirical realities and not by employing a preconceived ideology. Flanagan's critical incident technique has offered wonderful tools that are still useful to qualitative researchers, even though some are not comfortable with the overall positivistic assumptions of the method. Maslow's research on the healthy personality advanced psychological theory in an important area without philosophical attention and sophistication. The primary virtue of qualitative research is the commitment to persons over ideas, the response to concrete needs of human life outside of the ivory tower—what Allport (1942) called the "touchstone of reality" it offers to science.

As important and necessary as it is for human science to gain philosophical sophistication and achieve methodological coherence and unity, we are reluctant to characterize the philosophical dimensions of qualitative research and the emerging methodologies with any neat and simple scheme. The risks of oversimplification, distortion, and misleading prescription are too great. We have benefited from philosophical study and from reflections that clarify and guide our research. We attempt to move forward the confrontation with philosophical pluralism and its challenges by presenting and comparing qualitative research methods based on multiple methodologies with attention to their philosophical backgrounds. In our accounts of our orientations and in our comparisons of approaches, methods, and findings in this volume, we share a sensitivity to philosophical issues, questions, and knowledge that is befitting of contemporary qualitative research. We are grateful for the increasing attention to fundamental philosophical issues and the methodological debates surrounding empirical research today. We encourage qualitative researchers—including students, novices, and seasoned experts—to develop philosophical acumen, to reflect on the philosophical assumptions of their chosen methodologies, and to openly acknowledge philosophical influences guiding research as they understand it.

Reflexivity and Standpoint

The qualitative movement has developed and come of age during a period in which philosophers of science have dispelled the myth that science has been or can be devoid of human interests, social positioning, and subjectivity (Habermas, 1971; Kuhn, 1962). The human presence in science, including values, practical aims, theoretical orientations, and social affiliations, has been acknowledged in philosophy and across the physical and social sciences. The reformulation of positivist approaches to psychology by way of neopositivism acknowledges the presence of human subjectivity and values in science (Polkinghorne, 1983), as have quantitative psychologists (Messick, 1975). One commonly accepted tenet of the contemporary qualitative movement is that research is radically relational; that although its thematic focus is on the subject matter and the aim is knowledge, research inevitably includes and expresses the orientation, methods, values, traditions, and personal qualities of the researcher. Therefore, part of the rigor of qualitative research involves self-disclosure and reflexivity on the part of the investigator. This dimension of the research has been developed as a genre of qualitative research in its own right, called "autoethnography," in which the researcher focuses on and transparently reveals his or her own experience in the course of doing research as a part of the research (Chang, 2008). Qualitative researchers in psychology often emphasize the importance of incorporating into normal scientific practice, in all phases of research, a self-critical disclosure of the researcher's interests, traditions, preconceptions, and personal relationship with the subject matter. Rather than undermining the legitimacy and validity of science with skepticism, the acknowledgment of science as a *human enterprise* and the call for reflexivity have extended scientific research by including unprecedented transparency, self-criticism, and social accountability.

Ethics, Power, and Politics

Qualitative research has introduced new perspectives not only in science but in research ethics. Of contemporary interest is how politics and power relate to research. Interdisciplinary scholarship—for instance, by critical theorists and feminists—has shown that each research method involves not only intellectual assumptions but also social positioning that is often taken for granted. Drawing on interdisciplinary and psychological traditions of participatory, partnership, and liberation research, qualitative researchers have raised issues beyond the usual principles of informed consent, anonymity, and confidentiality (Watkins & Schulman, 2008). Whereas in traditional science, the researcher is the center of power, qualitative research has relinquished one-way control in favor of sharing power and undertaking a more dialogical and collaborative relationship with research participants and lay communities

(Watkins & Schulman, 2008, p. 300). The ethical codes developed for natural scientific research methods involve a hierarchical distance between researcher and participant. Critical and participatory approaches have reflected on these implicit power relations and have raised questions of who defines the research topic and problems; which methods are considered appropriate and legitimate; who owns the data; whose interpretation counts; who has the power to challenge findings; and who does the reporting to whom (Mertens & Ginsberg, 2009)? Some qualitative researchers, critical of the power inequities in traditional research, have advocated a shift in privilege from the researcher to the participants and have sought new kinds of relationships with participants. Consequently, participants have been invited to play increasingly key roles in defining research problems, designing research, collecting and owning data, conducting analysis, and disseminating findings—in some cases, even becoming coresearchers (Silka, 2009).

Following from qualitative researchers' attentive engagement with the experiences and interests of research participants, concerns about the protection of individual participants and of communities have been raised (Marecek et al., 1997; Silka, 2009). Miles and Huberman (1994) documented belated realizations of ethical dilemmas on the part of researchers. Ethical models involving extended collaboration and dialogue have been advocated. It is increasingly assumed that unanticipated ethical issues will arise in research and are best addressed collaboratively in an ongoing process rather than only being anticipated, addressed, and resolved by the researcher alone based on abstract principles prior to conducting the research. Paolo Freire (1968/1992) urged researchers to ask: Does our work mirror the researcher's dreams or the community's dreams? "Dynamic questioning and response" in the company of others is suggested by Watkins and Schulman (2008, p. 302). Even anonymity, as a protection for participants, has been reconsidered in light of the meaning of this practice for participants themselves. Watkins and Schulman (2008) wrote:

> For some . . . the offer of anonymity re-inscribes the asymmetry of power in the research relationship, where authorship goes to the researcher and anonymity goes to the participants. Let your participants know they have a choice in this matter, thinking through with them any potential downsides. . . . [They] may wish to claim their own words and perspectives as their own. (p. 306)

Some qualitative researchers emphasize the ethical practice of addressing all dilemmas and challenges with others, not alone, and insist on including participants and other members of their communities in the research process from start to finish. Other qualitative researchers have implored researchers to enable participants to "talk back" to them (Oakley, 1981). "One of the deepest discernments for a researcher in this [liberation] tradition is determining what our witness requires from us" (Watkins & Schulman, 2008, p. 312). Although there are not always clear answers, more radical considerations of the perspectives and the roles of research participants, as well as the full spectrum of stakeholders in research, are being undertaken. Dialogical discernment of how to best serve the spectrum of human interests is increasingly viewed as an ethical imperative.

Education in Research Methodology and Praxis

Course curricula for learning qualitative methods has received considerable attention throughout this period (Churchill, 1990; Hoshmand, 1989; Josselson, Leiblich, & McAdams, 2003; Poulin, 2007; Stabb, 1999; Wertz & van Zuuren, 1987). Stoppard (2003) noted the need for research on mentor development and the impact on faculty and students. Describing her graduate course curriculum, she recommended survival strategies for those conducting qualitative research in graduate school. Walsh-Bowers (2002) interviewed students and faculty to discuss the challenges of integrating qualitative methods, with their pluralistic methodological contexts, into curriculum, research, and careers. Onwuegbuzie and Leech (2005) argued that debate between qualitative and quantitative methodology advocates has been divisive, counterproductive, and has led to an unnecessary divide among researchers, instructors, and students. They, echoing McMullen (2002), argue that all graduate students should learn both kinds of methods, and the methods should not be separated in curriculum but be taught in comprehensive research methods courses that include both. Dickson-Swift et al. (2007) interviewed 30 qualitative health researchers and explored the personal challenges of this kind of research. Yet Poulin (2007) observed that the literature on teaching qualitative methods in psychology remains limited. She argued that exposure to multiple traditions of qualitative research is essential for student learning.

Criteria and Guidelines for Best Practices

As qualitative methods are learned and creatively employed for various purposes, concerns about standards of education, mentoring, and publication have arisen and are also being addressed. Stiles (1993) provided one of the earliest articulations of the need for and means of quality control. Elliott, Fischer, and Rennie (1999) detailed seven guidelines for journal editors and referees pertaining to all research and seven additional guidelines pertaining specifically to qualitative articles submitted for publication. For instance, the latter guidelines include the need for researchers to explicitly acknowledge their philosophical, theoretical, and personal perspectives; to describe the sample of participants and situations researched; to provide examples of concrete data in order to delineate the analytic procedures used and illustrate the conceptual findings; to provide credibility checks with the research participants, with multiple analysts, and with multiple perspectives; to demonstrate coherence and integration of findings; to use methods and provide findings that accomplish the level of generality intended by the research; and to provide material that resonates with readers. They also describe examples of both good and poor practice. Yardley (2000) emphasized the need for contextual sensitivity, rigor, transparency, coherence, impact, and importance. Shank and Villella (2004) and Morrow (2005) reviewed the criteria of trustworthiness as they have emerged within various epistemological frameworks and added additional criteria. Parker (2004) provided guidelines for supervisors of research projects. Complaints about the inadequacies of training and quality assurance have continued to be voiced. For instance, Hodges et al. (2007) lamented that the specific methods used by qualitative researchers to analyze data are often not reported.

Although we recognize the importance of reflecting on the characteristics of excellent qualitative research, we also have reservations about potential downsides of such criteria. We have noted that students are often overwhelmed by the obscure terms used to describe criteria. We are also concerned that externally imposed norms may inadvertently stifle creativity and overburden researchers. External concerns may detract from valuable contributions that fall short of criteria or fruitfully violate guidelines. We hope that journal editors will welcome bold, innovative, and unconventional work, as Allport encouraged. We also hope that the growing codification of norms does not lead to rigidity or foster a guild mentality that discourages creative forms of qualitative work such as those provided by Freud, James, Maslow, and Kohlberg.

The Typical Organization
of the Qualitative Research Project

Formulation of a Research Problem

Good scientific research involves not only an important topic but a research problem. Research methods follow precisely from the goals of the research and from the way research problems are approached. In contemporary qualitative research, there are many starting points and ways to define research problems. One continuum is that ranging from prescientific common sense to the world of science. Real-world events—prescientific human suffering and human interests—may provide the motivation for research. Research problems may emerge from theoretical or disciplinary issues already recognized by scientists-scholars; in the researcher's critical reflections on the shortcomings of current knowledge; or in a fresh, open-ended collection and analysis of data. An overlapping continuum concerns whether the purpose of research seeks knowledge for its own (theoretical) sake or knowledge for practical change. In any case, research always addresses a gap between what we know as scientists and the world beyond science.

A *critical* review of the literature allows researchers to identify such a gap between what is known and the portion of reality that exceeds our knowledge. The goal can then be identified and the structure of the research organized in relation to this gap. Grounded theorists have shown how research problems may emerge in the process of grappling with data and only later, on that basis, are gaps between the extant literature and the subject matter identified. Traditionally, the scientist has defined the research problems, but qualitative researchers have begun to emphasize partnerships between researchers and persons researched even in the early stages of the work (Silka, 2009). Scientists have begun to include nonscientists in topic identification, critical literature review, and problem formulation, especially when research has practical or emancipatory aims.

Qualitative research problems typically involve determining the "what" and the "how" of the subject matter. Freud asked questions concerning the meaning (the purpose, aim, and role in psychic continuity) of psychopathological symptoms and dreams. James set out to determine the essence and typical variations of religious experience as well as their value in human life. Maslow took on the problem of defining the characteristics of the healthy personality and humans' best experiences. Kohlberg sought knowledge of the basic principles organizing the development of moral reasoning. Flanagan set out to discover, for instance, the best practices of combat leadership and the teaching of psychology. A researcher may use a qualitative investigation to gain knowledge of a subject matter in order to unify, or at least relate, fragmented or contradictory theories or to illustrate and draw attention to taken-for-granted understandings and practices. Another aim of some qualitative research is to identify the basic categories of a subject matter for the construction of a measuring instrument for basic or applied research.

In the current project, we loosely selected a topic that has been extensively researched—trauma (called "misfortune")—for our demonstration. Our purpose is primarily methodological—that is, to discover the similarities and differences among our methods of analysis—but in our attempt to simulate our typical practices, each researcher developed his or her own purposes for this research in accordance with his or her chosen methodology. Each researcher had his or her own conceptualization of the subject matter, utilization of literature, goals of analysis, relative emphases on theory, and individual sensibilities in crafting and designing the analytic method.

Participants, Situations, and Data

One of the greatest contributions of the qualitative movement is the expansion of the empirical data base of psychology and other human sciences to the full range of personal human expression. The capacities of written, graphic, artistic, auditory, kinesthetic, and verbal expressions to disclose lived experience are tremendous. The rich diversity of data we found in the work of Freud, James, Maslow, and Kohlberg has been widened and systematically extended by contemporary critical incident researchers, phenomenologists, grounded theorists, discourse analysts, narrativists, intuitive inquirers, and others. These empirical data, properly understood, provide very different types of information than the measurement of external events and include many ways in which people express their personal lives, verbally and nonverbally.

Like quantitative researchers, qualitative researchers first define the topic, the nature of the problem, and the purpose and scope of the research. On this basis researchers ask such questions as these: Which sources would best provide access to this topic? What criteria define these sources? What data are already available? How might the researcher best collect new data? Ecological validity is primary, in that qualitative research aims to encounter human life genuinely, as it is lived outside the research situation. Although the research topic and problem provide focus, qualitative research typically requires diversity and variability of data. Often, researchers define a coherent and yet diverse group of people who live through the subject matter, allow fulfillment of research goals, and are credible to the audience of the research. The sample can include the living and the dead, seek new expressions, or utilize archival ones.

The overarching criteria for qualitative data are relevance to the research problem and fidelity to human existence. Optimal qualitative data may involve "thick" or "rich" description—for example, detailed personal accounts of lived experiences directly related to the topic. However, as we learn from discourse analysts, the in-depth interview is a limited (and in some ways, contrived) form of talk; much may also be said for other kinds of expressions occurring in natural contexts. There is no one standard for qualitative data, for the data must serve the particular aims of the research as it confronts its topic. Given the common interest of qualitative researchers in studying in detail the complexity of lived experience and human practices, thick descriptions are often sought or elicited through reports of personal life events, stories, biographical accounts, or other types of original expressions collected in writing, in interviews, and in focus groups. If a qualitative researcher chooses to collect interview data with individuals or groups, a great variety of interview approaches and procedures now exist within the qualitative movement. Some of these are structured and formal, with some using preconceived questions and others using a sensitizing guide for solicitations and probes of relevant descriptions. Other interview procedures are more or less open-ended and informal, allowing the interviewee and interviewer a more spontaneous exploration of the topic at hand. Choices made from among these options depend on the topic and goals of a study.

Too often interview data are identified with qualitative research. Although interview data are one valuable kind for qualitative research, interviews are by no means the only source or the most appropriate one for a particular study. Descriptions of other people and their situations, as well as naturalistic encounters, may be relevant in addition to or as an alternative to first-person expressions. Qualitative researchers should not uncritically assume that data of a certain sort are required by a qualitative research project without regard to the topic or scope and nature of the research problem. Archival data from contemporary and even popular media and historical records, as well as journal excerpts, personal possessions, photographs, audiovisual media, and creative works may also be included in qualitative research, on their own or in combination with other kinds of data. Although qualitative researchers tend to rely on verbal and descriptive accounts, graphic and artistic media may also have great value, including photography, sound and video recordings, film, art, dance, and drama.

Freud used very open-ended interviews with close behavioral observations in his studies of psychopathology, and he developed a much more structured interview method in order to study dreams. In research on both topics, he collected data from many different kinds of participants and on highly varied symptoms and dreams. He used written materials such as journals, letters, and even a shopping list. In his study of jokes, he used archival materials. Freud made extensive use of literature and art in almost all of his studies and kept all these data in sight as he approached each given topic. James deliberately used archival materials in his study of religious experience, and he collected reports from individuals in various cultures, periods of history, and stations in life, ranging from saints and martyrs to a coal miner whose prayer made him less violent and alcoholics who achieved abstinence through conversion. Maslow's research on the healthy personality began with observations of his mentors, and he used increasingly sophisticated means to select and exclude participants, including tests of psychopathology. His means of data collection, including behavioral observation and interview, were quite flexible and called for special discretion when he found that participants' expression became stilted when they became aware of the topic of his research. The creativity of qualitative data collection is equally evident in Kohlberg, who collected thinking on a variety of hypothetical situations from children of many ages. He supplemented these data with those he collected in focus groups, in which he was able to observe moral reasoning in the social context of interactions aiming to achieve consensus. These pioneers all realized that participants are not of equal value and that some situations, participants, and forms of human expression afford special opportunities for analysis and general insight.

In the current project, the participants were given instructions to write a description of a personal misfortune and how they lived through it. Written descriptions like these, also used by James, Flanagan, and Maslow, can be quite rich and revealing. In the current demonstration, the interview was also used in order to clarify aspects of participants' experiences in relation to particular knowledge interests, including the role of social support and spirituality in resilience. Procedures like these were used by Freud, Maslow, Kohlberg, and Flanagan, as they have been used by many others throughout history (Kvale & Brinkmann, 2009).

Analytic Methods

Qualitative analyses include many varieties, including categorical, thematic, structural, interpretive, narrative, and eidetic forms and can also incorporate contexts in the research project and in the real world. We are taught that the starting point of science is the description of the subject matter; description is an important analytic activity in qualitative research. There is some debate and controversy over the nature of description and its role in analysis and in human knowledge. Some qualitative researchers believe that all description is interpretation, and they question the claim that description can provide fidelity ("objectivity" in the broad sense) to the matter under investigation. Other traditions in qualitative research argue that descriptive ideation is not only possible but also necessary, sufficient, and even privileged in human science. "Pure" phenomenology involves describing the essence of phenomena (by "eidetic analysis," which involves conceptualizing what is invariant through all imaginable examples of a phenomenon). Phenomenologists claim that eidetic description provides knowledge that faithfully reflects lived experience.

Qualitative analyses rooted in phenomenology also utilize reflection, that is, the process of turning attention to previously lived experiences in an attempt to focus on their processes (called "noeses"; the "how" of experience) and meanings (the "noemata"; "what" is experienced). Other analytic methods seek to apply predetermined categories or to determine new ones. These categories may be of many types, depending on the interests of the researcher. Interpretive analytic processes utilize a movement (called the "hermeneutic circle") back and forth between parts and whole, and between the whole and its context, in order to achieve a fuller grasp of its meaning. Variants of hermeneutic methods have been articulated by such thinkers as Schliermacher, Heidegger, Gadamer, and Derrida. Interpretive analyses may also explicitly use a framework or established meanings that are initially relatively independent from the data, in order to discern meanings in the data. These frameworks can be of many sorts, including theoretical orientations (e.g., psychoanalysis, behaviorism, family systems, ecology, critical theory) or social movements (e.g., feminism, Marxism, humanism, liberation). Qualitative analytic methods may also involve inferences, such as inductive, abductive, and deductive reasoning. Induction is the process used to establish empirical generalizations that hold among diverse data within a research project and even beyond the data collected by the researcher. Abduction is a process of analysis that moves beyond the data collected in order to freshly generate theory; that is, to construct models that yield explanation, prediction, or interdisciplinary connections to natural (neuroscience, evolutionary biology), cultural (anthropology, history), or formal (mathematics, computer) sciences, for instance. Using deductive reasoning, qualitative researchers may explore the validity of general theories or principles by means of the concrete specifics of their data. Analyses may also be intuitive, drawing on the researchers' most private, intimate, and mysterious experiences.

Qualitative analysis can achieve surprisingly general insights and knowledge by analyzing a single case in depth. One of the most significant contributions of the qualitative movement is the revival of interest in and the legitimization of the single case analysis (Fishman, 1999; Stake, 1995; Yin, 1994). Comparative analyses are evident in the practices of the pioneers and in virtually all the systems of qualitative research that guide contemporary researchers. Comparison is implicitly involved even in the analysis of the single case, and the systematic use of comparative analyses is indispensible to the achievement of general qualitative knowledge. Freud, James, Maslow, Kohlberg, and Flanagan employed the identification of similarities and differences among widely varying examples of the subject matter as a central analytic procedure for the production of general knowledge. Systematizers such as Flanagan and the others have delineated specific procedures for carrying out analyses of general trends. The analytic methods briefly touched upon above are not entirely distinct, and they can be combined.

The nature of and relations among these modes of analysis are currently under discussion and debate. The centerpiece of this volume is a detailed focus on and concrete exploration of these procedures. Examples of such analytic procedures that are in depth, comparative, thematic, structural, interpretive, and narrative, using inductive, abductive, deductive, and eidetic varieties of reasoning, are explored in detail in the subsequent chapters of this volume. One of our main interests is to identify how these different procedures are concretely carried out, what kinds of findings they make possible, and how they compare and relate to each other, including their potential compatibility and integration.

Report of Findings

Researchers' reports of analytic findings and their modes of presentation are important issues. The language used to express qualitative knowledge ranges from the specialized terms of the researcher—whether received or invented technical terminology—to that of ordinary language, including that of the participants themselves. Findings follow from the modes of analysis; the researcher's discourse may be descriptive, interpretive, structural, categorical, predictive, explanatory, or evocative—even poetic. The values guiding the form of presentation again concern the relevance to the research problem and fidelity to the subject matter as revealed in the analysis. Qualitative researchers often struggle to present very complex findings, whose intelligibility requires continual references to concrete life, in a coherent, internally differentiated, and comprehensive manner. Findings cannot be summed up as easily as can be the results of quantitative research, and so achieving a balance between conciseness and richness is a great challenge for the qualitative research writer. Findings may also take different forms depending on the audience of readers. One marvels at the masterful writing of Freud, James, and Maslow, whose reports have informed and challenged psychological scientists, researchers, and theoreticians across the spectrum of humanities and other social sciences, and are edifying and delightful to an educated lay readership. This resonance is possible because the findings of qualitative research take on important problems, attain a closeness to the life we live and observe every day, and offer new knowledge that is illuminating for and enhances the sensitivities of those who are interested in human affairs.

Good qualitative findings are profoundly data-based; therefore, the presentation of analytic findings almost always makes abundant references to concrete life situations regardless of their level of generality. Generally, in qualitative research reports, as initiated by the practices of pioneers such as Freud, James, Maslow, and Kohlberg, findings and claims are extensively explicated and generously illustrated by direct quotations from participants or excerpts from archival material. Because the focus is on the meanings, themes, and structural organization in psychological life, the context of concrete examples is important and must sometimes be carefully presented in illustrations of qualitative knowledge included in findings. Quotations may require background context as an introduction. Multiple examples and discussions of their similarities and differences are often necessary in order to communicate important general features and variations of the subject matter. These necessary strategies in reporting qualitative research findings often require manuscript lengths that exceed the limits of journals that have traditionally published quantitative research. Some qualitative venues, such as the *Journal of Phenomenological Psychology*, have no limits for manuscript length for this reason. Some new journals, such as *Qualitative Research in Psychology*, do not list page limits in their instructions to authors. Edited volumes and books may offer more fitting and necessary venues for the extensive and detailed nature of qualitative findings. As the qualitative movement develops along with new forms of communication such as online journals, more appropriate and flexible vehicles for presenting research that requires lengthy exposition with illustrations from data of many sorts may become increasingly prevalent.

Delineating the Implications of Research

The last task of the researcher is to return to the literature and the larger world in order to explicitly identify the fruits of the research in that context. Discussion sections in qualitative reports are typically similar to those in quantitative research in that they begin by reminding the reader of the purpose of the research, the research questions, and how the findings address them. Discussion generally involves relating the research findings to the world beyond the research project, including previously established knowledge presented in the literature, practical problems that the findings may address, and issues found in the larger ecology. One important implication of new qualitative knowledge is how the findings compare to previous knowledge claims about the subject matter and how the new findings are relevant to the problem area of a complex body of literature. Explaining the convergences and divergences between the findings and those of other researchers and scholars allows the researcher to contribute in a systematic way to that body of knowledge. The researcher asks: How do the findings correspond to, cohere with, contradict, and/or freshly disclose new features of the subject matter as it presents itself in everyday life and in other scientific works? The implications for theory, research, and practice are made explicit, in accordance with the original aims of the research. Finally, a self-critical perspective is adopted in order to identify the limits of the study, the horizons of the unknown, and the remaining gaps between knowledge (including the current study) and the world beyond the study. In this context, with an eye toward the future possibilities of research, additional and alternative participants, data sources, situations, modes of analysis, and so on, are considered. Directions for addressing the remaining gaps through future research, with reference to specific methods, are addressed.

Contributions of Qualitative Research Methods to Psychology

As we have seen, the qualitative movement is not limited to merely adding new tools for research in an otherwise unaffected discipline. Qualitative research involves special attitudes, approaches, and a new worldview in psychology. With the formalization and adaptation of qualitative methodology on a large scale and the acceptance of methodological pluralism, psychologists have gained increasing philosophical sophistication, new ways of conceptualizing human beings, increased reflexivity, and extended scientific accountability. The contributions of qualitative methods can be summarized as follows:

- ♦ The concept of science is extended to become more inclusive.
- ♦ The philosophy of science, including epistemology and ontology, is developed.
- ♦ Uniquely human matters such as meaning, agency, language, and values are focal.
- ♦ Methodological pluralism is accepted and advocated.
- ♦ Empirical data bases are broadened; evidence-based research is extended.
- ♦ New analytic methods and forms of knowledge are utilized.
- ♦ Critical reflexivity in research is promoted.
- ♦ The position of the scientist is acknowledged.
- ♦ Greater closeness to local, concrete human life is achieved.
- ♦ Holistic findings about a subject matter unify disparate forms of knowledge.
- ♦ The gulf between research and practice is bridged.
- ♦ New standards for knowledge are introduced.
- ♦ Disciplinary boundaries within and between the humanities and social sciences are opened.

The Five Ways Project

What follows is a demonstration of five ways of doing qualitative analysis using the same data. In the next chapter, we provide a written description and an interview from a pedagogical project in a qualitative research class that undertook the study of living through misfortune or trauma. We have called this written description and interview about an unfortunate event "the Teresa texts," using the pseudonym we gave the participant. A second description, offered by another research participant, "Gail," is included in the Appendix. In the five chapters that follow, researchers representing each of five traditions of qualitative research identify the origins, typical applications, and key procedures of his or her approach, followed by a demonstration of how it was carried out using the Teresa texts. These five demonstrations illustrate how contemporary researchers have appropriated the traditions described in the last chapter. These analyses serve as a basis for comparing various methods and as an effort to address general issues posed by the methodological pluralism that currently characterizes qualitative research in psychology.

References

Allport, G. W. (1942). *The use of personal documents in psychological science* (Prepared for the Committee on the Appraisal of Research; Bulletin #49). New York: Social Science Research Council.

Banyard, V. L., & Milller, K. E. (1998). The powerful potential of qualitative research in community psychology. *American Journal of Community Psychology, 26*(4), 485–505.

Camic, P. M., Rhodes, J. E., & Yardley, L. (Eds.) (2003). *Qualitative research in psychology: Expanding perspectives in methodology and design.* Washington, DC: American Psychological Association.

Cassell, C., & Symon, G. (2006). Qualitative methods in industrial organizational psychology. *International Review of Industrial Organizational Psychology, 21,* 339–380.

Chang, H. V. (2008). *Autoethnography as method.* Walnut Creek, CA: Left Coast Press.

Churchill, S. D. (1990). Considerations for teaching a phenomenological approach to psychological research. *Journal of Phenomenological Psychology, 21*(1), 46–67.

Chwalisz, K., Shah, S. R., & Hand, K. M. (2008). Facilitating rigorous qualitative research in rehabilitation psychology. *Rehabilitation Psychology, 53*(3), 387–399.

Denzin, N. K., & Lincoln, Y. S. (Eds.) (1994). *Handbook of qualitative research.* Thousand Oaks, CA: Sage.

Denzin, N. K., & Lincoln, Y. S. (Eds.). (2000). *Handbook of qualitative research* (2nd ed.). Thousand Oaks, CA: Sage.

Dickson-Swift, V., James, E. L., Kippen, S., & Liamputtong, P. (2007). Doing sensitive research: What challenges do qualitative researchers face? *Qualitative Research, 7*(3), 327–353.

Dilthey, W. (1977). Ideas concerning a descriptive and analytical psychology (1894). In *Descriptive psychology and historical understanding* (R. M. Zaner & K. L. Heiges, Trans.). The Hague: Martinus Nijhoff.

Elliott, R., Fischer, C. T., & Rennie, D. (1999). Evolving guidelines for conducting qualitative research studies in psychology and related fields. *British Journal of Clinical Psychology, 38*(3), 215–229.

Fischer, C. T. (Ed.). (2005). *Qualitative research methods for psychologists: Introduction through empirical studies.* New York: Academic Press.

Fishman, D. B. (1999). *The case for a pragmatic psychology.* New York: New York University Press.

Freire, P. (1992). *Pedagogy of the oppressed.* New York: Continuum. (Original work published 1968)

Giorgi, A. (2010). A history of the International Human Science Research Conference on the occasion of its 25th annual meeting. *Humanistic Psychologist, 38*(1), 57–66.

Goldman, L. (1993). Reaction: A broader scientific base for professional psychology. *Professional Psychology: Research and Practice, 24*(3), 252–253.

Greene, J. (2007). *Mixed methods in social inquiry.* San Francisco: Jossey-Bass.

Griffin, C., & Phoenix, A. (1994). The relationship between quantitative and qualitative research: Lessons from feminist psychology. *Journal of Community and Applied Social Psychology, 4,* 287–298.

Habermas, J. (1971). *Knowledge and human interests.* Boston: Beacon Press.

Havercamp, B. E., Morrow, S. L., & Ponterotto, J. G. (Eds.). (2005). Special issue on qualitative and mixed methods research. *Journal of Counseling Psychology, 50*(20).

Henwood, K., & Parker, I. (1994). Qualitative social psychology. *Journal of Community and Applied Social Psychology, 4,* 219–223.

Hodges, S., Hernandez, M., Pinto, A., & Uzzell, C. (2007). The use of qualitative methods in systems of care research. *Journal of Behavioral Health Services and Research, 34*(4), 361–368.

Hoshmand, L. (1989). Alternative research paradigms: A review and a teaching proposal. *Counseling Psychologist, 17,* 3–79.

Hoyt, W. T., & Bhati, K. S. (2007). Priniciples and practices: An empirical examination of qualitative research in the *Journal of Counseling Psychology. Journal of Counseling Psychology, 54*(2), 201–210.

Josselson, R., Leiblich, A., & McAdams, D. P. (Eds.). (2003). *Up close and personal: The teaching and learning of narrative research.* Washington, DC: APA Books.

Kidd, S. A. (2002). The role of qualitative research in psychological journals. *Psychological Methods, 7*(1), 126–138.

Krahn, G. L., Holn, M. F., & Kime, C. (1995). Incorporating qualitative approaches into clinical child psychology research. *Journal of Clinical Child Psychology, 24*(2), 204–213.

Kral, M. J., & Burkhardt, K. J. (2002). The new research agenda for a cultural psychology. *Canadian Psychology, 43*(3), 154–162.

Kuhn, T. (1962). *The structure of scientific revolutions.* Chicago: University of Chicago Press.

Kvale, S., & Brinkmann, S. (2009). *InterViews: Learning the craft of qualitative research interviewing* (2nd ed.). Thousand Oaks, CA: Sage.

Leech, N. L., & Onwuegbuzie, A. J. (2008). Qualitative data analysis: A compendium of techniques and a framework for selection for school psychology research and beyond. *School Psychology Quarterly, 23*(4), 587–604.

Marecek, J., Fine, M., & Kidder, L. (1997). Working between worlds: Qualitative methods and social psychology. *Journal of Social Issues, 53*(4), 631–644.

Mark, M. (2001). Evaluation's future: Furor, futile, or fertile? *American Journal of Evaluation.*

McMullen, L. (2002). Learning the languages of research: Transcending illiteracy and indifference. *Canadian Psychology, 43,* 195–204.

Mertens, D. M., & Ginsberg, P. E. (2009). *The handbook of social research ethics.* Thousand Oaks, CA: Sage.

Messick, S. (1975). The standard problem: Meaning and values in measurement and evaluation. *American Psychologist, 30,* 955–966.

Michell, J. (2004). The place of qualitative research in psychology. *Qualitative Research in Psychology, 1,* 307–319.

Miles, M. B., & Huberman, A. M. (1994). *Qualitative data analysis* (2nd ed.). Thousand Oaks, CA: Sage.

Morrow, S. L. (2005). Quality and trustworthiness in qualitative research in counseling psychology. *Journal of Counseling Psychology, 52,* 250–260.

Oakley, A. (1981). *Subject women.* Oxford, UK: Martin Robertson.

O'Neill, P. (2002). Tectonic change: The qualitative paradigm in psychology. *Canadian Psychology, 43*(3), 191–194.

Onwuegbuzie, A. J., & Leech, N. L. (2005). Taking the "Q" out of research: Teaching research methodology courses without the divide between quantitative and qualitative paradigms. *Quantity and Quality, 39,* 267–296.

Parker, I. (2004). Criteria for qualitative research in psychology. *Qualitative Research in Psychology, 1,* 95–106.

Polkinghorne, D. E. (1983). *Methodology for the human sciences: Systems of inquiry.* Albany, NY: State University of New York Press.

Polkinghorne, D. E. (1994). Reaction to special section on qualitative research in counseling process and outcome. *Journal of Counseling Psychology, 41,* 510–512.

Ponterotto, J. G. (2002). Qualitative research methods: The fifth force in psychology. *Counseling Psychologist, 30,* 394–406.

Ponterotto, J. G. (2005). Qualitative research training in counseling psychology: A survey of directors of training. *Teaching of Psychology, 32,* 60–62.

Poulin, K. L. (2007). Teaching qualitative research: Lessons from practice. *Counseling Psychologist, 35,* 431–458.

Powell, H., Mihalas, S., Onwuegbuzie, A. J., Suldo, S., & Daley, C. E. (2008). Mixed methods research in school psychology: A mixed methods investigation of trends in the literature. *Psychology in the Schools, 45*(4), 291–309.

Rabinowitz, V. C., & Weseen, S. (1997). Elu(ci)d(at)ing epistemological impasses: Reviewing the qualitative/quantitative debates in psychology. *Journal of Social Issues, 53*(4), 605–630.

Ratner, C. (2008). Cultural psychology and qualitative methodology: Scientific and political considerations. *Culture and Psychology, 14*(3), 259–288.

Rennie, D. L., Watson, K. D., & Monteiro, A. M. (2001). The rise of qualitative research in psychology. *Canadian Psychology, 43*(3), 179–189.

Ricoeur, P. (1970). *Freud and philosophy: An essay on interpretation* (Denis Savage, Trans.). New Haven, CT: Yale University Press.

Russell-Mayhew, S. (2007). Key concepts from health promotion evaluations: What psychology needs to know. *International Journal for the Advancement of Counseling, 28*(2), 167–182.

Shank, G., & Villella, O. (2004). Building on new foundations: Core principles and new directions for qualitative research. *Journal of Educational Research, 98*(1), 46–55.

Silka, L. (2009). Partnership ethics. In D. M. Mertens & P. E. Ginsberg (Eds.), *The handbook of social research ethics* (pp. 337–352). Thousand Oaks, CA: Sage.

Smith, J. K., & Heshusius, L. (1986). Closing down the conversation: The end of the quantitative–qualitative debate among educational inquirers. *Educational Researcher, 15*(1), 4–12.

Stabb, S. D. (1999). Teaching qualitative research in psychology. In M. Kopala & L.

Suzuki (Eds.), *Using qualitative methods in psychology* (pp. 89–104). Thousand Oaks, CA: Sage.

Stake, R. E. (1995). *The art of case study research.* Thousand Oaks, CA: Sage.

Stiles, W. B. (1993). Quality control in qualitative research. *Clinical Psychology Review, 13*, 593–618.

Stoppard, J. M. (2003). Navigating the hazards of orthodoxy: Introducing a graduate course on qualitative methods into the psychology curriculum. *Canadian Psychology [Psychologie canadienne], 43*(3), 143–153.

Walsh-Bowers, R. (2002). Constructing qualitative knowledge in psychology: Students and faculty negotiate the social context of inquiry. *Canadian Psychology, 43*(3), 164–178.

Watkins, M., & Schulman, H. (2008). *Toward psychologies of liberation.* New York: Palgrave Macmillan.

Weinberg, R. S., & Gould, D. (2007). *Foundations of sport and exercise psychology* (4th ed.). Champaign, IL: Human Kinetics.

Wertz, F. J., & van Zuuren, F. J. (1987). Qualitative research: Educational considerations. In F. J. van Zuuren, F. J. Wertz & B. Mook (Eds.), *Advances in qualitative psychology: Themes and variations* (pp. 3–24). Lisse, The Netherlands/Berwyn, PA: Swets & Zeitlinger/Swets North America.

Yardley, L. (2000). Dilemmas in qualitative health research. *Psychology and Health, 15*, 215–228.

Yin, R. K. (1994). *Case study research.* Thousand Oaks, CA: Sage.

Yin, R. K. (2006). Mixed methods research: Are the methods genuinely integrated or merely parallel? *Research in the Schools, 13*(1), 41–47.

PART II

FIVE APPROACHES TO
QUALITATIVE DATA ANALYSIS

CHAPTER 4

The Teresa Texts

Thick Description of Living through Misfortune

The occasion for this data collection was a graduate class in qualitative research methods for psychology. The class undertook a group project in which students decided on a topic. Each wrote a first-person description that would provide data relevant to that topic. Students then formed pairs and conducted interviews with each other, focusing on the life events about which they had written.

After discussing possible topics for the research, the class settled on that of trauma and resilience. In order to avoid technical terms, students decided to refer to their subject matter as "a situation in which something very unfortunate happened and how the person responded." The class formulated instructions for the written description that follow below. Each student wrote one description and submitted it to the class anonymously. After reading all 12 descriptions and considering possible themes for further investigation, the class decided on two relevant issues of interest that would guide the gathering of interview data: the roles of "social support" and "spirituality." Students were free to pursue any other topics of individual interest, including specific ones present in the written description. Interviewers were asked to write a short introduction describing the interview situation and their approach.

The participant, whom we have called Teresa, was 26 years old, the daughter of a Venezuelan father and Filipino mother, and a developmental psychology doctoral student. Although the researchers did not have this information during their analyses, Teresa has subsequently reported, for our readers, that her ethnicity is Philipino-Chinese-Venezuelan-Scottish. The interviewer was a 28-year-old male doctoral student in a psychometrics doctoral program, and this was his first experience conducting an interview.

Instructions: *Describe in writing a situation when something **very** unfortunate happened to you. Please begin your description prior to the unfortunate event. Share in detail what happened, what you felt and did, and what happened after, including how you responded and what came of this event in your life.*

Written Description

I'm afraid that the time "just prior to the event" is a little long, but I'll do my best to be brief, for what it's worth. About two weeks before my unfortunate event, I was a vocal performance major on the verge of beginning my junior year. I had recently been cast in my first main-stage opera role, was finishing up a one-act opera for which I'd landed the lead, had just finished preparations for my junior recital, and was in rehearsal for a musical. I had even lined up a couple of sizable auditions which, despite my age, were looking very promising. I was nineteen, and it was early July.

I was in my car and stopped at a red light on my way to musical rehearsal one afternoon. I dropped my visor to look in the mirror and put on some lipstick, when I noticed a large, two-or-so-inch long bump along the front left side of my neck.

It wasn't there the day before, I was positive of that. I touched it, and it didn't hurt. I poked it, even thumped it . . . it was hard as a rock, and I didn't feel a thing. I got to rehearsal and noticed during the course of the evening that I was finding it a little difficult to sing, as though I was singing against something that was causing pressure on my vocal apparatus. Naturally, I was concerned, so I visited a local doctor the next day. He told me it was a goiter, though he found it strange that I should have one. Not satisfied, I went to another doctor two days later, this time back in my home town, for a second opinion. The second doctor gave me the same diagnosis . . . a goiter. He referred me to a throat specialist, reportedly one of the best in the business, a favorite of superstars who came from all over the world to see him. I got an appointment with him three days later, and, once again, received the same diagnosis, along with the advice to visit an endocrinologist who could address my odd thyroid goiter situation. When I met with the endocrinologist, he ordered a scan of my neck, the results of which he said came back as a "cold scan." He didn't seem bothered; "Come back tomorrow," he told me, "and we'll do a quick biopsy to have a better look at this thing." The biopsy was scary . . . the syringe they used was the big metal sort you might expect to see in a horror movie (I can see why now), and the needle itself was certainly impressive. Of course, the worst part of the experience was that this massive contraption was going to be in my neck, so I kept calm by taking nice, deep breaths and reminding myself that local anesthesia can do wonders. And, as it so happens, it can.

The next day, I received a phone call from my endocrinologist; the results of my biopsy were "inconclusive." Still, I was going to have to go into surgery to get "the mass" removed, no matter what it was, and, by the way, to pack a bag because this would be taking place in two days. The day after that phone call, I was in a surgeon's office, ready to go over the next day's surgical game plan. I'd never had surgery of any kind before; heck, I'd never even broken a bone or gotten stitches. However, I was sure this was no big deal. After all, this was just a thyroidectomy, and only affecting one lobe . . . people have their thyroids taken out all the time. I was actually just taken up in the whole strangeness of suddenly being on the verge of surgery. "Wow," I thought. "My first surgery . . . weird."

The surgeon asked me who had found "the mass," at which point I almost laughed, as I moved my hair aside to show him the rather sizable lump on my neck. "Oh . . . I guess you found it, then," he said, matter-of-factly. Then he asked me what the endocrinologist had told me, and I gave him as accurate a report as I could . . . that the scan came back cold, that the biopsy was inconclusive, that it had to come out. At this point, the surgeon seemed to have gotten very angry with something I'd said. "Damn it," he grumbled. "I hate when they do this. I hate when they make it so that I'm the one that's saying this right before surgery." For the first time, I was stunned, confused. There wasn't anything that made sense for me to say, so I couldn't say anything. Then, the surgeon sat down across from me at his desk. "Do you want your mother to come in?" Instantly, I declined. He asked me again, looking a bit puzzled. Again, I said no. Then he shifted a little in his seat and leaned in, resting his elbows on the desk and looking intently at me. "I don't know why your endo didn't tell you this. Your biopsy wasn't inconclusive. You have anaplastic carcinoma. That's thyroid cancer. We've got to get that thing out of there right now."

Then there was silence, and he just sat there, staring at me, waiting for who knows what. I sat back in my chair a little, let out a big breath, and stared back at him. "Okay," I said. "What're we going to do about it?" In an instant, he was fumbling around on his desk, grabbing a pen and notepad, clearing a space in the midst of the odd clutter. He drew a picture of what seemed to be the two lobes of the thyroid gland (which looked rather like a weird kind of bow tie), then drew out the incisions and various possible mishaps that could occur. I took it all in very methodically, as though we were talking about someone else entirely that he'd be cutting into the next morning. After that was done, he leaned back in his chair and asked me if I had any questions, and I didn't. Then, perhaps in an effort to make small talk, he asked, "So, you're a college student . . . what's your major?" I told him it was vocal performance, and his face went white. He looked grimmer now than he had at any point in our conversation. "Look," he said very gently, "because of where this thing is and what we're going to have to do, there's a chance you won't be able to even speak the same way again. You may not be singing anymore after this."

I froze. I couldn't breathe, couldn't move, couldn't even blink. I felt like I had just been shot. My gut had locked up like I'd been punched in it. My mouth went dry and my fingers, which had been fumbling with a pen, were suddenly cold and numb. Apparently picking up on my shock, the surgeon smiled a little. "We're going to save your life, though. That's what counts. And you know what? The other surgeon working with me is a voice guy. We're going to do everything we can not to be too intrusive." I started to breathe a little, very little, and I felt myself trembling. I tried to say something meaningful, expressive . . . all that I could manage was, "Man . . . I was actually pretty good."

Then, all of me let loose. I was sobbing, but there was no sound; just a torrent of tears, and the hiss of crying from my open mouth, pushing through the pressure from the accursed mass. The surgeon hastened to my side, armed with a tissue and a firm, reassuring hand on my shoulder. I heard him speaking softly from beside me as I heaved in my silent wailing. "You're going to beat this. You're young, and you're going to beat this thing. And you'll get your voice back, and you'll be singing at the Met. And I want tickets, so don't forget me." Slowly, I came back to myself, began to breathe again, and listened to the surgeon as he told me that he was going to use the smallest breathing tubes possible, even make the cleanest possible work of the incision. By the end of the visit, I was completely drained, like a ghost of my former self. I felt as though the biggest and best part of me had died in that office. Cancer wasn't as frightening to me as never being able to sing again. Singing had been my life for as long as I could remember; the one thing I could excel at, the only thing I knew. It had been my solace in all my times of distress, through every hardship . . . this would be the most grueling hardship of all, and I wouldn't be able to sing my way out of it. Literally. Worst of all, I still had to tell my mother.

That meeting in the surgeon's office is what, for me, qualifies as my most unfortunate event to date. The next day, I went into surgery, and it went very well. It took a bit longer than expected, since the mass, a large and exponentially growing tumor, had already begun spreading to my lymphnodic tract and the muscle tissue on the left side of my neck. When I woke up from surgery, I no longer had any thyroid at all, and had also lost some muscle tissue in my neck and two parathyroids. My voice was indeed changed, and it was very hard to speak for a few weeks. Later, my speaking voice returned, but my singing voice wasn't as quick to reemerge; I was left with no choice but to leave the music school at my university and give up all of my singing projects. I had been a cantor at three area churches, and found that I could no longer bring myself to go to church at all . . . it was too painful to go if I couldn't sing. All my friends had been fellow singers, and I knew that they couldn't bear the discomfort of being around me under the circumstances; my voice teacher, who was like another father to me, greeted me in tears each time he saw me afterwards . . . he was there for my surgery, and was the last person I saw before my anesthesia kicked in. Seeing the dreams we had built together go to pieces the way they did was just too much for either of us, and we spoke very little after that.

Many suggested that I take a break from school, that no one would think any less of me, but I was determined to move on as if nothing had happened. When I met new people, I no longer introduced myself as a singer, which was strange for me. Now, I was a psychology major, and I told people this as though I had always been. I suddenly had nonmusician friends, which was also odd, yet strangely refreshing. I was having conversations that I never had the opportunity for in my previous life; my friends now were philosophers, scientists, poets, and historians, and I was learning of a life beyond the hallowed catacombs of practice rooms, voice studios, and recital halls. On top of that, I took up fencing, motorcycling, rock climbing, and theater acting, and seemed to do pretty well. Frankly, I just wanted to live as much as I possibly could, and do everything imaginable while I was at it. Meanwhile, I had also become acquainted with the intricacies of cancer treatment, undergoing a series of radiation bouts and long days alone in clean isolation rooms so I wouldn't contaminate anyone while eradiating. Just when I could fool myself into thinking I was normal again, I'd be back in the hospital.

It took an extra year to get through my undergrad work due to the change of major, during which I met and married my very nonmusical, very academically inclined husband. I began contemplating what to do with my bachelor's degree in psychology when, three years after my surgery, my singing voice began to come back. Ridiculous timing. While holding down my nine-to-five job, I bean working slowly toward getting my voice back in shape, and eventually maintained my own voice studio of around sixty students, serving as my own poster child for the miracles of good voice technique. I sang with two opera choruses, got back into singing at weddings and church services a bit, even visited my old voice teacher a few times for a few lessons. Still, I loved my newfound intellectual life, and I didn't want to give it all up and go back to the grind of full-time classical singing. Besides, I had discovered that, while my voice was still misbehaving (and often does, to this day), I could sing other kinds of music pretty well, particularly rock and blues. I began tinkering with writing my own music, and eventually acquired my own regular gigs at night clubs and live music venues. I continued in my psychology work, as I do now, for I love it dearly, particularly in that it brought forth in me a part of myself I never knew I had, one that seems to hold its own well enough with the more intellectual crowd. The intensive opera chorus work still makes me an opera singer, but that doesn't seem so important to me anymore. I can sing my own music now, so I'm a singer in an entirely new way. I've officially been in remission for over a year now, and, since my type of cancer is an angry sort, I have to go in for scans twice a year. As I see it, though, if I could get through that day in the office with that surgeon (who, by the way, I fully intend to invite to my first breakthrough gig, whatever style of music I'm singing at the time), I suppose I can get through just about anything.

Interviewer's Introduction

The following is the interviewer's retrospective notes, in which he reported the context, his goals and plans, and some thoughts after he conducted the interview.

"This interview was conducted face to face in a teaching assistant's office. My goal was to explore the details of the story in an attempt to look more closely at resilience. After conducting the interview, I realized how I had 'conceptualized' the idea of resilience. My questions were geared towards trying to find sources of support because I believed that resilience cannot happen without a source of strength or support.

"Another idea that I wanted to look at was betrayal. Throughout the story there were people who I thought did not support this participant or who may have appeared as nonsupportive. Since I thought of resilience as a function of support, I thought that that was a relevant topic. Those individuals were friends, doctors, and God.

"I also looked at the areas where resilience occurred. This participant initially had to recover from the news of her urgent surgery. The physical recovery from surgery is involved, and there are the effects that the surgery had on her life as a whole. Because the surgery took away her voice, which was the center of her life, the surgery almost took everything from her life. Hence, she had to recover socially, academically, and in every other aspect of her life.

"The interview gave me insight into the tragedy as well as the participant herself. Along with obviously being smart, the participant showed that she is also strong and courageous. It was an honor to conduct the interview."

Interview Transcript

INTERVIEWER: The first thing that I want to ask is about how, in your story, you didn't make any mention about your father. Do you have a relationship with your father, and, if so, what is it?

PARTICIPANT: That's a very interesting question. I do not have a good relationship with my father. Um . . . my parents are married, and I'd always lived with both of them, but the relationship with my dad is such that we don't get along very well at all. So, in terms of all of this happening, he was probably the furthest from my mind in terms of somebody I would have wanted to go to for support. What's interesting is that, the day before the surgery, when he found out about the surgery, and at that point still didn't know exactly why I was going in, he had a moment of . . . of . . . uncharacteristic emotion. He just came up to me and started crying, and he hugged me . . . and I found that a little odd. Not comforting at all . . . not remotely. Because it was so uncharacteristic. He was never very emotionally demonstrative as a father, and, uh . . . you know . . . as I said, he and I had a rocky dynamic, for as long as I can remember. That's why the occurrence was a little bizarre for me.

INTERVIEWER: You said that he's not demonstrative with his feelings. Is that due, maybe, to the coolness of his character, because he's not the type to demonstrate emotions, maybe one of those typical guys . . . or do you think it's more of a personal thing, due to the relationship that you two have?

PARTICIPANT: Oh, I think it's definitely akin to the fact that he and I don't get along. Um . . . he's actually a very hot-blooded, passionate person. We just don't like each other. And when it comes down to being demonstrative, he's demonstrative, all right, but in other ways, the least of which seemed to be affection. He's always been sort of belligerent towards me . . . it's unfortunate. And I think that, as time has passed, he's gotten older, and I've gotten older, and that animosity has definitely tempered somewhat, which is nice. Besides, he had a heart attack, and ever since that heart attack, he's been sweet as molasses to me . . . I mean, relatively speaking. I've always made more of an effort to get along with him, but . . . he's an interesting guy. He probably qualifies as childish . . . he's very temperamental, has to have his own way . . . in my view if he has to lie or cheat to get it, he'll do it. And that was a little tough for me to grow up with. So yeah, ever since the heart attack, he's been a puppy compared to what he once was.

INTERVIEWER: I don't want to stray too far off the subject, but I have one more question about that. Do you think you might know the source of the bad relationship? Was it just one event that sort of catapulted things and then they just never calmed down, or was it more of "I am who I am, you are who you are, and we just don't mix well"?

PARTICIPANT: I think a lot of it is "I am who I am, you are who you are." What I feel that it really comes down to is the fact that he is of Latin American descent, that he was raised as the one male child in a Venezuelan household. Not to mention, a white man growing up in Venezuela. So he regarded himself very highly, and has always had a very machismo take on male–female relationships. My mother, on the other hand, is very submissive, very "yes, sir, no, sir." I came into the picture, I suppose, as not being a very submissive person, taking more after my father than my mother in that regard, I'm sure. It's not so much that I was looking to pick fights with him . . . it was just a clash of ideals. He thought that, by the time I'd hit the age of 11 or 12, that I should be doing a lot more around the house, when previous to that, I hadn't done a *thing* around the house. As far as this particular event and our relationship . . . my father has a tendency toward the dramatic . . . which I think, to an extent, I share, only I think I temper it a little better than he does. So for a little while after the surgery, and during my first round of radiation treatments, he was very open, and was lavishing gifts on me . . . buying me lots of things. I got a new TV, I got new furniture . . . I got a new apartment! I mean, I got *stuff*! That's just the way he operates. He wanted to demonstrate his affection and his concern by buying me things, and well . . . a 19-year-old college student is certainly going to take advantage of that, no doubt. And then, after . . . I think after the cancer became old news, you could say . . . it tapered off, and he was back to his old belligerent self again. But, for a little while there . . . for about a month, maybe, it was, you know . . . it was kid-in-a-candy-store time for me.

INTERVIEWER: Let's see . . . you made mention that you told your mother . . . no, you told your voice teacher the news before your mother?

PARTICIPANT: I didn't tell my voice teacher before my mother, but, for whatever reason, it was a lot harder to tell him. Where my father lacked, my voice teacher sort of picked up the slack. He was very supportive, he was about the right age to be my dad . . . he was, um . . . he understood my passion for singing, and believed in it, whereas my father, quite frankly, thought it was a pipe dream, and I ought not give money and time to a university to learn how to sing. To him that was ridiculous. My voice teacher thought it was a noble art form, and I found that really comforting. I told him . . . the day before my surgery, almost the same time I told my mother . . . just after.

INTERVIEWER: So, after you told your mother?

PARTICIPANT: Yeah, but just barely. I mean, I didn't have very much time to disclose this news. I found out I had cancer. I had surgery the next day . . . I had to just tell people. And naturally, he drove up to see me the next day, was at the hospital, held my hand, the whole nine yards. But it was harder for me to even conceive of telling him, because our relationship hinged solely on the fact that I was a singer. My mother would have been there for me. But as far as my voice teacher? If I couldn't sing, I was going to lose this guy. As far as I was concerned, not being able to sing would destroy not only everything that we'd worked toward that past 2½ years, but also our relationship . . . professionally, personally, you name it. And I just couldn't deal with that.

INTERVIEWER: How would you describe your relationship, in general, with your teacher?

PARTICIPANT: What . . . now?

INTERVIEWER: No, then.

PARTICIPANT: Oh, then. I used to spend every possible moment in the voice studio with him. What I had in that teacher was gold. To this day, I swear by him. He has something very special in his technique. That's a very typical thing for a voice student to say about a teacher. Voice people tend to build up this sort of cult mentality about their voice studios, particularly undergrads. But this particular teacher really does have something. And the proof's in the pudding; his students do phenomenal things, and his technique is very scientifically based . . . it's not just this artsy intuition that you see so much in the field. Of course, you need to be an artist, but, if you look beyond that, you have a body and an apparatus, and a means by which it physically operates . . . and that's very important to him. I saw firsthand, so many times, that his studio was the place to be. And I wanted very much to be an opera singer, and do it well, to the best of my ability . . . the only way to do that was to be around this man 24/7. On top of which, he was just a great guy. But I had very monocular vision when it came to my goals in life, which contributed to me being very intimately involved with working in the studio and with my teacher . . . and which is why it was so devastating when all of this happened.

INTERVIEWER: You said your teacher kind of filled in the gaps your father didn't. What were some other areas, other than being supportive of your voice and vocal career . . . in what other ways did he fill in the gaps?

PARTICIPANT: Well, I guess you have to think of it in terms of my being 17 and going off to school, and experiencing the world on my own terms for the first time when I met him. He stood for the beacon of wisdom that I think every kid sort of looks for in situations like that. He had invaluable knowledge of the campus, of the people there, of the politics . . . and in the music school, there are *politics.* In any program, there are politics, but in the music school, you've got a whole different kind of ego that you're dealing with. There are performing faculty, with different studios and factions . . . not to mention, the auditions, the recitals, and all levels of performance. There's this heightened sense of "I need to be part of a team, or I'm going to just float around until I totally lose it!" And that's where he came in, and he provided me with that kind of grounding. He did that for a lot of people. And I don't think that he sought to be anybody's father figure. I don't even think that he'd look fondly on my calling him a father figure, but it can't be helped . . . he was.

INTERVIEWER: When you got the news that the results weren't as good as the previous doctor had said, that it was cancer, and that it had to be out ASAP, you were very, very cool about that. Why was that?

PARTICIPANT: I . . . still don't know. I mean, I . . . I remember thinking that panicking wasn't going to do any good. I remember thinking that the best thing to do at that point was to be just as methodical and professional as he had to be, and sort of remove myself from my physical self, as it were . . . to look at the problem as though I was a cohort of his, trying to analyze the problem . . . trying to take on my own role in this cancer battle we were about to embark on. It was the best possible thing I could do to, for one, maintain my sanity at that moment in time, because that's a little heavy, and two, to just get it done. I mean, it didn't seem . . . I reverted completely to logic at that point. I do that. In moments of stress, or anxiety, or tension, or grief . . . you name it. Um . . . I don't try to avoid the emotion, but I do try to temper it . . . by at least maintaining some degree of practical reasoning and logic as the basis of what I'm thinking and doing, just so I don't go completely off kilter and start looking like a moron. I think that, in part, has a great deal to do with growing up with my father, who doesn't have a lever to control that with. So, um, that's what I think contributed to my oddly cool demeanor upon getting the news.

INTERVIEWER: In some ways, does that kind of logic conflict with your artistic personality?

PARTICIPANT: Strangely enough . . . no. Though, at the time, I would have thought so. That was the interesting thing about being in the voice studio I was in. I had never had a voice teacher prior to that. Nobody would want to touch me, because a lot of voice teachers say that, as long as you're doing things here and there that are good, then, by and large, they let you do your own thing technically. At the time, I was pretty damn good, and they just left me alone. And I did sing from my guts, and I was very emotional . . . and of course, being in a very emotional household also contributed to the emotionality of my performance. When I got to college and entered the voice studio, I was told to restrict that emotion and to focus more on the physicality of what I was doing, on releasing tension. When you're emotional, you get physically tense. And when you get physically tense, that kind of messes with what you're doing vocally . . . and that's what was happening to me. So getting away from that emotionality and reminding myself why . . . which, of course, takes logic . . . was actually very instrumental in the long run, not in quashing my emotions . . . I still listen very much to my emotions . . . but understanding that they're just a part of what needs to take place in order to help me function in a given scenario.

INTERVIEWER: Do you remember how you felt towards the previous doctors that didn't tell you how serious it was?

PARTICIPANT: After the fact? Or . . .

INTERVIEWER: After, and, maybe, during?

PARTICIPANT: Okay. During the fact, I just sort of thought, "Well, there are better doctors, I guess." I didn't hold it against them personally, I didn't have any animosity toward them. I mean, how could they know? Nobody could possibly know that. And it was so bizarre. I mean, even after they took it out, they kept that thing in pathology for a long time because they couldn't figure it out. It's still one of those cases where everyone just sort of stood back and thought, "Okay . . . well . . . that was weird." After I realized that I'd been . . . um . . . misled . . . a couple of doctors, the first two . . . no grudges whatsoever. I have no problem with either of them. The third doctor, the doctor who treated all the famous people . . . okay. He was flippant. He was arrogant. And I trusted him because he was flippant and arrogant. Our consultation was all of 5 minutes. He looked at it and said, "Ah, it's a goiter." And I believed him . . . how do you not believe something like that? Especially with his credentials . . . I mean, he had pictures of Cher and Bono on the walls of the waiting room, for crying out loud. So, I mean, I didn't think anything of it.

After the fact, almost instantly after I found out, I think most of my animosity was directed toward him. I couldn't even understand the fact that he was allowed to practice because of his flamboyance . . . and, in the end, was entirely wrong. And if he had tried a little bit and gotten it right . . . we could have stopped this thing from growing quite a bit. It had just started spreading to other parts of my neck . . . it was already on my lymphnodic tract . . . that's scary. That happened in the last couple of days. I could have caught that a week previous if that doctor hadn't been such a jerk and hadn't done what he'd done, and maybe looked into it a little more. That really made me mad. To this day, he's a highly esteemed throat specialist for many of my friends who are still singers. I tell them, time and again, "Be careful with this guy." And they don't listen. They say, "Oh, but he's the best. So he messed up with you . . . that was just once." Well, what can you do? Maybe he is good, but what he did to me, I really can't forgive. As for the endocrinologist, the fact that he sort of deceived me and told me the results were inconclusive . . . I think I understand where he was coming from, and I don't have any hard feelings toward him. I don't feel, you know . . . bamboozled by that deceit. It's probably a greater transgression than that of the other doctor, but the fact that the endocrinologist was the one that took the steps that no one else had taken, and since he found the problem and acted on it, I think he's pretty much made up for it. I stayed with him for my treatments and my scans, so yeah, I don't hold it against him. That other doctor, though? Forget it.

INTERVIEWER: Could you talk about the ease . . . maybe . . . or difficulty . . . in the actual physical recovery?

PARTICIPANT: It was horrible. I remember the instant I woke up from the surgery. And the surgery was supposed to take, maybe, 3 hours . . . it ended up taking something like 6, maybe 7 hours, because they didn't expect to find the spreading. I woke up . . . and . . . well, anesthesia has an interesting effect on people. I'd seen people come out of anesthesia before, and it's funny sometimes . . . people just start bawling and talking gibberish. Naturally, I wake up and I just start wailing, crying. But I realize, first thing, that my voice is coming out much better than it had before surgery, so I thought, "Yeah, this is great!" The following weeks, I was in a lot of pain, primarily because of the nature of the surgery. For a thyroidectomy, there's a period of healing, of course, but my surgery was different because they had to go to the side of my neck where the tumor had begun to spread. As a result, I couldn't walk, could barely move. I was in bed for a good 3 weeks. I'm not the sort that can be bedridden easily. So I was miserable, and more unfortunate, I had to stay with my parents. My mother was fine . . . she doted on me a bit too much for my taste, but it was no surprise. But I could have done without my dad being there, and he was there plenty. And my condition didn't mean we didn't argue, which just complicated things with my voice. Following the surgery, there was a notable inability to speak well for about a month, when my phonation was very definitively affected. Slowly, it started coming back here and there, but something had definitely changed. I got everything checked, but no one could tell what changed. It's been theorized that the surgery was responsible for shifting some things around, so things were just going to be different from that point on. That was difficult . . . healing physically and coming to terms with the fact that things would have to be so different from then on. I wasn't even myself anymore after that. My voice was gone, so I was gone, and I'd never been anything but my voice. So, yeah, that was really hard.

INTERVIEWER: Since you did a lot of singing with yours and other churches, how did this affect your relationship with God?

PARTICIPANT: That's an interesting question.

INTERVIEWER: I mean, you worked for the church, and you were no longer able to . . .

PARTICIPANT: Yeah. That's a very interesting question. Well, for as long as I can remember, I've been a Catholic cantor, so I knew the Mass parts backward and forward, and I always had to stand at the front and lead the congregation, and everybody looked at me and thought, "Oh, isn't she a good Catholic," bla bla bla, and that's great. To be honest, if I wasn't singing, I wouldn't have gone to church. My relationship with God back then was . . . um . . . a casual, conversational one. I mean, it was, "Hi, God, how are you . . . I'm fine . . . that's good . . . how've you been . . ." and it suited me. And I was grateful for things, and I'd offer prayers of thanks. And then when this happened, and I couldn't sing . . . obviously, I was initially grateful . . . grateful to be alive, grateful we'd caught it. Still freaked out, though, because the doctors kept telling me they hadn't gotten it all, that I had to be eradiated and have things burned out, and so forth. And then I couldn't be in the clear because of scans and such, and I would have to be on hormones for ever and ever until I die. So it was hard to be 150% thankful. There was always a bunch of "what if-ing," and it never really went away. With cancer, it doesn't goes away. So you always have to wonder . . . you know, if it's going to come back. Or if it never left. Or if they haven't caught it all. I mean, when you have a bunch of doctors telling you that you have a goiter when it's really a massive tumor growing out of your neck, you start to wonder if any doctor knows anything.

The funny thing is that none of the churches I sang at were actually *my church*. They were paid jobs. I sang at a Catholic church, a Jewish temple, an Episcopal church, and a Baptist church. I tried to go to church after surgery, just to go, but would have to leave during the opening hymn because I couldn't handle it. And then I started asking questions . . . not so much questioning God . . . but questioning religion in general. I got into studying East Asian philosophies, I got into studying all kinds of religious systems and beliefs . . . and I came to the conclusion that my relationship with God, as far as I'd always known it, was very much centered on my voice and being able to sing. And it was very real to me. Singing was my prayer. That was my connection. That was my big gift. I was a fat kid with no friends for as long as I could remember, but I could sing! That was the "in" for me. When I lost that, I lost my connection with God, I lost all my friends, I lost my calling in life, I lost my passion in life, I lost my trump card . . . the thing that was gonna get me out of being that fat kid with the oppressive dad, and whatever . . . that was going to be my ticket out. I lost my ticket! So I lost my connection to God. Gone.

I began to understand things in a very logical, philosophical way, and I took to logic because passion hurt too much. Because music was passion for me. If I had a problem in life . . . seriously . . . I would sing. That's how I fixed it. Always. And I've had problems. Um . . . because I'm lucky like that. But I couldn't sing, even though things would happen. Like, uh, if I was dating a guy . . . and it wasn't like I would just date a guy. I would date a guy who'd beat me up. I was good like that. If I could sing, that would go away for me. Yeah. Couldn't sing. That was bad. Eventually, as my voice started trying to come back, I realized . . . I wasn't angry at God . . . I just really didn't think there was a God working on things for me out there. I don't have any animosity toward religion, nor do I have any judgments on people who have religious beliefs. I respect spirituality, I believe myself to be spiritual . . . yet I can't say that I now adhere to any one given faith. Qualifiedly agnostic, you could say. I'm open . . . if the deity of choice wants to zap me and give me a moment of epiphany, I'm fine with that. But as of yet, it hasn't occurred, to my knowledge. I'm waiting for whatever. In the meantime, I'll keep reading my Lao Tsu, and my Baghavad Gita, and my Koran, and my Book of Mormon. I've got an interesting collection at home. But I keep myself abreast of the thoughts out there, and I think about it a lot. I do feel that spirituality is a big part of what I do, like in my writing, my music now . . . yeah. A huge part of it. I'd rather think of how I live and how much I live, though, rather than whether or not there's a greater being. Is there a God I'm giving it all up to? No, I don't feel that way. I feel that, honestly, if there's a God, and I end up in heaven, the first thing I'd like to hear is "Okay, you were wrong . . . I exist. But it's okay." I think that, if there is a God, he'll totally understand where I'm coming from. I think he'd be okay with it.

INTERVIEWER: You mentioned your friends not being able to stand being around you because they knew how much pain you were in. Describe how that manifested itself, in terms of their actions or their relationships with you.

PARTICIPANT: They disappeared from my life. And I think that was on both our parts; we're talking about dear, dear friends, of which I've retained one . . . I think we were so close that nothing was going to drive a stake through that. But you have to remember that we're dealing with a voice studio and a voice school where everything is very competitive, and everybody knows who's who and what they're capable of, and voice parts having their different animosities between themselves . . . there's always a queen bee. I was the freak *wunderkind* mezzo-soprano at the music school that got the auditions, got the solos, got the favoritism from directors. I didn't really want things like that, because it sucked. By default, people started hating me. I had graduate students come up to me in the halls and threaten me . . . it was weird. But it was my calling . . . it was me, it was what I had to do. To hell with the grad students. It was me, who I was . . . and everyone just kind of knew I was going to be something someday. So when this happened to *me*, it scared the crap out of everybody . . . scared the *crap* out of everybody. And I even had a couple of them tell me how tragic it was . . . like I was dead, and they were telling me about it. It was weird. But essentially, I *was* dead. To them. I mean, if I wasn't a viable musical threat, then what was the point of knowing about me, knowing of me at all . . . knowing *me* . . . because the only reason I was an entity in their lives was because I was a dominant singer. When I was out of the picture, I think they put it out of their minds, because for that to happen to someone where I was . . . was just scary. I think I put myself in their place a lot . . . I didn't hold it against them. I think if that had happened to someone else, and I'd watched it happen, I would have probably done the same thing.

INTERVIEWER: Why?

PARTICIPANT: It's scary!

INTERVIEWER: Why is it scary?

PARTICIPANT: Because singers tend to be kind of insecure. Because I'm not the only one walking around, thinking, as a singer, "That's my voice, and without my voice I have nothing." It's a huge step for a singer to say, "Eh . . . maybe I'll try *this* career change." That's huge. It's almost as big as religion. It may be bigger. Because for musicians to devote themselves that completely to their art and to even consider the thought of straying from that path, even for a moment . . . that moment is very pivotal for a singer. Whenever you hear about people who have degrees in music and do completely different things . . . there was a big choice that took place there. In my case, it was forced on me. But if I were confronted with that situation, and there was someone I knew to be particularly talented with high hopes, then suddenly felled by a disease and not being able to sing anymore . . . I don't think I'd be able to carry on being around them too much. Not only that, but they'd feel uncomfortable talking about what was going on at school, in the field . . . because that's all we talked about! And I couldn't do it anymore, so what would they talk to me about? That had to have been difficult for them. I mean, it was difficult for me, but it was easy for me to put myself in their place.

INTERVIEWER: I guess the next logical question would be, looking back now, would you consider these people to be real friends?

PARTICIPANT: No . . . but, then again, a lot of friends in college aren't *friends*, but you don't know that at the time. They're people that you know from the department, people that you hang out with by default, people with similar interests . . . and that helps to segue into social circles forming. But, for the most part, in times of crisis, those aren't always the people you run to. Still, they're what I had. So I showed up on the first day of the next semester looking like I'd been in a crazy knife fight . . . and word travels fast. And especially since I'd been cast in an opera . . . they had to recast it. I had to reschedule my recital, because at the time, I was still in the music school and was going to try to get my voice back. Which didn't happen.

INTERVIEWER: Did you actually try to get back on track?

PARTICIPANT: Oh, yeah . . . oh, yeah. For a whole semester.

INTERVIEWER: How did that go?

PARTICIPANT: That was painful . . . painful. Having been called in by every single professor and conductor in the music school, to sit down and have a moment with me in their offices . . . just to reflect on life, and how tragic it is for this 19-year-old kid with so much promise to be taken out by cancer. I mean . . . again, being spoken to as though I was already dead. And these were professors who I thought never really liked me. Some would even tell me, "Yeah, I've got this lump over here," and I'd want to say, "Um . . . I don't care!" It was so strange and morbid . . . everybody kept looking at me like I was already death warmed over. Even now, people find out about my medical history, and I still get those looks. But in the music school at the time, with a big gash in my neck? That was priceless! Not only that . . . of course, my voice teacher would just openly cry in front of me. I just couldn't handle that, you know? I mean, I really cared about this guy, and I was just bringing him way down. And then one day, I was leaning on the piano in the studio, and he was sitting at the keyboard, and we were having this sad lesson . . . and he just looked at me and said, "Why don't you just stop coming?" And I said, "You're right." And that's the last time I went to the studio. It was like that. It was like that. Plus, I was in every top choir in the school . . . and this was a school with a pretty hard-core choral program . . . recordings, international tours, the works. I was a member of the elite chamber choir, the youngest member, so it was a big deal. This thing was like lightning when it hit. So I became like this weird kind of ghost, like a pariah . . . the untouchable one that everybody talked about.

INTERVIEWER: Did you have any resentment for your teacher?

PARTICIPANT: No . . . well, a little bit, a little bit. Because, even though I expected us to drift apart because of this, I harbored this secret hope that there was more to it than just the singing . . . that we could find common ground as people. I thought we did. Or maybe we did, but it was just too painful, and we couldn't get past the pain. And I understand that now. I mean, he had a full studio, and a lot to deal with, and people were talking about me a lot when I wasn't in the studio, which he had to deal with. And since then we've talked . . . he's very supportive of what I do now. He actually just retired, and all of his old students got together for a big party. Then people saw me and were, like, "_____, _____, what are you up to now?" And I'd tell them, "Um . . . I'm starting work on my PhD in psychology." "Oh, my God, you're smart? We didn't know!" I was like, "I know! I didn't either!" Which is true . . . I didn't know I was smart. How could I have? I was an intelligent singer, sure, but you don't have to be intelligent to be a good singer, really. Look around sometime at a few singers . . . a lot of jokes go around about sopranos, but we won't go there. My point is that I didn't have an opportunity as a vocal performance major to explore that area of myself. As soon as the voice was gone, I had to find something or I was going to die. I really felt that I was going to have to die, or kill myself . . . or hold my breath until it ended. Anything but feel like that. It was miserable and painful, and terrible. I can't explain in words how awful it was. I guess I know a little of how the Katrina people feel, in my own way. They lost everything. I lost my identity. I lost myself. And now I didn't have a leg to stand on, like, with my dad, because I'd always fought him on being a good enough singer to make a living. Well, now he had me. So that was horrible.

It took me . . . wow . . . it took me. I think, even now, I struggle with it a lot. But I fight it . . . I fight it tooth and nail. Because I'm still a singer, damn it. You're not gonna stop me. I have a sick passion to fight odds . . . I take pride in it, because . . . I don't know why. I don't know that I'm a prideful person. But I'm proud of what I've done, kind of, in an American way. Not in, like, an arrogant bastard kind of way. Feeling like, "Okay, for a cancer patient, I'm kind of doing okay." I'm doing stuff. And as soon as I get started on that, I gotta go do more stuff. I gotta go be a fencer, go rock climbing, get a PhD. I have to keep going, like I'm obsessed with it. There's a spare moment? I could be studying . . . I could be working on a song. I need to just keep doing. Because what if this thing comes back? I won't have done anything important if it were to come back today. I better get on with it. Yeah, it took a long time to come to terms with not being an opera singer . . . Maybe 2 years of straight misery. Then, in my senior year of undergrad, my voice started coming back. And that was terrible. Because I used to say, "I'd give anything to have my voice back," when it first happened. And I meant it. I'd have killed somebody, I think. But then it came back, and I was like, "Oh . . . great." And I was on the verge of finishing my psych degree, and I thought, "Ugh . . . you gotta be kidding me." I was mad, at nobody . . . just pissed. I mean, you gotta be kidding me. What are the odds?

I went in and talked to my voice teacher, and he let me in on the secret that I didn't need a voice degree to sing. That's when I started doing auditions, doing the professional opera chorus gigs . . . and still, I realized I had kind of gotten used to the idea of not being an opera singer . . . and it wasn't that bad. And I *was* kinda smart . . . and my friends who weren't musicians were a little less vapid. I mean, not that all musicians are vapid, but a good many are. And I still had a couple, like my friend who tried to be there for me throughout . . . we're still very close. I don't know what I'd have done without him. Oh, and by that point, I'd already gotten married, and this guy didn't know me as a singer. He met me a week before I found out about the cancer, so my voice was already headed downhill. So he never really heard me sing. But he did see me perform eventually . . . and he was a part of my starting to fence. He was a big-time academic . . . still is. I mean, he must be one of the smartest people I know. So he only knows me in a certain respect. Becoming a musician again, in a new way . . . that was a ride in itself.

INTERVIEWER: I have a couple more. Describe your mom throughout the whole process.

PARTICIPANT: Wow. My mom was a wreck. She's a worrier by nature. She's always been very timid and skittish. I think that my dad being such a tyrant made her very nervous all the time. I remember her getting in trouble all the time for doing things wrong. Like the coffee was too hot or too cold . . . ridiculous things like that. So I always saw her as this cowering person, despite the fact that she really is a very strong individual . . . but I saw her throughout my childhood as cowering under the shadow of this overbearing presence of my dad. She's always attributed this attitude to her ethnic background, being Filipino, and being raised in a very dogmatic, Catholic understanding of wifely duties to one's husband . . . being a good, subservient wife. And that the wife's duty is to the husband first, and to the children second . . . and she told me that, a lot. So, needless to say, that didn't do good things in terms of my animosity toward my dad, nor did it help things in terms of my religiosity. That's probably my biggest thing with the Catholic Church . . . the position of women. And I've tried to talk to monsignors and cardinals about this. That's another thing that's changed . . . now I don't care who I talk to . . . no shame. But my mother's role in the situation . . . she became even more nervous, and more worried, and more concerned. And that was dreadful. When I told her, we were driving from the office, after I had just found out. It was about an hour drive, and it wasn't until right before we got home. I didn't want to tell her.

INTERVIEWER: And you felt you knew how she was going to take it, how it was going to go?

PARTICIPANT: I knew *exactly* how it was going to go down! I knew this woman was going to freak out. She was going to pull over, start crying, get worried, call a bunch of people, make them worry too. I thought, "Crap . . . why don't I just go through the surgery and not tell her?" And, in a sense, I did. I told her some things . . . not everything. I didn't tell her what kind of cancer it was . . . she's a med tech, so she knows things. I told her they might have to do a full thyroidectomy, and that the lump . . . I basically pulled the same game that the other doctor did . . . that the lump was *probably* cancer. That they didn't know exactly what it was. I left it at that, but that was enough . . . she lost it. She was so nervous, and so freaked out. I understood, but I waited until after the surgery before I gave them all the details. I felt like, since I was going into surgery, that I couldn't exactly deal with all of that just then. I care . . . I mean, she's a saint, and I prize her above all human beings on the planet . . . but I made the executive decision to moderate her amount of knowledge at that point. She did not do well. But she did go into overdrive as soon as it was time for me to recover. She was in charge of getting me to treatments, getting my medications, my creams, my food, my blood work, my insurance, my scans, my weird schedules and appointments. She was the master hub. In that regard, I think she and I share that need to pop things into logical overdrive and do what needs to be done, rather than succumb to the prospect of becoming completely pathetic under the weight of your emotions. And she functioned, and that helped me get through. But, you could see it. She was falling apart.

Even now, there are the questions that come with every phone call. "Are you taking your meds? Do you have enough meds? Have you taken your meds today? Are you sure you're taking your meds? Are you taking care of yourself? Take care of yourself. Have you taken your meds?" I guess she has good reasons. I've had trouble ever since the diagnosis. I end up in the hospital for one thing or another. The last year of my undergrad, they found another tumor, and this time it was a pituitary tumor . . . this time, it was a freakin' brain tumor. And it was inoperable, so we just sit around and watch it. It doesn't do any tricks . . . it just kind of sits there. I mean, it grows, and it shrinks, but it's not doing anything amazing. But what can you do? So that sucked. "Here we go again," is what that was. It was a little scarier, because of it being in the brain, but whatever. What can you do? Me, I turned to logic. So I ended up doing my undergrad thesis on the psychological side effects of pituitary tumors. I figured that, if I had to have this thing, I may as well get something out of it.

INTERVIEWER: Describe the role of your fiancé, now husband. Describe his role, I guess, in your healing, during that 2-year-period.

PARTICIPANT: Interesting role. We got engaged, got married, moved to California for a year, then moved back to Texas, when I finished my undergrad. In that 2 years . . . anyone who's been married will tell you that the first year is a doozie, no matter who you are. But that, on top of having to go through radiation . . . and the therapy I was undergoing has nothing on chemo, thankfully, but it still sucked. I only lost a little patch of hair about that big . . . I could cover it up with the rest of my hair. But I think it was all a little too much for him to handle. I mean, we've talked about it since. But this man's got as much ADHD as 10 little kids that are high on pixie sticks.

The cancer stuff is not something a guy like that needs to have to deal with in his first year of marriage, I think.

Our relationship has been very egalitarian . . . he and I are both firm believers in an equal partnership in our relationship. The thing is that he's always been really committed to considering me an equal in every sense, which I love. That only becomes a problem when I get sick. I mean, we have our differences, but they're differences that we have equally. He's a nondenominational Christian, I'm agnostic, and we talk about it and have some good conversations . . . that's an example. But with cancer and my radiation . . . there was no parallel for him. And I think that he tried very hard to see me as strong . . . I wanted to be seen as strong. But whenever I was falling all over myself because of the radiation, he didn't know how to deal with it. He would just kind of look at me and say, "Come on, get up." And I couldn't get up. So then he thought that I was trying to milk this whole thing for attention. He didn't think it was that bad, I guess, because I tended to downplay things. It hasn't been till recently that he's started to realize that, despite my strengths, which are relatively okay, given the nature of things, my weaknesses tend to be pretty bad. And whenever I'm sick, I'm sick with a vengeance. But now, I think he gets it. And we've been married almost 7 years now, so it took him, what, 6 years? So that's been a long process. Those 2 years? He was kinda worthless then. But we sure grew from it. I mean, strength through adversity? Absolutely. And I think it comes with age . . . age and experience. We've both grown a lot. Besides, when you go through something like that, it's very lonely, very isolating, no matter what you do. I mean, even other cancer patients didn't know what it was like, because the cancer I had was so weird. Anaplastic carcinoma is a weirdo cancer that can kill you in a couple of weeks. And then the thing in my brain . . . well, that's just a lot for a new spouse to handle. So I certainly don't hold it against him . . . he was definitely standoffish. But then his mother passed this summer, of colon cancer. And that's when I think it clicked. Because he saw me kind of connecting with her, and she opened up to me. I wrote her a song, and she really opened up to it and liked it. Then, our discourse began from there. I think he saw that, and then saw where I could have ended up. He watched her die, and it was pretty gruesome the way she suffered in those last days. I think he finally realized that the same thing could have happened to me . . . that it might still happen to me. And I think it may have helped him take stock of how severe things can get, even though I try to play things off like there's nothing wrong.

INTERVIEWER: And what exactly is a goiter?

PARTICIPANT: A goiter is an inflamed thyroid gland. One of the lobes, maybe both lobes of the gland, will have gotten big and scary. Typically, they're due to a deficiency of iodine, which is why it's so flippin' rare for a young American female to get a goiter in this day and age. I mean, we get plenty of iodine. Salt is iodized, for chrissakes. We don't have a lack of iodine in our diets anymore. This mass was sticking out about an inch or so from my neck, but you really had to really look to see that things were bigger on one side. And it was rock hard. I mean, it was weird. But hey . . . what else could it be, right? The weird cancer wasn't even on the list of possibilities. That's what's so scary. Matter of fact, my thyroids were working perfectly well . . . one lobe just had a big, fat tumor sitting on top of it.

INTERVIEWER: So, did they come to a conclusion that it really did inflame that quickly, or was it slower but didn't show up as big at first?

PARTICIPANT: There are different kinds of thyroid cancer. What I have is a faster type. If you're going to have a cancer, make sure it's thyroid cancer. It's great, because you can get rid of it . . . the survival rate is best . . . well, Renquist didn't do so well, but whatever. The thing about my type, anaplastic carcinoma, is that it's an extremely fast-growing type. The cells are so advanced that it can grow overnight . . . my tumor *did* grow overnight, and the spreading took place in less than a week. It's the fastest growing of all the thyroid cancers, and there's something like a 15%, maybe 20% survival rate in the first couple of months. It seems like most everybody who gets this thing dies from it. My case was very different for several reasons. First of all, I'm not dead. Second, I was 19 . . . that sort of cancer typically doesn't hit people until their late 40s, early 50s. Third, the cell structure was a little weird . . . not to mention, I have no history of cancer on either side of my family. I mean, there's one distant relative with hypothyroidism, so she's a little overweight, but that's not even close to cancer. But, yeah, this thing grew overnight, while I was sleeping. Boom . . . tumor. Just like that.

INTERVIEWER: There's no chance that maybe you were really busy the day before, or you just didn't see it . . .

PARTICIPANT: Nope . . . we were in dress rehearsals for a show, so I was in the mirror for makeup every day. I would have seen it. Besides, it was *Nunsense*, which meant we had to wear nuns' habits, including a neckpiece. I would have definitely seen it, felt it. But, yeah, just like that. It can happen to anybody, at any time. I think they wrote me down, the weirdo case of the girl with the weirdo tumor. The whole thing took less than two weeks to go that far . . . creepy.

CHAPTER 5

A Phenomenological Psychological Approach to Trauma and Resilience

Frederick J. Wertz

I n this chapter, I explore a phenomenological approach to psychological research. I provide a brief introduction to the approach, history, methods, and applications of phenomenological research with an emphasis on psychology. Then I describe the practices that I employed in the current demonstration. My analysis of Teresa's experience of trauma and resilience (and the themes of social support and spirituality) was too lengthy to be fully included here. Therefore, I present the forms of my findings with samples of my reflections and of the kinds of knowledge generated by my analysis. I spell out the procedures I used in moving toward general findings, including a comparative analysis involving the experience of the second participant, Gail. Finally I mention some characteristics of typical research reports. Although I limit the use of technical terms, I introduce and employ some basic phenomenological vocabulary in order to promote understanding and literacy among psychological researchers.

The Phenomenological Approach

The phenomenological approach to research has its roots in the work of Edmund Husserl at the turn of the 20th century. Husserl (1913/1962) developed the research method he called "phenomenology" for use in philosophy and the human sciences. In psychology, this method is a descriptive, qualitative study of human experience. The aim is to faithfully conceptualize the processes and structures of mental life, how situations are meaningfully lived through as they are experienced, with "nothing added and nothing subtracted" (Giorgi, 2009). Phenomenology sets aside such theories, hypotheses, and explanations as refer to biology or environment and investigates *what* is experienced and *how* it is experienced.

The Phenomenological Attitude: Focus on Lived Experience

Husserl (1936/1954) adopted two fundamental procedures as necessary for the study of experience: the *epoché of the natural sciences* and the *epoché of the natural attitude*. *Epoché* (from the Greek ἐποχή, pronounced "ĕ-pō-kā'") means abstention. These epochés distinguish phenomenological from mainstream and contrasting methods. The first epoché involves putting aside natural scientific and other knowledge—theories, hypotheses, measuring instruments, and prior research about the topic under investigation. As Husserl (1900–1901/1970, p. 252) famously said, "We must return to 'the things themselves' (*zurück zu den Sachen selbst*)." Abstaining from or "bracketing" prior knowledge of the subject matter allows the researcher to attend to what Husserl called the "lifeworld" (*lebenswelt*) and to freshly reflect on concrete examples of the phenomena under investigation.

The second epoché, that of the natural attitude, is sometimes called the "phenomenological reduction" (Husserl, 1936/1954). The researcher abstains from the natural tendency of consciousness to unreflectively posit and focus on the existence of objects independent of experience. This procedure enables the investigator to closely examine how situations present themselves through experience. The *psychological* phenomenological reduction (in contrast to the transcendental reduction used in philosophical investigations) is a partial epoché of the natural attitude, in which the psychologist continues to posit the existence of persons and of the experiences under investigation but takes no position regarding the existence of their objects of experience (Husserl, 1925/1977, 1936/1954). For instance, in studying experiences of automobile accidents, the psychologist focuses on the way drivers attribute fault to themselves and to others, including all the meanings and consequences of fault as experienced by drivers, without investigating or judging the objective existence of fault, which is the focus of judges and insurance adjusters. The phenomenological attitude is reflective. It selectively turns from the existence of objects to the processes and meanings through which they are subjectively given. Although this attitudinal focus is called a "reduction," the field of investigation is not narrowed but rather is opened up and expanded to encompass all the complexities and intricacies of psychological life that come into view.

It is important to understand that these epochés do not involve doubt or disbelief about natural science (or any) theories and research, let alone about the objective existence of the world around us. These are *methodologi-*

cal procedures that aim is to extend science into the realm of subjectivity. These epochés are similar to the "bracketing" performed by natural scientists (e.g., methodological behaviorists), when they set aside personal meanings and values in order to investigate the purely physical. Husserl (1936/1954), who was himself a mathematician and admired the successes of natural science and technology, held that methods borrowed from the physical sciences cannot answer all important scientific questions. Husserl criticized the universalization of the methods of the physical sciences (called "scientism") and advocated different but equally rigorous methods tailored to study subjectivity and matters human. In his view, science enables human beings to freely shape their destiny by means of rational, unprejudiced knowledge that is true to each kind of subject matter. Investigation of subjectivity, human meanings, values, and culture requires uniquely suitable methods. For Husserl, the prosperity of humanity depends on methodological pluralism in our sciences.

Phenomenological Method: Intentional and Eidetic Analysis

The two other procedures that Husserl (1913/1962) developed are called *intentional analysis* and *eidetic analysis*. Intentional analysis is the procedure of reflecting on, gaining insight into, and describing the "how" and the "what" of experience—*how* experiential processes proceed and *what* is experienced through them. *Intentionality* denotes the transcendental quality of consciousness, that consciousness is *of something* (beyond itself). Psychological processes are irreducibly relational in that they meaningfully illuminate *the person's world*, including experiences in the same or other persons' mental lives. For instance, I see a blackbird, I turn the knob to open a heavy door, I imagine a centaur, I fondly recall my childhood home, I remember how I felt when I was laughing, I anticipate enjoying a delicious lunch with my friend, I am struck by my neighbor's horror when he hears the bad news, and so on. Experience is intrinsically relational in that by perceiving, behaving, imagining, anticipating, and so on, the person—as center of passivities, activities, possibilities, and habitualities—relates to the world. Phenomenology investigates the person's ways of being-in-the-world by descriptively elaborating the *structures* of the I ("ego" or "self"), the various kinds of intentionality (ways of experiencing), and the meaningful ways in which the world is experienced. Phenomenological reflection, called "intentional analysis," shows that human experience is embodied, practical, emotional, spatial, social, linguistic, and temporal.

As a scientific undertaking, phenomenology seeks *general knowledge* on the basis of evidence. Its form of rationality, which is qualitative rather than mathematical, utilizes a general human capability that Husserl called the *intuition of essences* (*Wesenschauung*), which he developed as a scientific method known as *eidetic analysis* (Giorgi, 2009; Husserl, 1913/1962; Wertz, 2010). We are familiar with and continually experience essences (what things are) in everyday life. When I see a cat, I experience the individual as an example of the general kind, "cat." The essence, "cat," is intuitively (directly, with evidence) given in the experience of an individual cat. As an instance of a general kind, a concrete example includes all that is essential to that kind. The most basic question for qualitative methodology is: How can we know such essences? Phenomenology uses the procedure of eidetic analysis.

Eidetic analysis begins with a single example of the kind of experience or object under investigation. The investigator practices what Husserl called *free imaginative variation* of that example in order to conceptually clarify its essence (*eidos*, Greek εἶδος, meaning "form"). If, even after a particular characteristic of an example is imaginatively removed, the instance is nevertheless an example of the phenomenon, what was removed is not essential to the kind. By comparing many imaginatively varied individuals, an investigator can conceptualize what is invariably present in all examples of the kind in question. If it is impossible to imagine an example of the kind without a particular characteristic, that characteristic is essential. Knowing an essence involves conceptually clarifying the invariant characteristics and structure evident in a virtually limitless multiplicity of possible exemplifications. The use of free imaginative variations in understanding what is essential among individuals of a certain kind distinguishes eidetic analysis from induction, which in contrast infers empirical generality on the basis of a limited number of actually observed cases.

The generalizing procedure that clarifies the essences of phenomena is sometimes called the "eidetic reduction." Eidetic psychological analysis does not diminish or simplify its subject matter but opens up and highlights its vast richness and complexity. The procedure aims to conceptually clarify all that human beings live through in a particular kind of psychological phenomenon, including not only all its constitutive processes and meanings, but their distinctive holistic structure, including embodied, practical, emotional, spatial, social, linguistic, and temporal aspects. Human mental life entails *many levels and kinds of eidetic generality* that research can clarify and elaborate. Investigators can provide knowledge of various scopes of eidetic generality, including specific contextual parameters—at very high levels, at typical midlevels, and/ or at lower, more context-bound levels (e.g., "consciousness"; "emotion"; "disappointment"; "disappointment in New York City among illegal, adolescent, Mexican immigrants"). Inasmuch as psychology seeks general knowledge of real human beings, the investigator must clarify what is invariant among *realistic* examples of the phenomenon under study. The free imaginative variations used in psychological eidetic analysis are therefore informed and guided by numerous real examples of the subject matter. Numerous real examples of the subject matter are imaginatively varied in realistic ways, and their thick details are compared with each other in the acquisition of general knowledge. Eidetic knowledge may be improved as insights move from relatively partial to thorough, incomplete to complete, vague to clear based on the adequacy of examples, imaginative variations, and conceptual insightfulness. Like all science, eidetic analysis is not finalized in a single study and moves forward through complementary investigations that describe the similarities and differences among the structures of phenomena.

A phenomenological study of "trauma" begins with an example such as Teresa's and identifies in that individual experience its essence: *what trauma is.* Teresa's trauma involved a life-threatening thyroid cancer, but by imaginatively varying her situation, it becomes evident that many other unfortunate events could also be traumatic, such as a different illness or a natural disaster. Thyroid cancer is not generally essential to the experience of trauma. We begin to clarify what is essential to trauma by discovering those qualities that, when imaginatively removed, yield instances of experience that are not traumatic. One might find that without suffering the destruction of something crucially important in a person's life, there is no traumatic experience. Perhaps the experienced destruction of something crucial, on which personal existence depends, is invariant or essential to trauma. Although research begins with the study of Teresa's example, eidetic analysis is not limited to this. The analysis of various real and freely imagined examples of trauma is necessary to clarify "what trauma is"—that without which the lived experience of trauma is unimaginable, inconceivable. Research may address the highest level of generality—the invariant characteristics all traumatic experiences— but psychological researchers are often interested in more specific types and context-bound manifestations of trauma. Perhaps distinguishing types of trauma involved in "illness," "accidental injury," "violent crime," "domestic violence," "war," or "natural disaster" would be significant—analysis would be required to know. Phenomena can be known and described eidetically at various levels of generality, ranging from the lower limit—a particular *individual's experience* of trauma, such as Teresa's—to various *types* or typical kinds of traumatic experience, and to the most *highly general* characteristics of all types of traumatic experience.

The Phenomenological Movement

Philosophical and Transdisciplinary Directions

Husserl's work entailed nothing less than a radical and comprehensive study of consciousness with all its various kinds of processes, meanings, and objects. His initial interests in epistemology and the philosophy of science led to studies of mind–body relations, language, time, intersubjectivity, the person, culture, and history. His publications, primarily on epistemology and the philosophy of science, represent only a small portion of the 45,000 manuscript pages he wrote in his lifetime. Much of Husserl's published works focus on the programmatic delineation of phenomenology, though they contain some of his brilliant and painstaking concrete analyses, for instance, of perception and time consciousness. Husserl viewed himself as a perpetual beginner and returned to revise his analyses throughout his career. His assistants, students, and followers extended and developed this philosophical work in such areas as ontology, ethics, language and symbol studies, social sciences, and environmental studies. Their work took a series of turns, including the existential (Heidegger, 1927/1962; Merleau-Ponty, 1942/1963, 1945/1962; Sartre, 1943/1956, 1936/1948b, 1939/1948a), hermeneutic (Gadamer, 1960/1989; Ricoeur, 1974), social construction (Berger & Luckmann, 1967; Schutz & Luckmann, 1983.1989; Schutz, 1932/1967), narrative (Ricoeur, 1981), and ethical (Levinas, 1961/1969) . Others such as Marcel (1965) and Bachelard (1938/1964a, 1958/1964b) also contributed to the effort. The phenomenological movement extended into virtually all fields in which consciousness is relevant, including the spectrum of social sciences, humanities, and fine arts studies. With its broad transdisciplinarity, phenomenology has also contributed to such practical professions as education, health, social service, and business.

Phenomenological Psychology

No other discipline is closer to phenomenological philosophy or has received greater attention in the movement than psychology. Husserl wrote about psychology starting in his first phenomenological publication (in 1900–1901/1970) and continuing through his last (1936/1954). He provided meticulous analyses of perception, speech, thinking, time consciousness, imagination, emotional life, social experiences such as empathy, ego habitualities, and many other intentional processes. Many phenomenological philosophers have addressed disciplinary issues in psychology and have performed psychological analyses. For instance, studies of the emotions, imagination, personality, behavior, psychophysiology, human development, and social interaction have been conducted by Sartre (1939/1948a), Merleau-Ponty (1942/1963, 1945/1962), Gurwitsch (1964), Schutz (1932/1967) and Gendlin (1962). The movement had considerable impact on European schools of psychology as well as psychiatry (Giorgi, 2009; Halling & Dearborn Nill, 1995; Spiegelberg, 1972; Wertz, 2006). The work of phenomenological psychiatrists, beginning with Jaspers (1913/1963) and Scheler (1913/1954), became known in America with the popular publication of *Existence* (May, Angel, & Ellenberger (1958). Other important psychiatric research has been conducted by Binswanger (1963), Minkowski (1933/1970), Boss (1963), Straus (1966), van den Berg (1972), and Laing (1962; Laing & Esterson, 1963). Phenomenology is a broad, adaptable movement that includes many different topical interests, talents, sensibilities, and unique styles of its investigators. It often involves creative modifications of the methodological attitudes and analytic procedures outlined above (Spiegelberg, 1972, 1982; Valle, 1998).

Learning Phenomenology

The multifaceted and broadly influential history of phenomenology presents an educational opportunity and also a challenge for psychological researchers. Although familiarity with phenomenological scholarship in philosophy, sociology, communications, theology, literary criticism, art history, and other disciplines is invaluable, psychological research may be undertaken without extensive study of the movement. The phenomenological literature, much of which touches on psychology, offers researchers a philosophy of science that contrasts sharply with others ranging from positivism to constructivism and helps establish a crucial foundation for research focused on the essential characteristics of human experience. This literature contains detailed elaborations and illustrations of methodological principles and procedures as well as a wealth of descriptive conceptual tools and terminology relevant to the rigorous investigation of human experience. These writings sensitively focus on familiar phenomena of human experience and consequently often evoke an immediate resonance and recognition on the part of readers who, as Merleau-Ponty noted, may experience phenomenology as "what they had been waiting for" (1945/1962, p. viii). Merleau-Ponty characterizes phenomenology as a "manner or style of thinking" prior to a formal discipline, and therefore this approach may be readily accessible and embraced by researchers with various styles and interests.

Phenomenological procedures were not invented but discovered in practice by Husserl. Husserl (1925/1977) credited Brentano, who identified the intentionality of mental life, and Dilthey, who brilliantly enumerated many essential qualities of mental life, as achieving phenomenological insight prior to the formal specification of its methodology, showing that such basic procedures as the epochés and eidetic intentional analysis can be practiced spontaneously without formal training. Without calling themselves "phenomenologists," others carry out these practices in meeting the demands posed by the scientific study of consciousness. Husserl and his followers have articulated, systematized, and legitimized procedures that are required for the rigorous study of consciousness and experience. Phenomenology is neither a doctrine nor a contrived method but a diverse, living movement that is still changing. Phenomenological research utilizes the full sensitivity, knowledge, and powers of comprehension of the researcher and is consequently quite personal. Merleau-Ponty (1945/1962) wrote that one learns phenomenology *by making it one's own*. The flexibility of the method allows its creative adaptation to diverse topics, research problems, and styles of researchers.

Psychological Research Method
Using Lifeworld Descriptions

Since the 1960s, specific, formal procedures for conducting phenomenological psychological research have been used as a guide for researchers and as a framework for scientific accountability (Giorgi, 2009; Wertz, 2005). After demonstrating how phenomenology offers a broad approach capable of providing a foundation for psychology (Giorgi, 1970), Giorgi developed, articulated, and justified phenomenological research methods that are applicable to the full spectrum of psychological subject matter (Cloonan, 1995; Wertz, 1995). Perhaps most influential was Giorgi's (1975, 2009; Giorgi & Giorgi, 2003) description of procedures for collecting concrete, lifeworld examples of psychological phenomena and for analyzing their processes, meanings, and structures. Giorgi (1985, 2009) delineated the various phases of phenomenological psychological research, including the formulation of the topic and research problem, the constitution of research situations, the various sources of description, the steps of analysis, and the formulation of results.

General Analytic Procedures

Giorgi made the procedures of phenomenological psychological analysis explicit, systematic, and accountable, in contrast to the informal way phenomenological research in psychology had been done by the earlier pioneers in philosophy, psychiatry, and other disciplines. Giorgi (1975, 1985, 2009) delineated four essential steps of protocol analysis: (1) reading for a sense of the whole; (2) differentiating the description into meaning units; (3) reflecting on the psychological significance of each meaning unit; and (4) clarifying the psychological structure(s) of the phenomenon. In the first step of *open reading*, the researcher follows the expressions of the participant without any agenda, aim, or even attention to the research phenomenon. This holistic reading is similar to what Freud called "evenly hovering attention" in that it involves no judgment, no selectivity, and an openness to all details that provides a background for the next steps. In the second step, discriminating *meaning units*, the researcher differentiates segments of the description that are relevant to the research interests and whose size and content lend themselves to fruitful analytic reflection that answers the research question. There is no standard size, and meaning units can range from a sentence to a much longer expression. One determines units with psychological sensitivity to meaning that is relevant to the research and according to the researcher's sensibilities. There is no single correct performance of this step, and in the next step of reflection, a researcher may find it necessary to further differentiate or combine the meaning units established in this second step in order to facilitate fruitful analysis. The third step, *psychological reflection*, is the most difficult one. In this step, the researcher attends to what the expressions in each unit reveal about the psychological processes under investigation. If the research involves multiple questions, they are all systematically posed to each meaning unit in turn, and the researcher answers those questions in light of the meaning unit. The researcher explicates what each meaning unit reveals about individual examples of the phenomenon with the help of free imaginative variation and begins to develop general knowledge. The fourth step, *structural understanding and description*, involves the integration and statement of insights that were gained in all the various reflections on meaning units. This final step entails an articulation of the meaningful organization of the investigated psychological phenomena as a structural whole.

The following attitudinal constituents and active operative procedures have been identified in the practice of phenomenological reflection (Wertz, 1983a, 1985):

Constituents of Basic Attitude

1. Empathic immersion in the situations described;
2. Slowing down and dwelling in each moment of the experience;
3. Magnification and amplification of the situations as experienced;
4. Suspension of belief and employment of intense interest in experiential detail;
5. Turning from objects to their personal and relational significance.

Procedures of Reflection on Individual Examples of the Subject Matter

1. Identification of the "existential baseline" or temporal background of the experience;
2. Reflecting on the relevance of each moment of the experience, what is revealed about the phenomenon;
3. Explicating implicit meanings that are not thematically clear;
4. Distinguishing the various constituents that make up the entire experience;
5. Understanding the relations among constituents and their roles or contributions to the whole experience;
6. Thematizing recurrent modes of experience, meanings, and motifs;
7. Interrogating opacity—extending and acknowledging the limits of comprehension;

8. Imaginatively varying constituents in order to identify their mutual implications and essential, invariant structures;

9. Formulating descriptive language for psychological knowledge (using everyday parlance, received scientific terms, or philosophical discourse);

10. Verifying, modifying, and reformulating findings after returning to data;

11. Using received concepts as a heuristic to guide descriptive reflection.

Procedures for Achieving General Findings

1. Identifying potentially general insights in individual structures;

2. Comparing individual examples of the experience for general, even if implicit, invariant characteristics;

3. Imaginative variation of individual examples to identify generally invariant features and organizations;

4. Explicit description of general psychological structure(s).

The general procedures formalized by Giorgi had already been used, though not made explicit, in phenomenological psychological research as well as in such research traditions as existential psychiatry and psychoanalysis. I have argued that these basic practices formally articulated by Giorgi are essential to all descriptive psychological analyses (Wertz, 1983b, 1987a). The researcher collects naïve descriptions in ordinary language from participants who have lived through situations relevant to the topic under investigation. The researcher then reflects on the persons' experiences of situations, explicating lived meanings, including each person's embodied selfhood, emotionality, agency, social relations, language, and temporality as evident in examples of the subject matter under investigation. When conducted methodically, this approach is characterized by meticulous and thorough description that achieves fidelity to psychological life by clarifying its processes, meanings, and general (eidetic) structures.

Phenomenology has offered resources for the development of various methods for researching psychological life. During the last 20 years, several research methods drawing on phenomenology have emerged, including those of Halling and Leifer (1991), van Manen (1990), Moustakas (1994), and Smith (1996). Each draws selectively on the phenomenological tradition. For instance, interpretive phenomenological analysis draws on phenomenology along with such related traditions as hermeneutics and idiography (Smith, Flowers, & Larkin, 2009). Although space does not permit a comparison of these methods in this chapter, readers are encouraged to compare the emphases and procedures of these methods, which continue to evolve with further applications.

Applications and Exemplary Studies

Phenomenological psychological researchers have studied topics in many areas of psychology. Some good illustrations of phenomenological psychological research using the analytic procedures featured in this volume include Aanstoos (1984) on thinking; Bremer, Dahlberg, and Sandman (2007) on the experience of a significant other's cardiac arrest; Churchill (2006) on clinical impression formation; Dahlberg (2007) on loneliness; Davidson, Stayner, Lambert, Smith, and Sledge (1997) on recovery among people with schizophrenia; Fischer (1978, & 1985) on anxiety and self-deception; Mruk (2006) on self-esteem; and Wertz (1983a, 1985, 1987b, 1997) on perception, criminal victimization, abnormality, and consumer behavior. Halling and Leifer (1991) have developed a "dialogal" method of research that is nicely exemplified in a study of forgiveness by Rowe et al. (1989). Along with the four-volume *Duquesne Studies* series cited in Chapter 3, exemplary studies can be found in edited collections by Pollio, Henley, and Thompson (1997); Valle (1998); Valle and Halling (1989); and Valle and King (1978).

Limits and Critical Evaluation

The phenomenological approach to psychology is at once broad and narrow. Its breadth stems from its applicability to research problems that require understanding and description of the essentials of lived experience. It also has strict limits. Phenomenological psychology is not an appropriate method for investigating physical (environmental, biological, evolutionary) phenomena and processes; for constructing abstract theories and models; for testing causal hypotheses; for estimating empirical magnitude, frequency, and prevalence; or for assessing quantitative relationships among variables. Criticisms of the phenomenological approach by mainstream psychologists assume the importance of these interests and goals. Although phenomenological psychology is capable of informing and complementing neopositivistic research, it is not capable of answering its questions or fulfilling its aims.

The following questions are appropriate in evaluating research projects and reports of phenomenological psychology. Does the research address a significant topic and research problem that require qualitative knowledge of lived experience? Did the data collection provide genuine and adequate access to sufficiently varied lifeworld examples of the phenomena under investigation? Were all relevant data reflected upon with conceptual fidelity to participants' experiential processes and meanings? Do the findings conceptually clarify the essence(s) of the research phenomena, including all constituents and themes in their holistic, structural relationships with each other? Are all knowledge claims supported by and illustrated with concrete evidence? Are the levels and kinds of generality achieved, the contextual limitations of

the study, and the remaining open issues and questions transparently articulated? Do the eidetic descriptions intelligibly illuminate and ring true of
all examples of the research phenomena both in the study's data and in the
literature, in the lifeworld, and in the reader's experience and free imaginative variation? Are the contributions of the phenomenological findings to the
theory and practice literature made explicit?

Personal Appeal

I am personally attracted to phenomenology's refreshing movement from
abstract theories, constructs, experiments, operational definitions, and cal-
culations to concrete descriptions of experiences lived through by persons in
actual life situations. I adore psychological knowledge that brings to light the
meanings of previously unreflective human experience. Good phenomenological knowledge has a genuineness and a fidelity to life that I do not find in
any other approach. My own characteristic attitudes of wonder and precision
in the face of the complexities, multiple dimensions, intricacies, depth, and
ambiguities of human existence draw me to phenomenology. I experience
research as a form of *love* in which I immerse myself in other people's lives. In
analyzing protocols, I am often surprised and as I reflect more carefully, I gain
deeper understanding and feeling of intimacy with human beings. I resonate
with the dark sides of existence, and I am drawn to the precious value and
dignity of real persons. I would characterize my individual reflective style and
analytic contributions as fascinated and meticulous. I am interested in the
tiniest details of experience and enjoy understanding them better by relating
them together in the ever-changing holism of experience. My reflections on
protocols are much longer and more expansive than those of many other phenomenological colleagues, whose conciseness I admire. For me, it is a terrible
challenge to convey my findings in the usual short research report.

I appreciate the many faces of phenomenology, which have allowed me
to move in very different directions. My style of description and the knowledge I have gained through research vary according to the research problem and subject matter. My analysis of the dramatic Teresa texts may be seen
as verging on the poetic. I believe that knowledge of highly implicit meanings requires creative language and that some important aspects of human
experience are best conveyed with evocative prose, which therefore qualifies
as genuine, scientific discourse. I view the accurately poetic description of
human experience as objective. However, I am not a poet; my aim is general
knowledge. I seek systematic, progressive contributions that answer scientifically posed questions about human psychological life. My research projects
have varied according to the research problems and subject matters. The current project contrasts most with my research on perception (Wertz, 1982),
which addressed problems in perceptual theory and quantitative research by

systematically distinguishing the constituents and structures of everyday perceptual processes, enumerating various types of perception, and detailing the relationships between perceptual and nonperceptual processes such as remembering, anticipating, thinking, and so on. In that work, the language, tables, and diagrams used to present my findings were designed to move traditional perceptual theory and research forward. My analysis and findings in this project about trauma and resilience are more dramatic inasmuch as they reflect the life and death struggles of the human being.

Method and Sample Findings of Teresa's Experience of Trauma and Resilience

In approaching Teresa's experience, I used the method developed by Amedeo Giorgi (1975, 1985), as I have elsewhere (Wertz, 1982, 1985, 1987b, 1997). The overall attitude I adopted in this work was first to put aside my knowledge of scientific theories and research on trauma and resilience in order to focus on the concrete example in Teresa's life. I also set aside ("bracketed") concerns about the objective reality of her cancer, her parents, her peers, her body apart from her experience of them, and remained disinclined to explain her experience with reference to her brain, heredity, environment, or any external factors. I focused exclusively, through her description, on the way in which situations were meaningfully experienced by her as she lived through trauma and resilience. This was an "intentional analysis" in that I reflected on her psychological processes with attention to the relational meanings inherent in Teresa's engagement with the world. This attempt at faithful explication was only a beginning; I do not claim that my knowledge is error free; it is open to critique and improvement. The shortcomings of my analysis can be corrected by more rigorously employing the phenomenological method.

Organizing the Data:
An Individual Phenomenal Description—Meaning Units

First, I read the written description and interview several times. Then, in order to prepare a well-organized data set for analysis, I integrated Teresa's written description with the interview material into a first-person, master narrative. With the phenomena of trauma and resilience in view, I organized this narrative in paragraphs, each a meaning unit ranging up to 15 sentences and coherently describing a moment in the temporal unfolding of Teresa's experiences. This narrative, called an individual phenomenal description, contains 55 meaning units and is about 15 single-spaced pages. My aim in constructing the individual phenomenal description was to render Teresa's original experience as readily accessible to reflection on trauma and resilience as possible.

Contexts, such as family and culture, which may at first appear remote from the topic, are included because they may have significant bearing on the psychology of trauma and resilience. The description begins with the temporal background (past) taken from the interview.

Meaning Unit 1. My mom's a worrier by nature. She's always been very timid and skittish. I think that my dad, being such a tyrant, made her very nervous all the time. I remember her getting in trouble all the time for doing things wrong. Like the coffee was too hot or too cold, ridiculous things like that. So I always saw her as this cowering person, despite the fact that she really is a very strong individual, but I saw her throughout my childhood as cowering under the shadow of this overbearing presence of my dad. She's always attributed this attitude to her ethnic background, being Filipino, and being raised in a very dogmatic, Catholic understanding of wifely duties to one's husband, being a good, subservient wife. And that the wife's duty is to the husband first, and to the children second, and she told me that, a lot. So, needless to say, that didn't do good things in terms of my animosity toward my dad, nor did it help things in terms of my religiosity. That's probably my biggest thing with the Catholic Church—the position of women.

Two later examples of meaning units follow. They were drawn from Teresa's initial written description of the situation after her doctor informed her that she had thyroid cancer.

Meaning Unit 16. I froze. I couldn't breathe, couldn't move, couldn't even blink. I felt like I had just been shot. My gut had locked up like I'd been punched in it. My mouth went dry and my fingers, which had been fumbling with a pen, were suddenly cold and numb. Apparently picking up on my shock, the surgeon smiled a little. "We're going to save your life, though. That's what counts. And you know what? The other surgeon working with me is a voice guy. We're going to do everything we can not to be too intrusive." I started to breathe a little, very little, and I felt myself trembling. I tried to say something meaningful, expressive; all that I could manage was, "Man." I was actually pretty good.

Meaning Unit 17. Then, all of me let loose. I was sobbing, but there was no sound; just a torrent of tears and the hiss of crying from my open mouth, pushing through the pressure from the accursed mass. The surgeon hastened to my side, armed with a tissue and a firm, reassuring hand on my shoulder. I heard him speaking softly from beside me as I heaved in my silent wailing. "You're going to beat this. You're young, and you're going to beat this thing. And you'll get your voice back, and you'll be singing at the Met. And I want tickets, so don't forget me."

Psychological Reflection on Meaning Units

The first step of my analysis was to reflect on each of the 55 meaning units in the individual phenomenal description in order to understand what it expresses about Teresa's psychological life. Then I focused more particularly on what it reveals about her trauma and resilient recovery, including the pre-selected themes of social support and spirituality. In such reflections, I aimed to grasp the psychological sense of each meaning unit in context, in relation to the others and to the experience as a whole. I tried to conceptualize what each meaning unit reveals as well as the distinctive role it plays, what it contributes to the overall psychological process through which Teresa lived. Immediately after reading each paragraph/unit of the individual phenomenal description, I wrote my reflections as they occurred, in their original free and spontaneous form, including my questions and uncertainties. These reflections included self-criticism and revision as they proceeded. Some reflections are up to four times longer than the original description, whereas others are relatively brief, depending on the relevance of the unit and the extent to which layers of significance and multiple meanings require explication. The document containing both the individual phenomenal description and my reflections, with the meaning units in italics and the reflections in regular font, is 33 single-spaced pages.

Below is my reflection on Meaning Unit 1, sampled above, involving Teresa's past, her childhood, family, and cultural background. In the first paragraph, I reflected on the meaning of the situation described in general. In the second paragraph, I reflected on its particular relevance for our knowledge of Teresa's trauma and recovery.

> *Reflection on Meaning Unit 1.* As a child in her family, Teresa experienced her father as a tyrant who unfairly diminished the status of and controlled her mother and who put Teresa in the lowest social position. Teresa experienced her mother as an anxious, subservient person with little self-confidence who underestimated, as prescribed by her husband's cultural and religious values that legitimized his empowerment and the females' disempowerment, her own strengths and capabilities. Although it is not possible to trace the development of Teresa's stance toward her parents, she appears to have opposed the oppressive authority of the father (and its legitimization by the church) and her mother's fearful subordination. At least implicitly, Teresa was angry at her father's treatment of her mother, which violated her mother's true reality as a strong person and led her mother to falsely cower beneath his dominance. It is as if, in her experience, "my childhood situation was all wrong: My father's exclusive power is unfair, my mother is not as weak as she often acts, and I oppose these injustices, including my being placed at the bottom of the family order."

These meanings are developmentally significant in the later trauma and resilience, when Teresa is in the process of establishing her own independent order in the world through her career and eventually in her own marriage and family. She is in the process of righting and repairing, creating a relational configuration in which she is empowered and gender roles are fair (equal). Perhaps the threat of her cancer (to herself as an emerging singer) is existentially akin to the disempowerment her father inflicted on her in the family. Both the father and the cancer oppose her singing career. Trauma throws Teresa back into her previous position of powerless suffering, echoing her childhood family trauma at the hands of her father. Recovery involves finding her way up and out of this disempowerment to a strong life of her own. Teresa's adulthood trauma recovery repeats the earlier trauma recovery in her striving to emerge from the unjust interferences of the family during her childhood by becoming a professional singer. Her illness places her back in the dependency of her childhood, subject to her father's cruelty and her mother's overly nervous but physically competent care. The childhood background is the original contingency of Teresa's life, and although she began the process of transcending it, the second contingency of traumatic illness throws her back into her parents' hands and requires a second upsurge of transcendence. Resilience is more than a battle to vanquish thyroid cancer; it involves overcoming the oppressive social structures surrounding Teresa as she attempts to establish an equal position as an empowered and thriving adult successfully choosing her own direction.

We now sample the reflection on Meaning Unit 16, in which Teresa describes her initial response to the physician's news of her cancer.

Reflection on Meaning Unit 16. As she stops breathing, Teresa's life comes to a screeching halt, to a cessation, to a kind of death. She is paralyzed and becomes cold and numb. Her strong sense of movement and transcendence, the high-velocity engagements of her singing, and her more recent practical efforts to remedy her medical problem all cease. She feels assaulted and the basic qualities of life—her moisture, her movement, her sentience—cease. In this death-in-life situation, Teresa experiences the doctor responding to her life cessation with counterassurance in the hopeful anticipation that Teresa will not die: He will save her life. In a dramatic and profound statement, her physician addresses the primary concern about the possibility of her death and the secondary concern about the possible destruction of her voice, by strongly proclaiming his commitment to preserving her life and to protecting her voice. His statement is an appeal to Teresa, inviting and urging her to join with him in this basic life-saving project. He tells her that he will save her life and preserve her voice as much as is possible, assuring her of his technical competence and capacity for success. This is an appeal to Teresa to rise from her paralysis by resuming her previous alliance with rational, practical, and competent medical practice. The doctor appears to Teresa not merely as an expert technician but as one who understands her as a person (a singer) and as a specially skilled carer for the human voice, thereby affirming Teresa's central and highest value as a person, her potential as an opera singer. This is a wonderful, moving, and very powerful reciprocal interchange.

In response to this invocation to live and her helper's assurance that her life and voice will be saved, Teresa begins to live again, to breathe again, first tentatively and trembling in fear. This situation is so primal that Teresa is quite unable to express its meaning by speaking, which she attempts in a micro-heroic effort. The meaning of her utterance, "Man," is difficult to articulate. It would seem to be an expression not only of shock and horror but of great wonder, awe, at her possibly of remaining alive through death, of surviving a nearing-death moment. I am not sure if her expression "I was good" was a retrospective evaluation or is a reflection of what she felt at the time—perhaps both—but this expression of "goodness" is a deep moment of self-esteem, for she has risen from a descent toward death, through an alliance with a person who was a stranger moments before but who offered her an intimate and effective, life-saving relationship. Teresa "was good" in that she was facing the truth (as given in the physician's diagnosis), absorbing its crippling emotional impact, and opening herself fully and unflinchingly to realization of the meaning and possibilities of the situation. To sum up, *traumatic misfortune means her death, and resilience means living through death. Social support involves understanding of the impending death and helping the death-bound person live well again, according to his or her ownmost values and aspirations.*

The following is my reflection on Meaning Unit 17 in the individual phenomenal description. Here Teresa weeps and experiences the comfort of her physician. The second paragraph of this reflection focuses more fully on the special theme of *social support.*

Reflection on Meaning Unit 17. In response to Teresa's expression of overwhelming vulnerability, her physician joins her with a compassionate commitment to her well-being. In weeping, Teresa lets her emotions flow in a global rhythm of life whose meaning is very difficult to articulate in words. I sense a certain duality, for it entails a strong life force, an affirmation of life, and yet a kind of reduction of life to a directionless, pulsing cry. So alone, so individualized, Teresa's is a cry of pain and despair, a cry in the face of death, and yet a cry that also embodies her expressive movement returning to life. This cry also undoubtedly has a social dimension, as a demand, as a *call* to her surgeon. It is an unabashed counterappeal to the person who has committed himself to saving her life. Teresa is trustingly open to him and shares her most basic life impulse and need with him. In dramatic micro-cosm, Teresa's life force, embodied in her expressive cry, pushes diametri-cally against and in opposition to the "accursed mass," the thyroid cancer that threatens her life. This forceful cry is understood and then modulated by the surgeon, who hastens closely to her side. He is beautifully in tune with Teresa's elemental life force, which was at first so trapped inside that it could not even escape from her lips. As its waves flow through her body, her doctor intimately joins her, entering closely alongside her bodily space and providing firm resuscitation. He is "armed" with a tissue, has the strength and wherewithal to remove her tears, her suffering, her agony; and he does so reassuringly. He touches her with his hand, his capability, and she feels his firm, palpable reassurance on her shoulder (helping her "shoulder" the burden of cancer), reassurance conveyed through the very part of him that will remove the accursed mass. His gestural softness is the same tenderness that promises to so gently remove the life-threatening tumor. The physician speaks where Teresa is silent, almost speaking *for* her and yet ahead of her, as an ally who will not only save her vital life but will free her for the fulfillment of her highest personal aspirations. In this very expression of commitment to help her achieve success in her opera career, he proclaims his own depen-dency on Teresa to fulfill his desire to share in her personal triumph. This is an encounter of the most life-affirming and personally supportive kind, a profound testimony to and engagement in human interdependency: "I want tickets, so don't forget me."

Thematic Reflection on Social Support. We learn something here about the role of the other in the face of trauma, in resilience. This physician's behav-ior is extraordinarily hospitable to and affirmative of his patient's highly personal situation, to Teresa's expression of emotions that bursts beyond the pragmatic, rational, problem-solving mode in which he and Teresa had previously been comfortable (and which Teresa had learned from and with her mother). Together at this moment, the physician–patient couple open themselves to a much fuller and deeper personal, emotional sharing and aspirational life. I am impressed by the surgeon's ability to shift among dif-ferent modes—from professional truth-saying and responsibility, to techni-cal problem-solving rationality; to personal dialogue; to emotional availabil-ity; to authentic personal expression of his own emotions; to an integration of warmth and practical competence; to clear, expressive, life-affirming and creatively ethical speech; and to a humble recognition of relational (doctor-patient) interdependency—all this synchronous with and responsive to the dynamically flowing need and passionate appeal of Teresa, his patient. Here she experiences *being in good hands*—the antinomy of trauma and the har-binger of recovery.

Summary of Findings:
The Individual Psychological Structure

After reflecting in this manner on each of the 55 meaning units in the 15-page first-person narrative, I attempted an integrative summary of my findings, called an "individual psychological structure." Not all phenomenological psychological researchers carry out this step (Giorgi, 2009). I find this procedure useful in focusing thematically on the psychological topic as it presents itself in an individual example, which has the potential to exhibit all the generally essential features of the phenomenon within its structure. In writing this document, I gave Teresa's experience of trauma and resilience a tentative name, "Toward a Fuller Life in the Face of Death." My aim was to express the knowledge I had gained about her experience of trauma and recovery as a whole, including its various interrelated constituents—temporal and otherwise—in the overall organization. I began this summary with a brief, introductory sketch in order to highlight its overall character and structural unity. This experience was extremely complex and changing; it extended through time and involved a series of dynamic restructurations. I distinguished 11 temporal moments (substructures) of Teresa's resilience in living through trauma. This single-spaced 16-page structural description is temporally organized, takes a narrative form, and explicates the substructures under each of the following 11 subheadings:

1. Childhood/Distal Background: Emerging from Family Trauma
2. Youth/Proximal Background: Singing as Initial Resilience
3. Dawning Young Adult Trauma: Discovery of an Unknown Illness
4. Actualization of the Trauma: Being Destroyed by Threatening Cancer
5. Initial Response to Misfortune: Averting Death with a Supportive Ally
6. Facing Trauma Isolated and Alone: Cognitive, Practical, and Social Intentionalities
7. Bodily Submission and Collapse as a Condition of Regeneration: Being in Surgery
8. Bodily Suffering, Constriction, and Beginning Recovery: Bedridden Hospital Life
9. Failure, Loss, and Relinquishing of Former Life: A Pariah Unable to Sing in Conservatory
10. Reorientation in the Face of Death: Discovering New Possibilities by Broadening Self–World Relations
11. Sustaining Life, Meeting Ongoing Challenges, and Developing a New, Wider Selfhood: Integrating Antinomies in the Face of Continuing Misfortune

Space does not permit the inclusion of the entire individual psychological structure here. However, I present several excerpts in order to illustrate this research step and form of knowledge. The introductory section, comprised of two paragraphs, offers a schematic overview of Teresa's experience that is elaborated in the sections that follow.

Structural Overview. Teresa's traumatic illness has the meaning of a destruction of possibilities so central to her ambitious personal life trajectory that it entails an existential death. Her vigorous (yet narrowly focused) academic involvements, social relations, and highest hopes for her singing career *collapse*. After undergoing a period of immobilization, recognition, horror, and mourning for a lost life and world, Teresa's acceptance of this "death" enables her to rise from the ashes of her former existence. In the face of continuing trauma (recurrence and spread of cancer) with its meaning of the possible end of her life, Teresa actualizes diverse new possibilities that rebuild and broaden her world. In this process a wider, more variegated self and world are realized, habituated, and inhabited. As traumatic illness continues to challenge her, Teresa strives to integrate initiatives of practical self-care with an expansive quest for a fuller, more complete life in the face of death. Teresa struggles for unity within several profound, paradoxical antinomies: emotional surrender and practical action; dependency on others and individual agency; vulnerability and power; fate and responsibility; and discontinuity and continuity in life.

The structure or essence of Teresa's living though her misfortune involves and exceeds her coming of age. Teresa's living through the experience of trauma is a life historical event that shows how the traumatic event, a serious life-threatening and career-ending cancer, disrupts the continuity of her upward trajectory from childhood into adulthood at a crucial point of transition. In this rise, Teresa is initially involved in making a life of her own by cultivating her greatest natural gift and value—her voice—by becoming a singing star in the opera world. Cancer strikes to the very heart of her being—her throat—and annihilates her developmental trajectory, engendering a near total collapse of her self and world. Confronted with the end of her singing and possibly of her life itself, Teresa, with the help of doctors, her mother, and later her fiancé/husband, rises from being undermined and seizes life with a vengeance. Against all odds she appropriates a widening breadth of personal possibilities. Teresa discovers new potentials—talents, friendships, recreation, scholarship, and love—in an expanding world that includes new forms of work, pleasure, and social relations. Teresa's new life is no longer based, as before, on a divine but narrow given—her voice, from which she had built the initial transcendence of suffering in her traumatic childhood and youth. Her present adult-bound resilience—her posttraumatic transcendence of cancer—is of her *own making*, a free and urgent striving for a broader and deliberately complete life in the face of the continuing possibility of her nonbeing. Teresa's resilience is spiritually animated: An intensely faith-based (grateful, charitable, and forgiving, though cognitively agnostic) embrace of a widening range of life prospects in the face of threats and suffering, including the continuing illness. The outcome of her resilient living through trauma is an expansive process of becoming a more complete person in the wider world. In this process, Teresa aims and begins to integrate and unite effective practical–rational action with emotional vulnerability and depth, to combine singing and an array of other activities, to own her suffering in passionate expression, and also to strive toward joy. In love and celebration of life, Teresa undertakes diverse and far-ranging projects aiming to make her special mark on the world in the continuing presence of the possibility of death.

Within each of the 11 sections describing the individual psychological structure, one temporal moment (substructure) of the experience is elaborated in detail. In order to illustrate this detail, below is one small sample, one paragraph from the larger, last (11th) substructure of the experience, "Sustaining Life, Meeting Ongoing Challenges, and Developing a New, Wider Selfhood: Integrating Antinomies in the Face of Continuing Misfortune." This section offers psychological knowledge of Teresa's extraordinary adventure into a wider life, which includes such activities as studying new subject fields, forming new friendships, traveling across the country, mountain climbing, and becoming engaged and married. Based on multiple examples with significant variations in Teresa's life, the psychological structure already begins to clarify essential (general) qualitative knowledge, though the extent of generality is not fully explicated and requires further comparative analyses. This section elaborates several psychological paradoxes within Teresa's life with which she struggled in her unique set of activities. The fulsome integration of these antinomies remained in the realm of possibility for her. The sample paragraph below (the 4th and final one in this subsection) focuses on her marital relationship.

> One of the facets of Teresa's struggle with trauma is her effort, as a spouse, to function competently as her husband's equal and also to receive his care as a vulnerable and dependent partner. This involves significant development in Teresa's marital relationship. She moves from initially battling cancer through solitary self-care (not wanting to burden her new husband with a sickly wife) toward sharing her illness and receiving the care from her husband. This transformation appears to begin in the context of the married couple's encounter with her mother-in-law's illness, suffering, and death. Although up until this point, Teresa's husband has been relatively indifferent to Teresa's suffering and struggle, she successfully communicates (similarly

to her cry in the physician's office) its meaning—the possibility of her own death as the same fate that befell his mother. Teresa's sharing of her husband's personal tragedy appears to be a turning point in the married couple's relational way of coping together with Teresa's suffering, and it potentiates a structural transformation in the marital relationship. Perhaps based on the increasing success of her own efforts to integrate logical practicality and emotional vulnerability, Teresa engages with her mother-in-law's condition and shares this experience in a poem with her mother-in-law and her husband. In poignantly bringing home the meanings of the loss of a loved one's life to her husband, Teresa experiences him as shifting his stance toward greater emotional openness and responsiveness to her by increasingly acknowledging her sickness, collapse, and potential death. Teresa begins to experience her husband as sharing the possibility of her death and of responding to her suffering with more dependable care, without her giving up their important mutual commitment to equal power and worth in the relationship. Teresa begins to expressively integrate "heavy" emotions, such as helpless need and passionate dependency, in her marital relationship, which begins to contrast significantly with past relationships. Teresa experiences her husband as understanding her more fully and deeply, including her horror of potential demise that even she is often inclined to deny and avert through her isolated, practical–rational mode of coping. Over a process of 6 years, Teresa and her husband become more able to see her as both strong and weak/sick, and to share a wider range of emotions, including pain, fear, and anger.

Individual Thematic Findings

Because a number of interesting themes emerged along with the two that were planned (i.e., social support and spirituality), I developed additional summaries of them within the structure. To report these findings, I collected the meaning unit reflections that addressed each of five themes and summarized each set sequentially in a document of seven single-spaced pages.

1. The Meanings of Trauma
2. The Varieties of Social Support
3. Practical Intentionalities of Resilience and Transcendence
4. Paradoxes: Life and Death, Reception and Creation, Dependency and Self-Sufficiency
5. The Role of Spirituality in Trauma and Recovery

In order to illustrate these thematic findings, I offer below a sample paragraph in which I summarize one of the various forms of Teresa's resilience, the practical–rational coping mode:

In it immediate aftermath, the meaning of the traumatic situation has two protentions (implicit anticipations of the future) for Teresa: emotional collapse and logical practicality. The emotions spontaneously arising in the course of traumatic experience are uncanny ones, that is, ones negating possibilities for action—anxiety, terror, and horror. Passively suffered, these emotions present doom, involve extreme vulnerability, and signify a hastening of Teresa's demise. Founded on these emotions and their presentation of imminent collapse, Teresa engages a practical intention to avert worsening sickness and the collapse (ultimately death) of life-furthering pursuits. Teresa experiences uncanny, frightening situations as a series of problems to be rationally assessed and solved by planned effective action that ensures her life. She throws herself into "logical overdrive" and strives to practically master the threats to her health. For Teresa, if she does not engage in effective action, she will become "an emotional wreck." Coping with overwhelming emotions by rational coping is a shared, general style rooted in her past that she continues to live. Teresa has observed both emotional collapse and effective rational coping on the part of her mother, and she retains these meanings of her current traumatic situation. Teresa's mother continues to be both emotionally threatening and practically resourceful to her. Once again, Teresa enlists her mother as an ally and capably engages with her mother in preventing and limiting her emotional panic in the face of health threats. By steeling herself emotionally and engaging in the well-learned rational, problem-solving habitual orientation, Teresa protects and soothes both herself and her mother, with whom she pairs and also acts independently. Teresa learns everything she can about cancer and its treatment; she seeks consultation with experts who can best help her survive and recover from her illness; and she engages in treatment situations and self-care practices that will best facilitate her recovery. The variation of this dynamic in surgery and recovery are telling. In these, Teresa surrenders and inhabits the position of collapse while others (her doctors and mother), assuming the position of executive problem solver, keep terror at bay and engender emotional calm and well-being if not enjoyment (of father's gifts). One may wonder if there already is, within Teresa's surrender and independent practical coping, another underlying functional emotionality—some kind of hope or faith: a life-affirmative emotion in the face of possible demise.

In order to demonstrate how phenomenological research can attempt to address subtle and elusive dimensions of experience, I take a final sample of individual findings from theme 5, the section that addresses the class-assigned theme of *spirituality*. This sample contains the most unexpected findings of my analysis and demonstrates that analysis is far from a passive summary of interview material. These reflections are a searching, tentative excursion into implicit meanings relating to a theme identified as important for research. This exploration probes the role of "spirituality" by drawing together all the relevant reflections on meaning units and risking conclusions that remain provisional without more descriptive data.

> The role of religion and spirituality in Teresa's experience of trauma and recovery is complex, difficult to understand, and challenges analysis. Although Teresa has not participated in religion as a formally committed participant and has difficulty conceiving of God with a certainty of belief (she considers herself an agnostic), Teresa identifies herself as a "spiritual" person, and the spiritual dimensions of her experiences can be explored. Although Teresa's spirituality appears to have little cognitive certainty (belief in God) or formal social engagement (church attendance), she embodies such emotional intentionalities as hope, faith, charity, humility, gratitude, redemption, and well-being in the face of the most difficult threats and challenges of her life. She is a seeker who opens herself to texts and situations that access the *sacred*.
>
> This mode of resilience, like all the others, is rooted in and continues her childhood and past, prior to her current calamity. Teresa states that her singing, done in many different churches, *was her "religion"* before she became sick. However, Teresa's "spirituality" is evidently not limited to her voice, for in the current situation when Teresa looses her voice, she continues other spiritual modes of experience in the course of suffering and in coming to terms with the tragic possibility if her death. Hope and faith are involved as Teresa eventually accepts the loss of her voice, sees the narrow limits of her peer relationships, and seeks greater fulfillment beyond what is immediately actual and visible. Teresa embodies a life force, an affirmative emotional well-being that sustains her through trauma, one that is not dependent on other people or anything particular in the world. She understands others generously and accepts many even in their fallible destructiveness. This presence may even be at the very core of Teresa's way of living through trauma.
>
> Teresa's spirituality may be grasped in various moments of her experience. The typical structure of these involves a widening intentionality, beginning with an acceptance, by virtue of faith, of inimicality that in some cases is also experienced as a bountiful gift. For instance, Teresa experiences the cancer itself as possessing a numinous quality of something other-worldly. Although threatening, destructive, and diminishing, cancer is also, less obviously, *a divine gift*. This cancer, an Other animated in a life of its own—a particularly "angry" (almost supernaturally so) form of cancer—becomes both foe and eventually also friend from an unseen world. As Teresa gets to know the cancer, it continues to present itself as unobjectifiable, as unknowable, as mysterious—much as "God" does for her—and she develops a certain

respect for its awesome wrathfulness. In a strange and paradoxical way, she accepts this cancer without being able to know or control it with certainty, and she appropriates this form of life "with a vengeance."

Teresa's spirituality has roots in her childhood, as do all her habitual ways of coping with trauma. Feeling disadvantaged in her family and teased as a "fat kid" in school, Teresa's voice became her consolation and means of ascendance, salvation, transcendence, and fulfillment: Her voice was her "religion," as she puts it. Her voice embodied a spiritual intentionality that could overcome the worldly adversity, abandonment, and forlornness of her childhood. Teresa's spiritual center was her voice. Through singing, Teresa became connected with a loving universe. She was graced with a gift, a means of salvation in the face of problems, of transcendence of the slings and arrows of worldly misfortune.

As a young adult, Teresa searched for consolation in religion, and her intellectual exploration gave rise to some insights, but with the loss of her singing voice, she lost her central connection with this source of well-being that had been more powerful than life's threats. This loss of her voice was therefore a loss of hope, of self—a loss of bountiful life itself. When Teresa loses her voice, she becomes spiritually lost, undergoes a spiritual crisis, perhaps even a spiritual death, in that her ultimate source of being and value is lost. One consequence of trauma is this crisis of faith. It is therefore understandable that Teresa emphasizes so pointedly the *absence* of God from her experience and reaffirms her agnosticism. However, her very "lostness" is a founding condition of faith and consequently a place where it may be reborn. In living through the traumatic loss of voice, Teresa experiences the possibility of a good life beyond her singing voice, and she is able to find consolation there. Teresa learns that her voice, a worldly gift, is not sufficient to animate her life in its completeness, not sufficient to protect her from the great horrors of the living and dying. In this way the loss of her voice—and with it the loss of her limited faith, based as it was on her voice—becomes the occasion for the emergence of a greater consolation, a deeper faith that embraces the world much more completely. Eventually she will experience the recovery of her voice itself as a gift regiven in time, in a widened world.

A spiritual experience of her cancer is involved in her equanimity toward the physicians who misdiagnosed her. Partly in view of the utter strangeness of this disease, which continues to manifest that original sense of the awesome, Teresa forgives them. In understanding them and accepting their fallibility, she adopts a kind of ultimate, beyond-this-world perspective, a compassionate (one could think, *divine*) grasp of life, even as endangered, fragile, and ugly, as also being mysterious and not lending itself to judgment or control. Teresa similarly forgives many partly deficient people in her life—her mother, her physicians (except for the flippant, arrogant, "favorite of superstars" whose minimal effort led to the spread of her cancer), her schoolmates, her teachers, and even her father. As a habitual way of being with others, Teresa puts herself in their shoes and embraces them with compassion, an attitude of respectful acceptance—love. This attitude is ego transcendent, in sharp contrast to her rational–instrumental modes of relating to others by means of what they have done or can do for her, which, through much of her traumatic experience, is *nothing*. This spirituality is an important part of how she gets along with others harmoniously and also how she transcends their impotence, indifference, and lack of support. Teresa's acceptance of others' failings is a crucial foundation for cultivating her own agency in the face of trauma while remaining engaged and connected with others.

Reemerging from the encounter with her own possible demise, Teresa's spirituality is also connected with thankfulness for being gifted with life. She mentions this thankfulness for being alive as a part of her postsurgery experience. Her gratefulness is not always complete or overflowing, and it vacillates with anger, forlornness, and bitterness. Despair is a precondition of her gratefulness for life, just as the destructive aspects of cancer and other people are the precondition for their acceptance and experienced value. That Teresa's thankfulness is not continual and can be shaken, even broken, does not invalidate our recognition that it concerns not merely a part but her life itself as a whole. Her gratefulness tends toward an all-embracing capacity and has an ultimate, transcendent quality that comes into even clearer relief when we see its discontinuity, its fragility, its relationship with what it is not.

Teresa's spirituality seems essentially to arise out of her sense of abandonment—the opposite of being gifted with life—of life being taken from her, with her being bound to become nothing. Teresa reads ultimate meaning through her life situation. As her life is increasingly enveloped in the threat of cancer, she rises in opposition. In living her very forsakenness in all its uncertainty, Teresa fights for and works toward affirming the value of living. She embraces her life as a blessing and a gift. Teresa's relationship with *the ultimate* is therefore ambiguous and embodies both its negation and affirmation. When initially struck by cancer, she is thankful to be alive at all. When she begins to feel betrayed, compromised, faulty, she battles to win a life redeemed. No doubt her anxious presence in the face of uncertainty and ongoing threat is at times bereft of grace. Yet recurrently, even after others have failed her, Teresa embraces her interdependency on them with hope.

Teresa's relationship to God parallels her relationship to her voice and to the redeeming world her voice opens up for her. Teresa feels more *abandoned by* than *angry at* God in this fateful loss, hence the very absence of God as a believable presence throughout her experience. If Teresa experiences God at all, she does so in the mode of God's abandonment, as a dynamic absence. She does not experience a personal God who is credibly there for her. With belief in God in suspense, Teresa remains open to being moved by or bring recalled by God's presence. Her search through various texts and traditions is open to a potential, prethematic presence of God, whose actuality is not yet proximate, not yet revealed in her life. Nevertheless what Teresa calls *spirituality* appears to be taking place below the level of any belief in a personal deity, and it pervades her life. This spirituality is about how and how much she lives and loves in the face of the bitterness and the possible negation of her existence. What she calls *spirituality* may be the deepest affirmative force in Teresa's life itself. As a transcendence toward completion, it is embodied in her struggle with cancer, her generosity toward those who fail her, her fencing, her rock climbing, her new studies, her marriage, and eventually her return to singing. But this secret, mysterious process is not manifest in a conception of God. It therefore makes sense that Teresa feels faithful even though she is not sure of the existence of God, that she imagines a final day of judgment when God understands and accepts her, even including her very lack of belief. Within her lived experience, deep in its implicit core of intentionality, Teresa is persistently in tune with divinity even though God is only imagined in a hypothetical, final dialogue. Perhaps we would not be going too far to say that there is a divine presence in Teresa's psychological life, at the very core meaning of her trauma and recovery.

Toward a General Psychology of Trauma and Resilience

Methods of General Analysis

Although a central focus of this chapter is the analysis of Teresa's individual experiences, phenomenological research aims at general knowledge through such individual examples. By "eidetic seeing," one identifies what makes each an example, that is, its concrete qualities that are also involved in other, many, even all examples. Such analyses are enhanced by the procedure of free imaginative variation of individual features with attention to those that are invariant. Teresa's experiences, which are already variable, may be imaginatively modified further, creating a virtually limitless series in which can be seen "what trauma is" and "what resilience is" in general. Examples from other people's lives, from the researcher's personal experience, from the scientific literature, and from creative works can also be collected, imaginatively varied, and studied to further explicate general processes, meanings, and structures of the phenomena. I cannot offer definitive general findings about the topics of trauma and resilience because my analyses in this demonstration are incomplete. I describe and sample some methical procedures that I used in order to move toward more general knowledge.

The first attempt at general knowledge involves work with a single example of the phenomenon. Teresa's experience as a whole can be taken as one instance of the general phenomenon of "resilient recovery from trauma." In principle, the general features of this kind of experience can be identified *in this example*. However, all features universally present in examples of this kind of experience are not necessarily clear to us in this example alone, because our access to Teresa's experience is limited by her description, by the interview context, and by the researcher's powers of comprehension. However, even with these limitations and especially with the aid of free imaginative variation, many general characteristics of this kind of experience can be identified in this one example. A sense of "what trauma and resilience are" was already present in my above reflections on, and structural description of, Teresa's experience.

It is important to understand that although Teresa is a single person with thyroid cancer, she describes dozens of individual experiences of trauma and resilience in her life, which offer numerous rich and varied examples of the phenomena under investigation. For instance, she experienced trauma when she was initially diagnosed, when she saw her mother react to the news of her cancer, when in the hospital bed after surgery, when unable to sing in her voice lesson, and as a "pariah" in the conservatory. She experienced resilience when cared for by her mother, when planning effective cancer treatments, when changing her major, when mountain climbing, and in her marriage. What might be viewed as a single case literally provided many, and with imaginative variations, literally hundreds of examples of the research phenomena. My comparative analysis of these examples, accessible through Teresa's thick description, already entailed extensive eidetic clarifications of psychological processes, meanings, and structures.

As a first explicitly generalizing procedure, I read through the individual psychological structure of Teresa's experience in order to clarify the general insights already gained. I enhanced my "seeing of essences" during this procedure with continuing imaginative variation of the individual structures and constituents in order to identify those psychological processes and meanings that are invariantly present in various general types and even all possible examples of trauma and resilience. I was able to tentatively identify and describe 40 potentially general insights, though in some cases my uncertainty and questions called for further investigation.

Second, as phenomenological researchers typically do, I turned to an additional example of the phenomenon through another person's written description. Researchers usually use *at least three* different sources of empirical examples and sometimes many more (Giorgi, 2009), along with others from personal experience and observations as well as from many literatures— scientific, personal, and creative—that describe lifeworld examples of the topic under investigation. All these actual and imaginative variations form the complete data set on which the general claims of phenomenological research are based. For this demonstration, I utilized the second protocol collected from the same class. The participant, Gail, described her experience as a competitive collegiate gymnast who suffered a dislocated and broken arm in a fall from the uneven bars during a practice (in the Appendix). Usually numerous protocols are freshly and comprehensively analyzed in their own right before an explicitly general analysis is conducted. In the present study, I used a novel procedure in order to more briefly address the issue of generality. First, I empathically read, became familiar with, and began to reflect on the psychological processes and meanings of Gail's injury and recovery (an informal analysis). Then, I read through Gail's protocol and, on the list of 40 possibly general insights drawn from the preliminary eidetic analysis of Teresa's experience, I made note of (1) moments of Gail's experience that exemplified the generalities based on the Teresa analysis; (2) constituents of Gail's experience that offered evidence of processes and meanings not previously identified but implicit in Teresa's experiences; and (3) aspects of Teresa's and Gail's experiences that are *different* and are therefore either idiosyncratic or typical, that is, present in multiple but not all individual examples of the phenomenon and therefore are not general at the highest level. One of the most challenging aspects of all psychological research is to determine the most fruitful level of generality of knowledge, ranging from the highest levels through common types, rare types, and relatively individual instances. To my surprise, all 40 tentatively postulated general insights gleaned from Teresa's example were found in Gail's example. Gail's example also contained 4 new constituents that had not previously been grasped in Teresa's example but were evident in it once clarified in Gail's example. Finally, many differences between Gail's and Teresa's examples were found that suggest various levels and kinds of generality and idiosyncrasy.

General Features in Teresa's Example

Teresa's lived experience can be viewed as an example of *what trauma most generally is.* Although in her example, thyroid cancer ended her emerging career as an opera singer and threatened her life, these particular details of her experience are obviously not present in every example of trauma. For instance, with regard to the traumatic event, *that which is traumatic*—thyroid cancer—could instead be liver cancer, another disease such as AIDS, or a car accident, a military attack, torture by terrorists, a ravaging hurricane, criminal victimization, stigmatic verbal abuse, the death of a loved one, food deprivation, and so on and on, in an infinite series of potentially traumatic events. We see more than one example of trauma even in Teresa's experience, for she was traumatized by her father's disempowering criticisms and by the other children who called her "fat." Trauma can be either physical or social. What makes these events *traumatic*?

As a psychological phenomenon, trauma resides in the *meaning* of these events, particularly in their *personal inimicality*, their destructiveness, their undermining of a *person's life*. In considering "that which is traumatized" (regarding the person), we may imaginatively vary Teresa's experience and see that trauma need not invariantly involve the destruction of a person's voice and could involve the destruction of sight, movement, trust, self-esteem, a significant other, or virtually any aspect of personal intentionality. In order to exemplify "trauma," these events must strike at and destroy a person's potential for centrally meaningful engagement in life situations. Trauma, as a psychological phenomenon, essentially involves destruction, or threatened destruction, of a meaningful world relation. On the world side of the traumatic relation, examples include an infinite series such as those listed above and so many others. However, in themselves, without destruction in a person's meaningful relational life, these events are not traumatic. Equally essential to trauma is "that which is suffered" through the trauma—the undermining of world relatedness. Trauma is the annihilation of intentional relations with the world, one's very personhood. The loss of intentional world relations covers a widely varied series of personally lived experiences involving, for example, not being able to go on fighting in a war; no longer inhabiting one's home, which was destroyed in the hurricane; not being able to be with a lost loved one; not being able to work after losing a limb in a car accident; being bankrupted by the stock market crash; starving; and so on. Invariant in these instances of "being traumatized" is that the very basis of one's psychological life—what one lives from, what one depends on—whether one's own body, one's motility, one's necessary supportive others, one's possessions, one's sustenance—is negated, removed, or destroyed. In short, trauma is the negation of human intentionality suffered through an event whose meaning annihilates central and significant world relations. The resilient living through of trauma in all these variations is evidently quite complex and involves bodily, social, and temporal horizons that can also be analyzed in their most general essence and in less general, typical forms. All involve the reactivation of intentionality, the restoration of world relations, which can take many individual and typical forms.

Space does not allow an account of the imaginative variations of all features of Teresa's experience or of all 40 constituents that I eidetically found to be highly invariant. Below I present part of my eidetic work pad, a list of brief, informal summary statements of 26 constituents present in many, if not all, instances of the trauma experience and therefore possibly essential at a high level of generality. As *constituents*, these are overlapping and interrelated moments of the unitary structure of this experience, not independent elements. However, a general structure of trauma and resilience has not been completed in this project. What follows is some of the analytic work that is beginning to move in that direction.

1. Initially, trauma is passively suffered. It happens to a person, was not intended, and therefore is experienced in cognitive shock and disbelief, through uncanny emotions such as terror, horror, dread, and anguish, in which a previously active agent becomes an acute sufferer.

2. The traumatic event is negative—inimical, destructive, reductive—and thereby inactivates and nullifies a core, centrally meaningful intentionality in the person's psychological life.

3. The traumatic is an Other, something alien and antithetical, fundamentally opposed to Self.

4. That which is destroyed or reduced is not only a person's actual existence, way of life, but his or her *possibilities* for world relatedness; trauma depotentiates the person.

5. Trauma is lived bodily by way of numbness, paralysis, diminishment, contraction, shrinkage, or withdrawal in relation to the world.

6. In annihilating central intentionalities and world relations, trauma implies the possibility of demise, of death. Even if a person's life is not literally threatened or in jeopardy, trauma involves an *existential* death, a negation of being-in-the-world.

7. The sufferer engages in a battle against trauma in an attempt to resume a relatively free, self-directed life, which is preferred to the traumatically reduced or lost life.

8. One midlevel typical but perhaps not highly general aspect of Teresa's trauma (and many imaginable others) is the *persistence* and even *spread* of trauma, meaning that the traumatic event does not end but continues, possibly expanding through time.

9. The meaning of trauma is not contained in an isolated event but involves the curtailment of the person's historical life movement; trauma undermines the person's ongoing efforts toward goal fulfillment and negates his or her future.

10. The present, actual experience of trauma draws its personal significance in part from a person's history of prior traumatic events, whose meaning is retained and echoed in the current trauma, which is implicitly in part a repetition and continuation.

11. The individual's stance toward trauma and strategies of living through and coping with trauma are also continuations of the habitual ways in which he or she has coped with past adversity, inimicality, or destruction.

12. The person makes a concerted effort to transcend victimhood and reopen the future, sometimes developing new forms of empowerment.

13. The process of recovery changes the person's life.

14. One typical but not always present general way of coping with trauma involves gathering knowledge about the unfamiliar situation and approaching it as a practical problem to be analyzed and to be solved.

15. Trauma is individualizing, isolating, lonely—the traumatized person is singled out and separated from others.

16. Other people are experienced (feared or trusted) as potential harmers or helpers, are scrutinized and evaluated with regard to their tendencies to further traumatize and/or to help the vulnerable, reduced person restore relatively preferred world relations.

17. Stigma and shame (self-devaluation) are intrinsic possibilities inasmuch as trauma involves the diminishment and failure of the person's existence; thus trauma entails the possibility of being devalued, rejected, and abandoned as an individual, with a concomitant loss of social and self-esteem.

18. Sharing trauma with others—disclosing the experience of trauma to other people—is important but risky and demonstrates typical variations ranging from truth telling to protectively concealing and deceiving others regarding the traumatic experience.

19. Trust or fear structure interpersonal relationships, which are typically enhanced or dissolved. Living through trauma saliently reveals relational qualities of others as true friends, enemies, and/or indifferents.

20. Valued qualities of supportive others include bearing witness, truthfulness, sharing, practical assistance, softness, recognition and understanding of personal goals and resources, alliance, care, encouragement, and accompaniment into the future.

21. Weeping is a horizon or possibility of trauma as an expression of its agony and its uncanny emotionality, a mourning of lost actualities and possibilities. Weeping is also an expression of the vitality of life and a call to others for recognition and help.

22. Collapse and surrender are not merely testimonies to diminishment but are necessary moments of resilient recovery, which requires acceptance of destruction and loss.

23. Trauma and recovery have the meanings of death and rebirth.

24. Trauma involves a supernatural meaning in its unfamiliar, uncanny, numinous, and un- or other-worldly qualities.

25. The person's existence as a whole can be experienced as being at stake in trauma, making its horizon far-reaching and vast, virtually ultimate in its meaning. Some attempt to address this extreme scope may be made via

expressions of prayer, humility, thankfulness, receiving grace, healing, and the completion of life.

26. The spiritual dimension of trauma is lived in the acceptance of suffering and fallibility through broadening, life-affirming intentionalities that may be called *faith*.

Broader Comparative Analyses and Levels of Eidetic Generality

Evidence of Actual Generality across Persons

Insights into the essences of psychological phenomena are corrigible and require real-world as well as imaginative evidence. In examining Gail's experience, all 40 of the features identified in the imaginative free variation of Teresa's example were evident. One example follows: *The meaning of trauma is not contained in an isolated event but involves the curtailment of the person's life historical movement; trauma undermines the person's ongoing efforts toward goal fulfillment and negates his or her future.* Teresa's and Gail's examples of trauma involve the interference with biographical progress. Teresa's progress involves her establishing a life independent of her parents as an opera singer. Cancer ends her progress toward becoming an opera singer and nullifies her fulfillment of that future goal. Gail's progress, in contrast, involves improving her athletic performance and successfully contributing to her NCAA Division I team during her junior season. Her injury prevents her from fulfilling this goal. Gail's broken arm immediately means to her that her entire competitive season may be ruined. As she attempts to move her fingers, Gail questions her future; she evaluates whether she will need surgery, which means her season is over. Gail had been recruited with high hopes on the part of coaches, her family, her teammates, and herself. She had been disappointed sitting on the bench during the previous season and was now rising to fulfill shared expectations of success. Injured, she takes a place on the sidelines and again becomes a spectator watching others compete.

In both of these examples, and many others, a person's movement into the future is struck down by the trauma; historical progress is curtailed. For instance, the individual does not reach a travel destination, does not win a war, does not earn a degree, or does not get married. A car accident, brain damage, the failure of comprehensive exams, and the death of a fiancé are further examples of traumatic experiences inasmuch as they undesirably short-circuit the fulfillment of significant life goals. Without this feature, an experience is inconceivable as an example of trauma; therefore, the undesired curtailment of the person's life historical progress is viewed as essential to the structure of this kind of experience. Additional lifeworld examples, such as Gail's, with imaginative variations, provide evidence of generality—eidetic law. If one were to measure this aspect of "trauma," one would find ways to quantify the severity and extent of the destruction of life historical movement into the future.

New General Insight from an Additional Lifeworld Example

One reason that phenomenological research requires more than one real-world example is that additional descriptions unburden, supplement, and guide the researcher's imagination. New, highly general and essential aspects, and even different general structures of the phenomenon, may be found in other lifeworld examples. Four constituents found in the analysis of Gail's example had not been grasped in the analysis of Teresa's experiences. For instance, Gail described the experience of *physical pain* and also *the vacillation between hope and despair* in her recovery process. Both appear to be at least somewhat general constituents of trauma, and it is likely that Teresa experienced both, even though she did not explicitly or extensively describe them. A follow-up interview with Teresa would help investigate. Physical pain may be essential to the structure of some general types of trauma, but not all—for instance, types involving social neglect, abuse, or oppression. One of the most striking individual features of Gail's trauma in my analysis was her *fall*. As she literally fell from the parallel bars, she symbolically fell from the pinnacle of her gymnastic competitiveness, and she figuratively fell from the great social esteem to which she was aspiring. One might wonder if a *fall*, despite the relative uniqueness of Gail's experience, is essential to all examples of trauma. In Gail's example, the *vertical* dimension of high and low came to light in a meaningful way. Gail said that she was in the best shape of her life and attempting the greatest and most challenging tricks of her gymnastic career before she fell. Gail said that she "cried because I was really *down*"—another reference to the lowliness of the traumatized. Although not explicitly revealed as a theme in the case of Teresa, a vertical descent may be seen in the lives of both participants, for trauma *dethroned* both from positions of relative height.

The general meaning of *trauma as fall*, with its metaphors of high to low and rising back up, seem to take place in both instances and to be quite general. Further imaginative variation informs us that people can suffer trauma when they are not at the *greatest* height of their game/career trajectory, as these two participants were. However, perhaps *relative height and fall* are very general dimensions of this experience, implicating the upright posture, human dignity, and intentionality itself as an *up*surge of transcendence. Trauma is a "beat down," a "downer" that can "bring one to one's knees" or "drive one to the ground," reversing the distinctively human intentionality of the upright posture, nullifying the freely empowering hands otherwise capable of agency. Gail's example enables us to clearly see this essential dimension of the experience as a theme, thereby illuminating features of Teresa's experience: for instance, the meaning of her lying on the surgical table, being bedridden, and having fallen from the audition circuit, opera stardom, and even God's grace. "Trauma as fall" also leads us to imagine various possibilities of being *downgraded* by others and *lowering* one's head in shame, of rejection, stigma, and loss of esteem in traumatic *downfall*.

Differences between Cases and the Grasp of Typical, Midlevel Generality

The differences between these two lifeworld examples suggest features that are not present in all instances. Imaginative variation shows evidence that some of these are not merely idiosyncratic and may be essential, invariant, among examples of a certain *type*. "Types" are general structures, the essences of which can be clarified in contrast to each other; examples of a type share the same essential structure with each other. Although examples of different types do not share the same typical structures, they do share the essential structure of the most general kind, of which they are *types*. Types are qualitatively distinguished by their processes, meanings, and structures of experience rather than by external objective characteristics of persons or environmental circumstances, though age (infant, child, adolescent, frail elderly), culture, environmental context (illness, natural disaster, racial discrimination), and characteristic behaviors may guide researchers to identify distinctive psychological types, which may be age-bound, culture-bound, etc.

One difference between our two participants' experiences is that for Teresa, the traumatic loss (of her opera career) was final whereas for Gail, the traumatic loss (of a healthy arm) was temporary. Whereas Teresa changed her life profoundly by accepting the loss of her voice and discovering new talents, opportunities, and social relationships in a successful transformative widening of her life, Gail successfully reestablished her previous engagements. Almost as soon as she was injured, Gail's psychological life narrowed in a relentless and successful return to competition. The analysis of additional examples might help clarify in detail two different types of resilient living through traumatic misfortune: expansive life transformation and resolutely focused recommitment. Gail's example shows us that such recommitment does not necessarily involve a return to life as it previously was, for there was a new, special sweetness in Gail's return to competition. Gail experienced her return to competition as "the most significant performance in 13 years," suggesting an enhancement of her enjoyment, courage, strength, and leadership as an athlete. She was voted captain in the season following recovery. Her hard work and motivation "had not just gotten [her] back on the apparatus" but to a place she'd never been before. In making the uneven bars her most successful event, "what had once been my weakness had now become my legacy." Teresa's and Gail's experiences are not only examples of the most general phenomenon of trauma and recovery but commonly involve positive life change.

Continuing our imaginative variation, positive change as occurred in Teresa and Gail is no doubt quite meaningful in many, but not all, instances of misfortune. One can easily imagine a person dying in surgery after a noble struggle with cancer or suffering a life-ending athletic injury without any struggle at all. Perhaps what we have called "types" are more accurately sub-types of the more general type, *growth through trauma*. I remember a partici-pant in another study who was damaged and disabled by a series of natural accidents and medical misfortunes and who became increasingly embittered, lived an increasingly constricted and narrowed life, and seriously contem-plated suicide. There are traumatic experiences that involve a continuing diminishment and death. We know from the psychological literature and clinical experience that posttraumatic stress disorder (PTSD) is a psycho-logical type of trauma experience. Various distinct meanings of trauma and recovery could be phenomenologically clarified in terms of their essential, invariant structures through the comparison of various examples of humans living through trauma. Comparative reflection on other lifeworld examples, supplemented by imaginative variation, would provide eidetic qualitative knowledge at increasing levels of generality, from the highly idiosyncratic, to the rare, to more general subtypes, to highly general types, and finally to the very most general processes, meanings, and structure of the psychology of trauma, which would be manifest in all examples of this phenomenon.

Completing the Research

The completion of research depends on the nature of the problem as well as the nature of the phenomenon. One most important open issue in this research is determining the most fruitful level(s) of generality and form(s) that the general structure(s) would take. To accomplish this requires more specifically determining the purpose of the research, from which a more par-ticular focus and scope on the topic of trauma and resilience would follow. For instance, if a critical review of prior research pointed to a need for the most highly general understanding of trauma and the findings could clarify it, then one highly general structure would be articulated. If, on the contrary, the research set out to compare posttraumatic growth to the development of PTSD, at least two different typical structures might be necessary. Midlevel generality involving several typical structures might also be appropriate for a project comparing practical–rational and psychospiritual ways of coping with trauma. Particular theoretical issues and/or practical interests make demands on, and afford many possible directions for, analysis and the com-pletion of research.

The most significant levels and sorts of generality also depend on the intrinsic reality of the matters under investigation as revealed in lifeworld data through analytic findings. Additional actual data and analytic findings along with the research problem drive decisions concerning the levels and number of general structures developed. This is why in phenomenological psychology, multiple lifeworld examples (at least three, according to Giorgi, 2009) are required. I have sometimes utilized more than 100 protocols (Wertz, 1985, 1987b). Researchers may also draw on their own personal experiences and observations as well as on additional examples of the phenomenon from previous research, media, art, and literature. In this way the researcher delineates with greater certainty and clarity the most important levels of qualitative (eidetic) generality based on examples of the phenomena themselves.

Although all findings are intended to be holistic and moments of the phenomenon are to be understood as interrelated constituents in a structure, research may also thematize certain general issues within the whole, delve into them in greater detail, and gain knowledge of important dimensions of variation. For instance, the current findings suggest that issues for further investigation may include variations in the traumatized person's historically rooted vulnerabilities, developmental position, habitual coping strategies, interpersonal relations, stigmatization by others, modifications of self-esteem, sharing and concealing discourse, subsequent retraumatization, and potential for psychological growth.

Analyses and findings are viewed by phenomenological researchers as corrigible and subject to critique and correction. For phenomenological researchers, the inexhaustible diversity, depth, complexity, and fundamental mysteriousness of lived experience always exceed our knowledge. The findings presented in this demonstration could be changed and improved by revisions in the analysis of Teresa's and Gail's experiences as well as by the collection and further analysis of new data. As scientific, this knowledge is based on evidence and open to critique and improvement. Whether the challenge, revision, and refinement of knowledge are performed by the same researcher or by other researchers, they entail the same procedures delineated above— reflecting on examples and drawing evidence-based conclusions. As research continues, researchers bring their own personal sensitivities, research questions, and powers of reflection to enhance understanding. As in all science, no one project, no one researcher, can claim to provide the final word on a research topic or problem.

The Final Report

Phenomenological psychologists can present research in many different ways. Raw data may be presented in their entirety or in excerpts, though page limits usually preclude the inclusion of the full data set. All methods are described and may be exemplified in order to help readers follow the procedures. Individual, typical, and more highly general structures—as well as extended findings regarding dimensions of variation and themes—may all be presented, depending on the purposes and readership. Expositions may be brief or extensive, and diagrams and tables may be used to elucidate findings. There is no one kind of language used by phenomenological researchers. The form taken by psychological language depends on the nature of the subject matter as well as the researcher's style, purposes, and audiences. All terms are variants of ordinary everyday language, and whether knowledge statements utilize participants' own words, technical terms from philosophy and/or psychology, original poetic writing, or other forms of discourse, findings involve the *description* of the psychology of the experience under investigation with concrete evidence. In virtually all reports, references to concrete data and lifeworld situations, using quotations of participants, are included in order to render psychological insights and psychological terms intelligible with reference to actual examples and to provide readers with intuitive understanding of the findings. The discussion of findings can also take many forms, depending on the purpose of the research. It always features original knowledge of "the things themselves" (*den Sachen selbst*). For instance, new knowledge may be compared and related to previous research, may be used to address theoretical issues, and may inform or guide practice and policy. As in all scientific reports, a critical appraisal of methods, the limits of the research, and fruitful avenues for future inquiry are highlighted. The discussion of findings brings to light the benefit of the present research to science and human life.

References

Aanstoos, C. M. (Ed.). (1984). *Exploring the lived world: Readings in phenomenological psychology.* Carrollton, GA: West Georgia College.

Bachelard, G. (1964a). *Psychoanalysis of fire* (A. C. M. Ross, Trans.). Boston: Beacon Press. (Original work published 1938)

Bachelard, G. (1964b). *The poetics of space* (E. Gilson, Trans.). Boston: Beacon. (Original work published 1958)

Berger, P., & Luckmann, T. (1967). *The social construction of reality: A treatise in the sociology of knowledge.* New York: Random House.

Binswanger, L. (1963). *Being-in-the-world* (J. Needleman, Ed.). New York: Basic Books.

Boss, M. (1963). *Psychoanalysis and daseinsanalysis.* New York: Basic Books.

Bremer, A., Dahlberg, K., & Sandman, L. (2009). Experiencing out-of-hospital cardiac arrest: Significant others' lifeworld perspective. *Qualitative Health Research, 19*(10), 1407–1420.

Churchill, S. (2006). Phenomenological analysis: Impression formation during a clinical assessment interview. In C. T. Fischer (Ed.), *Qualitative research methods for psychologists: Case demonstrations* (pp. 79–110). New York: Academic Press.

162 APPROACHES TO QUALITATIVE DATA ANALYSIS

Cloonan, T. F. (1995). The early history of phenomenolocial psychological research methods in America. *Journal of Phenomenological Psychology, 26*(1), 46–126.

Dahlberg, K. (2007). The enigmatic phenomenon of loneliness. *International Journal of Qualitative Studies on Health and Well-Being, 2*(4), 195–207.

Davidson, L., Stayner, D. A., Lambert, S., Smith, P., & Sledge, W. S. (1997). Phenomenological and participatory research on schizophrenia: Recovering the person in theory and practice. *Journal of Social Issues, 53,* 767–784.

Fischer, W. F. (1978). An empirical–phenomenological investigation of being-anxious: An example of the meanings of being-emotional. In R. S. Valle & M. King (Eds.), *Existential–phenomenological alternatives for psychology* (pp. 166–181). New York: Oxford University Press.

Fischer, W. F. (1985). Self-deception: An existential–phenomenological investigation into its essential meanings. In A. Giorgi (Ed.), *Phenomenology and psychological research* (pp. 118–154). Pittsburgh, PA: Duquesne University Press.

Gadamer, H.-G. (1989). *Truth and method* (2nd ed., J. Weinsheimer & D. G. Marshall, Trans.). New York: Crossroad. (Original work published 1960)

Gendlin, E. (1962). *Experiencing and the creation of meaning.* Chicago: Free Press.

Giorgi, A. (1970). *Psychology as a human science: A phenomenologically based approach.* New York: Harper & Row.

Giorgi, A. (1975). An application of phenomenological method in psychology. In A. Giorgi, C. Fischer, & E. Murray (Eds.), *Duquesne studies in phenomenological psychology* (Vol. 2, pp. 82–103). Pittsburgh, PA: Duquesne University Press.

Giorgi, A. (Ed.). (1985). *Phenomenology and psychological research.* Pittsburgh, PA: Duquesne University Press.

Giorgi, A. (2009). *The descriptive phenomenological method in psychology: A modified Husserlian approach.* Pittsburgh, PA: Duquesne University Press.

Giorgi, A. P., & Giorgi, B. M. (2003). The descriptive phenomenological psychological method. In P. Camic, J. E. Rhodes, & L. Yardley (Eds.), *Qualitative research in psychology* (pp. 242–273). Washington, DC: American Psychological Association.

Gurwitsch, A. (1964). *Field of consciousness.* Pittsburgh, PA: Duquesne University Press.

Halling, S., & Dearborn Nill, J. (1995). A brief history of existential–phenomenological psychiatry and psychotherapy. *Journal of Phenomenological Psychology, 26*(1), 1–45.

Halling, S., & Leifer, M. (1991). The theory and practice of dialogal research. *Journal of Phenomenological Psychology, 22*(1), 1–15.

Heidegger, M. (1962). *Being and time* (J. MacQuarrie & E. Robinson, Trans.). New York: Harper & Row. (Original work published 1927)

Husserl, E. (1954). *The crisis of European sciences and transcendental phenomenology* (D. Carr, Trans.). Evanston, IL: Northwestern University Press. (Original work published 1936)

Husserl, E. (1962). *Ideas: General introduction to pure phenomenology* (W. R. B. Gibson, Trans.). New York: Collier Books. (Original work published 1913)

Husserl, E. (1970). *Logical investigations* (L. Findlay, Trans.). London: Routledge & Kegan Paul. (Originally published in 1900–1901)

Husserl, E. (1977). *Phenomenological psychology: Lectures, summer semester, 1925* (J. Scanlon, Trans.). Boston: Martinus Nijhoff. (Original work published 1925)

Jaspers, K. (1963). *General psychopathology* (J. Hoenig & M. W. Hamilton, Trans.). Chicago: University of Chicago Press. (Original work published 1913)

Laing, R. D. (1962). *The divided self.* New York, NY: Pantheon Books.

Laing, R. D., & Esterson, A. (1963). *Sanity, madness, and the family.* New York: Penguin Books.

Levinas, E. (1969). *Totality and infinity: A study in exteriority* (A. Lingis, Trans.). Pittsburgh, PA: Duquesne University Press. (Original work published 1961)

Marcel, G. (1965). *Being and having: An existentialist diary.* New York: Harper & Row.

May, R., Angel, E., & Ellenberger, H. F. (Eds.). (1958). *Existence: A new dimension in psychiatry and psychology.* New York: Simon & Schuster.

Merleau-Ponty, M. (1962). *Phenomenology of perception* (C. Smith, Trans.). London: Routledge & Kegan Paul. (Original work published 1945)

Merleau-Ponty, M. (1963). *The structure of behavior* (A. Fisher, Trans.). Pittsburgh, PA: Duquesne University Press. (Original work written 1942)

Minkowski, E. (1970). *Lived time* (N. Metzel, Trans.). Evanston, II: Northwestern University Press. (Original work published 1933)

Moustakas, C. (1994). *Phenomenological research methods.* Thousand Oaks, CA: Sage.

Mruk, C. J. (2006). *Self-esteem theory, research, and practice: Toward a positive psychology of self-esteem* (3rd ed.). New York: Psychology Press.

Pollio, H. R., Henley, T. B., & Thompson, C. J. (1997). *The phenomenology of everyday life.* New York: Cambridge University Press.

Ricoeur, P. (1974). *The conflict of interpretations: Essays in hermeneutics* (D. Ihde, Trans.). Evanston, IL: Northwestern University Press.

Ricoeur, P. (1981). *Hermeneutics and the human sciences: Essays on language, action and interpretation* (J. B. Thompson, Ed. & Trans.). Cambridge, UK: Cambridge University Press.

Rowe, J., Halling, S., Davies, E., Leifer, M., Powers, D., & Van Bronkhorst, J. (1989). The psychology of forgiving another: A dialogal research approach. In R. S. Valle & S. Halling (Eds.), *Existential–phenomenological perspectives in psychology* (pp. 233–244). New York: Plenum Press.

Sartre, J.-P. (1948a). *The emotions: Outline for a theory* (B. Frechtman, Trans.). New York: Philosophical Library. (Original work published 1939)

Sartre, J.-P. (1948b). *The psychology of imagination* (B. Frechtman, Trans.). New York: Philosophical Library. (Originally published 1936)

Sartre, J.-P. (1956).*Being and nothingness: An essay on phenomenological ontology* (H. Barnes, Trans.). New York: Philosophical Library. (Original work published 1943)

Scheler, M. (1954). *The nature of sympathy* (P. Heath, Trans.). New Haven, CT: Yale University Press. (Original work published 1913)

Schutz, A. (1967). *The phenomenology of the social world* (G. Walsh & F. Lehnert, Trans.). Evanston, IL: Northwestern University Press. (Original work published 1932)

Schutz, A., & Luckmann, T. (1989). *Structures of the lifeworld.* Evanston, IL: Northwestern University Press. (Original work published 1983)

Smith, J. A. (1996). Beyond the divide between cognition and discourse: Using interpretive phenomenological analysis in health psychology. *Psychology and Health, 11*(2), 261–271.

Smith, J. A., Flowers, P., & Larkin, M. (2009). *Interpretive phenomenological analysis: Theory, method, and practice.* Thousand Oaks, CA: Sage.

Spiegelberg, H. (1972). *Phenomenology in psychology and psychiatry.* Evanston, IL: Northwestern University Press.

Spiegelberg, H. (1982). *The phenomenological movement: A historical introduction* (3rd ed.). Boston: Martinus Nijhoff.

Straus, E. (1966). *Phenomenological psychology: Selected papers* (E. Eng, Trans.). New York: Basic Books.

Valle, R. S. (1998). *Phenomenological inquiry in psychology: Existential and transpersonal dimensions.* New York: Plenum Press.

Valle, R. S., & Halling, S. (Eds.). (1989). *Existential–phenomenological perspectives in psychology: Exploring the breadth of human experience.* New York: Plenum Press.

Valle, R. S., & King, M. (Eds.). (1978). *Existential–phenomenological alternatives for psychology.* New York: Oxford University Press.

van den Berg, J. H. (1972). *A different existence: Principles of a phenomenological psychopathology.* Pittsburgh, PA: Duquesne University Press.

van Manen, M. (1990). *Researching lived experience: Human science for an action sensitive pedagogy.* Albany, NY: State University of New York.

Wertz, F. J. (1982). The findings and value of a descriptive approach to everyday perceptual process. *Journal of Phenomenological Psychology, 13*(2), 169–195.

Wertz, F. J. (1983a). From everyday to psychological description: Analyzing the moments of a qualitative data analysis. *Journal of Phenomenological Psychology, 14*(2), 197–241.

Wertz, F. J. (1983b). Some components of descriptive psychological reflection. *Human Studies, 6*(1), 35–51.

Wertz, F. J. (1985). Methods and findings in an empirical analysis of "being criminally victimized." In A. Giorgi (Ed.), *Phenomenology and psychological research* (pp. 155–216). Pittsburgh, PA: Duquesne University Press.

Wertz, F. J. (1987a). Common methodological fundaments of the analytic procedures in phenomenological and psychoanalytic research. *Psychoanalysis and Contemporary Thought, 9*(4), 563–603.

Wertz, F. J. (1987b). Abnormality from scientific and prescientific perspectives. *Review of Existential Psychology and Psychiatry, 19*(2&3), 205–223.

Wertz, F. J. (1995). The scientific status of psychology. *Humanistic Psychologist, 23*(3), 295–315.

Wertz, F. J. (1997). Toward a phenomenological consumer psychology. *Journal of Phenomenological Psychology, 28*(2), 261–280.

Wertz, F. J. (2005). Phenomenological research methods for counseling psychology. *Journal of Counseling Psychology, 52*(2), 167–177.

Wertz, F. J. (2006). Phenomenological currents in 20th century psychology. In H. Dreyfus & M. A. Wrathall (Eds.), *Companion to existential–phenomenological philosophy* (pp. 392–408). Oxford, UK: Blackwell.

Wertz, F. J. (2010). The method of eidetic analysis for psychology. In T. F. Cloonan & C. Thiboutot (Eds.), *The redirection of psychology: Essays in honor of Amedeo P. Giorgi* (pp. 261–278). Montréal, Quebec: Le Cercle Interdisciplinaire de Recherches Phénoménologiques (CIRP), l'Université du Québec.

CHAPTER 6

A Constructivist Grounded Theory Analysis of Losing and Regaining a Valued Self

Kathy Charmaz

Coding
memos
cmpt. comp
theor-samp
line-by-line
coding

G rounded theory enables researchers to unravel the complexities of doing qualitative analysis and to understand mysteries and moments of human life.[1] This method offers a set of flexible guidelines that demystify the analytic process and encourage researchers to stay involved in their projects. Grounded theory is a systematic yet flexible method that emphasizes data analysis, involves simultaneous data collection and analysis, uses comparative methods, and provides tools for constructing theories.

As grounded theory has gained acclaim, it has become a general method of analysis, and several of its key strategies, particularly coding and memo writing, have become part of the broader lexicon of qualitative inquiry. *Grounded theory coding* means applying a shorthand label to a piece of data that takes this datum apart and defines what it means. Codes *arise from* the researcher's interaction with the data; they are not preconceived and *applied to* the data, as occurs in quantitative research. Like other qualitative researchers, we grounded theorists code to summarize, synthesize, and sort our data, but moreover, we also use codes as conceptual tools (1) to fragment the data and thus take them apart; (2) to define processes in the data; and (3) to make comparisons between data. We begin our analyses with coding but soon start to write extended notes, called *memos,* to discuss and analyze our codes. Certain codes account for the data better than others, so we raise these codes to tentative analytic categories to elaborate and check.

Grounded theory categories become more abstract and theoretical as we ask analytic questions of them in our memos (see Charmaz, 2006a). We write memos to explore and record as much analytic detail about the cat-

Coding

Coding

memos

egory as we can provide. Memo writing is the pivotal intermediate stage of analysis between coding and writing the first draft of a paper or chapter. We write memos on topics such as the properties of our tentative categories, the conditions when a category is evident, how the category accounts for data, comparisons between codes and category. In grounded theory practice, we write memos throughout the research process and make them more analytic and precise as we learn about our topic and focus our research. We start writing memos during our early coding and continue until we reach our most sophisticated analysis of a category and its relationship to other categories. In short, grounded theory memo writing engages us in sustained and successive analysis of our emerging categories.

Grounded theory begins with gathering inductive data but relies on moving back and forth between data gathering and analysis. This iterative process aids in focusing data collection and in conceptualizing collected data in our memos. Thus, grounded theory strategies shape the kinds of data to collect and how and when to collect them, although this method emphasizes and explicates data analysis more than data collection. The major contribution of grounded theory to data collection is its emphasis on using tentative theoretical categories to inform subsequent data collection. Through collecting more focused data, we check and refine our nascent theoretical categories.

Through employing grounded theory strategies, we form successively more abstract, theoretical ideas about our data. The logic of grounded theory relies on its interactive character, systematic use of comparisons, and abductive reasoning (Charmaz, 2006a, 2008c). Using grounded theory guidelines keeps us interacting with our data and nascent theories by involving us in comparative analysis and writing each step along our research journey. As grounded theorists, we interact with the data, compare data with data as we code them, and check our emerging theoretical categories by collecting more data as we construct successively more abstract analyses. We use broad perspectives to begin inquiry and may start with "sensitizing concepts" (Blumer, 1969) to frame our studies, but we change our focus when these concepts do not fit what we find in the empirical world. Glaser (1978, 1992, 1998, 2003), in particular, warns researchers against preconceiving their data by drawing on existing theories and research literatures. However, few researchers, including grounded theorists, can avoid earlier theories and empirical studies in the areas of their research interests. Grounded theorists increasingly concur with Henwood and Pidgeon's (2003) proposal of adopting a stance of "theoretical agnosticism" rather than aiming to enter their research as a *tabula rasa* untouched by earlier ideas. Henwood and Pidgeon's stance demands that we subject our ideas and earlier theoretical interpretations to rigorous scrutiny. As such, theoretical agnostism shares some similarities with abductive reasoning, a type of reasoning that takes grounded theory beyond a purely inductive approach.

theoretical agnosticism

abductive

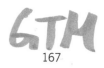

Abductive reasoning involves considering all possible theoretical explanations for a surprising finding and then returning to the empirical world and checking these explanations until the researcher arrives at the most plausible explanation to account for the finding (Charmaz, 2006a; Peirce, 1958; Rosenthal, 2004; Reichertz, 2007). Glaser's strategy of theoretical sampling invokes an abductive logic. *Theoretical sampling* means sampling to fill out and check the properties of a tentative category, not to achieve demographic representation of those chosen for the study. Thus, theoretical sampling does not involve initial sampling of relevant populations or of the distribution of population characteristics. How do grounded theorists conduct theoretical sampling? After developing a tentative category, we return to the field setting(s) to gain specific data to illuminate the category. In an interview study, we revise our interview guides to build in focused questions about this category to develop its properties; compare it with data and codes, and assess its robustness and usefulness in analyzing the data. Theoretical sampling is a novel strategy for increasing the power and usefulness of an emergent theoretical category and constitutes a pivotal step in theory construction (Charmaz, 2006a; Hood, 2007).

What stands as a genuine grounded theory study is contested. Hood (2007) argues that a grounded theorist must engage in theoretical sampling, but few researchers appear to conduct it. Many qualitative researchers who misunderstand the method or aim to legitimize their studies claim to use grounded theory. Whether or not other scholars accept their claims, researchers need to be clear on which grounded theory strategies they use and how they use them.

Glaser and Strauss's method for conducting qualitative research in sociology has become a general method of qualitative analysis for multiple disciplines and professions, including academic and clinical psychology (Bryant & Charmaz, in press; Charmaz & Henwood, 2007; Tweed & Charmaz, in press). The method is particularly useful for qualitative psychologists who study topics such as self, identity, and meaning. Grounded theory provides tools for developing theoretical analyses of psychological data from intensive interviews, personal narratives, case studies, and field observations. To date, almost all researchers have used the method to conduct qualitative analysis, although Glaser (see, e.g., 1978, 1998, 2008) has consistently contended that grounded theory strategies may be adopted in quantitative research.

Developments in Grounded Theory

Over the years Glaser and Strauss constructed independent, but inconsistent, versions of grounded theory. Glaser (1992, 1998, 2003) maintains that his version of grounded theory is the classic, that is, true version of grounded theory. In *Theoretical Sensitivity* (1978), Glaser (1) makes his concept-indicator approach explicit; (2) shows how to develop qualitative codes and theoretical categories through comparative analysis; and (3) introduces the notion of theoretical codes as analytic codes that form vital links for integrating the researcher's emergent theory. Strauss's approach to grounded theory began to diverge from Glaser's with publication of his 1987 book, *Qualitative Analysis for Social Scientists.* Strauss's coauthored 1990 book with Juliet M. Corbin, *Basics of Qualitative Research: Grounded Theory Procedures and Techniques,* diverged markedly from Glaser and Strauss's (1967) initial statement in *The Discovery of Grounded Theory* and Glaser's (1978) *Theoretical Sensitivity,* although most researchers treated *Basics* as an extension of these earlier books and as the major manual for learning grounded theory.

Thus by 1990, two distinctive versions of grounded theory had emerged, Glaser's positivist version and Strauss and Corbin's postpositivist version. Glaser (1992) contended that Strauss and Corbin's new techniques forced data into preconceived procedures, thus losing the fundamental grounded theory emphasis on emergent analyses. Several other researchers also saw these procedures as preconceived and rule-bound (see, e.g., Atkinson, Coffey, & Delamont, 2003; Charmaz, 2000; Melia, 1996). Since then, Corbin (Corbin & Strauss, 2008) has modified her stance on procedures and avers that they had not intended for readers to view their method as rule-bound.

During the past decade, Antony Bryant (2002, 2003) and I (see, e.g., Charmaz, 2000, 2006a, 2007a) wrote a number of works on grounded theory separately and together (Bryant & Charmaz, 2007a, 2007b). We developed "constructivist grounded theory," a version of the method that explicitly moved it into a social constructionist paradigm. In essence, constructivist grounded theory adopts 21st-century epistemological assumptions and methodological advances and treats earlier grounded theory strategies as flexible guidelines rather than rigid rules. Bryant and I argued that earlier versions of grounded theory were built on positivist assumptions of (1) an external reality, (2) an objective, authoritative observer, (3) a quest for generalizations, and (4) a treatment of data as given without acknowledging the participation and standpoints of the researcher in shaping these data. In contrast, our constructivist approach emphasizes multiple realities, the researcher and research participants' respective positions and subjectivities, situated knowledge, and sees data as inherently partial and problematic.

Constructivist grounded theory adopts the methodological strategies of Glaser and Strauss's (1967) classic grounded theory but does not endorse its epistemology. Our constructivist version adopts a relativist epistemology and seeks interpretive understanding rather than a variable analysis that produces abstract generalizations separate from the specific conditions of their production, as Glaser (1998, 2003) advocates. He aims to create abstractions removed from the particularities of time, space, and situation. Constructivist grounded theorists aim to create interpretive understandings located in these particularities and to take into account how the researcher and research participants' standpoints and positions affect our interpretations. Constructivists also reject Glaser's (1998, 2003) stance toward data, which does not take into account the research situation and how data are produced within it. On an epistemological level, Glaser's view assumes a neutral observer and a conception of truth as residing in, and discoverable in, an external reality.[2] In this view, data reside in this external world; representation of research participants is unproblematic, and reflexivity is optional. In contrast, constructivist grounded theorists view data as mutually constructed by the researcher and the researched. Neither data nor the subsequent analyses are neutral. Rather they reflect the positions, conditions, and contingencies of their construction. Constructivist grounded theorists engage in reflexivity throughout inquiry. Engaging in reflexivity and assuming relativity aids us in recognizing multiple realities, positions, and standpoints—and how they shift during the research process for both the researcher and the research participants.

The constructivist quest for interpretive understanding aligns the method with Strauss's (1959/1969, 1961, 1993) legacy of symbolic interactionism, which informs his early writings and last theoretical treatise, *Continual Permutations of Action* (1993), more strongly than his coauthored methods manuals with Corbin (Strauss & Corbin, 1990, 1998). Like Glaser (1992), constructivists disavow Strauss and Corbin's (1990, 1998) prescriptive technical procedures because they undermine creating emergent theoretical categories. Glaser emphasizes emergent categories but has also become prescriptive in how to develop them. Constructivist grounded theory treats methodological strategies as heuristic devices that researchers may adapt, and thus rejects prescriptions in both of the earlier versions (see Charmaz, 2006a, 2008a).

Adele E. Clarke's (2003, 2005, 2006) extension of grounded theory complements the constructivist approach and demonstrates that researchers can use it to study organizations, social worlds, and policies beyond the individual level of analysis. Constructivist grounded theory has gained proponents among researchers in diverse fields (see, e.g., Galvin, 2005; Hallberg, 2006; Madill, Jordan, & Shirley, 2000; Mills, Bonner, & Francis, 2006a, 2006b; Reich & Brindis, 2006; Scott, 2004; Torres & Hernandez, 2007; Ville, 2005; Whiting, 2008; Williamson, 2006). Consistent with recent trends in qualitative inquiry, constructivist grounded theory places the researcher as well as the researched within the field of inquiry.

Constructing a Grounded Theory of Loss and Regaining a Valued Self

My portrayal of using grounded theory strategies to analyze our project data aims to fulfill the following objectives: (1) to show how I developed initial ideas about the data through using grounded theory methods; (2) to link these ideas to my subsequent analysis of losing and regaining a valued self, the two major processes that I defined in the project data; and (3) to present the product of my analysis, a grounded theory of losing and regaining a valued self. Here the term *self*, refers to an unfolding social and subjective process, the experienced self, as contrasted with the self as stable structure, the self-concept (Gecas, 1982).[3] *Self-concept* refers to an *organized* set of consistent definitions of self, attributes, sentiments, values, and judgments, through which a person knows him- or herself (Turner, 1976). A self is fluid, multiple, and emergent in experience. In contrast, the self-concept has relatively stable boundaries but may become permeable under certain conditions (Charmaz, 2006b). Throughout the following analysis of losing and regaining a valued self, I emphasize the experienced self but note relationships between self and self-concept at telling points.

My analysis of losing and regaining a valued self arose from using grounded theory guidelines to construct an inductive analysis of our project data. I addressed meanings, actions, and processes that I defined in these data. In order to construct a fresh theory from the data, using grounded theory necessitates being as open as possible to what is happening in the data and beginning inductive inquiry from that point. Hence, grounded theory leads the researcher to ask: What is most significant in these data? When I read the data for our project, loss of self jumped out as the overriding issue these women faced.[4]

Grounded theory directs researchers to study the most fundamental process in the field setting and to construct a fresh theoretical analysis of it. A Glaserian (1978) ground rule of grounded theory is that extant concepts must earn their way into the analysis; they should not be applied to it. Thus, I could not begin analysis with the concept of resiliency; it was too specific. As a constructivist grounded theorist, however, I am keenly aware that my standpoints and starting points influence *how* I see the project data and *what* I see in them. Chronic illness has touched my life through myriad personal and professional experiences (Charmaz, 2009). During a brief sojourn as an occupational therapist in physical medicine, I saw firsthand the havoc that serious illness can cause. What I witnessed decades ago still lingers in memory. In addition, my background in sociological social psychology informed how I viewed the project data, and my earlier research about the experience of chronic illness (Charmaz, 1983, 1991, 1994, 1995, 1999, 2002) influenced the analysis below. The data we analyze here fits the kind of illness experience that Ciambrone (2007) calls an assault on the self and Scambler and Scambler (2010) view as assaults on the lifeworld. Both of these conceptions contain assumptions about the relative stability of prior selves and worlds and presuppose that consistency is possible. In addition, Teresa's illness amounts to a "biographical disruption" (Bury, 1982) yet occurs within the conditions of her life. As an independent young American woman, Teresa long struggled against her South American father to have a voice, while her traditionalist Filipino mother did not. Such struggles may foster articulation of one's views and actions long before taking command of medical decisions.

Our data for this project consist of written stories and interview accounts about a marker event, rather than direct observations of it. Giving the two research participants names accentuates their distinctive voices and assists readers in envisioning them and their worlds. We don't know what Teresa and Gail left unstated or how they experienced the original event, yet they give us compelling retrospective accounts of their experiences. A major difference between my analysis here and conducting a full-scale grounded theory study is in having sufficient data for checking the analysis against new data and developing the ideas. Such checks enable a researcher to see patterns in the responses and to make comparisons between them, as well as to discern variation in the studied process. If interviews were the only source of data, a sample of 30–40 interviews would provide a solid foundation for a detailed analysis.

Had my analysis drawn on a larger grounded theory study, I would have returned to Teresa and Gail and included other participants to follow up on key ideas that emerged in this analysis. As it turned out, I did make some comparisons with data from people I had interviewed for earlier projects, but not as many nor as systematically as I would be able to do in a grounded theory study in which I had conducted the data collection and focused it as the analysis ensued. I did interview Teresa once after writing the following analysis, although none of the data from our interview informs this analysis. By that time, all five researchers had decided to stick with the original data. Had we included further data, I would have liked to clarify blurred chronology, such as the extent to which Teresa was involved in and committed to her new intellectual life when her voice returned. Additional interviews would have also helped me to follow up on the unstated—to the extent that each woman expressed feeling comfortable in delving into it. What did gymnastics mean to Gail in her life after college? How central a place did it hold in her life? Was Teresa so rational as her statement suggests when her beloved voice teacher said, "Why don't you just stop coming?" What happened when her pituitary tumor was discovered? What did Teresa think, do, and feel then—and now?

Further questions could have also extended and deepened the analysis. How might the ways in which Teresa and Gail reconstructed their pasts influence their present selves? Time is an elusive phenomenon for which we have a limited language. I would have liked to have gone back to Teresa and Gail and asked questions about their turning points and telling moments. What more can these telling moments in their stories teach us about intentionality and transformation? If each woman remained willing to explore her experiences, I would have also attempted to gain further information to make my analytic categories more precise.

These data gave us much to think about and demonstrate that a respectful, receptive, but inexperienced interviewer can draw out important themes. If I had conducted follow-up interviews, I would have tried to keep my questions more open-ended than this interviewer's queries. I aim to learn about research participants' concerns from their perspectives rather than to impose a preconceived structure on them and, thus, would listen to their stories and use more "Tell me about" and "How" questions to foster open-ended responses.

By being as open as possible to what we discern in our data, we grounded theorists cannot ascertain in advance where our analysis will take us. Using grounded theory is an emergent process that relies on interacting with our participants, the data we gather, and how we develop our nascent ideas, as well as what we know and who we are. Grounded theorists move across data and compare fragments of data with each other, then data with codes, codes with categories, and categories with categories. Each comparative step successively raises the level of abstraction of the analysis. The category below, "loss of self," is considerably more abstract than many of my codes, such as "drawing on lessons from the past."

Grounded theory favors constructing theoretical analyses of significant processes in the data, rather than analyzing a participant's narrative in all its richness (although it certainly is possible to compare and categorize whole narratives, if a researcher has a substantial number of them). I used line-by-line coding (Charmaz, 1983, 1995, 2006a; Glaser, 1978) as a tool for early analysis. Line-by-line coding entails coding each fragment of data. Researchers use it as heuristic device for becoming involved in the analysis, shedding their preconceptions, and seeing the data anew. When conducting line-by-line coding, grounded theorists look for what is happening in the data and, to the extent possible, label in it short, active terms. We use gerunds, the noun form of the verb, because gerunds preserve action and promote seeing processes that a language of topics and structures minimizes. I had read Gail and Teresa's accounts earlier, as we all had, but my initial line-by-line coding forced me to engage these data in detail (see Figure 6.1).

Note that many of the codes in Figure 6.1 describe and summarize what I defined was happening in the data. I viewed the last codes in Figure 6.1 as having overriding significance for rendering these data and thus pursued as the categories of losing and regaining a valued self. Grounded theory relies on the researcher's grappling with the data and interpreting them. Other grounded theorists might have developed similar or somewhat different categories from the data, depending on the content and direction of their coding.

Some grounded theorists conduct incident-by-incident coding as their first analytic step. I have, however, found initial line-by-line coding helps to illuminate processes and problems that I had not otherwise seen in interview

Examples of Codes	Initial Narrative Data to Be Coded
	Could you talk about the ease . . . Maybe . . . or difficulty . . . in the actual physical recovery?
Enduring recovery Remembering first instant of consciousness Measuring surgery in hours Finding unexpected (?) spread of tumor Explaining effects of anesthesia	It was horrible. I remember the instant I woke up from the surgery. And the surgery was supposed to take, maybe, 3 hours . . . it ended up taking something like 6, maybe 7 hours, because they didn't expect to find the spreading. I woke up . . . and . . . well, anesthesia has an interesting effect on people. I'd seen people come out of anesthesia before, and it's funny sometimes . . . people just start bawling and talking gibberish. Naturally,
Waking up wailing Hearing a better voice Feeling jubilant about surgical results Being in pain	I wake up and I just start wailing, crying. But I realize, first thing, that my voice is coming out much better than it had before surgery, so I thought, "Yeah, this is great!" The following weeks, I was in a lot of pain, primarily because of the nature of the surgery. For a thyroidectomy, there's a period of healing, of course, but my surgery
Increasing the excision Stopping the spreading tumor Being immobilized	was different because they had to go to the side of my neck where the tumor had begun to spread. As a result, I couldn't walk, could barely move. I was in bed for a good 3 weeks. I'm not the sort that can be bedridden
Feeling miserable Being forced to stay with parents	easily. So I was miserable, and more unfortunate, I had to stay with my parents. My mother was fine . . . she doted on me a bit too much for my taste, but it was no
Wanting distance—dad	surprise. But I could have done without my dad being there, and he was there plenty. And my condition didn't
Continuing conflict complicating voice problems Externalizing her inability to speak coherently Experiencing altered speech Defining certain impairment Receiving no definitive explanation; not asking why; info withheld? Reciting possible loss Implying distress	mean we didn't argue, which just complicated things with my voice. Following the surgery, there was a notable inability to speak well for about a month, when my phonation was very definitively affected. Slowly, it started coming back here and there, but something had definitely changed. I got everything checked, but no one could tell what changed. It's been theorized that the surgery was responsible for shifting some things around, so things were just going to be different from that point on. That was difficult . . . healing physically and coming to terms with the fact that things would have to be so different
Defining permanent loss Experiencing forced loss Voice and self merge; losing valued self Acknowledging suffering	from then on. I wasn't even myself anymore after that. My voice was gone, so I was gone, and I'd never been anything but my voice. So, yeah, that was really hard.

FIGURE 6.1. Initial grounded theory coding.

data and personal accounts. The line-by-line coding in Figure 6.1, for example, explicates the progression of events and of loss. Throughout the analysis, I attempt to connect specific data with larger substantive processes and theoretical interpretations. By invoking comparisons, I also position analytic points against other possible interpretations. In a full-fledged grounded theory study, the iterative logic of the method would take me back to the field (or further in subsequent data collection) to check out these interpretations.

The following analysis reflects what I found to be most significant in these data. Other qualitative researchers or grounded theorists might stress other areas of significance. My analysis rests on an interpretive rendering of key points in the data, rather than an objective report. As a grounded theorist, selecting the most significant and/or most frequent codes served as my criterion for defining an analytic focus. In this case, I saw *losing a valued self* as the most significant code that brought other codes together in a coherent analysis. When I coded Teresa's statement, "My voice was gone, so I was gone, and I'd never been anything but my voice," I was struck by its power and poignancy. I had to pursue Teresa's loss of voice and, by extension, loss of self, which was the central category in a fundamental process.

From that point, I constructed an analysis of the category "loss of self" and the process of losing self. I began writing memos to explore, define, and analyze this category. Memo writing is a pivotal grounded theory strategy that prompts the researchers to engage in early data analysis and writing about their emerging categories. Memo writing also helps grounded theorists to see what kind of additional data they need to seek to fill out the category. The following early memo in Figure 6.2 gave me a direction to pursue and shaped the entire analysis.

In the memo, I began to examine Teresa's statement and to explore its meanings. She connected *voice* and *self*; I tried to explicate these connections and their magnitude. I also tried to situate her statement in time. Grounded theorists delineate the properties of their categories and define the category from these properties. In this case, the properties constituting the connection between voice and self in Teresa's narrative included (1) its essential merged nature, (2) the degree of this merging: voice and self are indistinguishable, and (3) the necessity of voice for the unity and expression of self.[5] Teresa's story also told of regaining another valued self. I saw connections between the two processes, but the accounts provided more material about losing self. Loss of self in serious illness is a topic that has long engaged me. Might I have imposed it on these data and preconceived the subsequent analysis? Perhaps. If, however, this analysis renders our project data in useful ways and resonates with these women's stories, then a focus on losing and regaining a valued self is worthwhile.

Rather than beginning my analysis with Teresa's agonizing moment in the surgeon's office, I began with what happened to her after surgery. Poten-

---

Losing and Regaining Self

It's been theorized that the surgery was responsible for shifting some things around, so things were just going to be different from that point on. That was difficult . . . healing physically and coming to terms with the fact that things would have to be so different from then on. I wasn't even myself anymore after that. *My voice was gone, so I was gone, and I'd never been anything but my voice.* (emphasis mine)

In her statement above, Teresa (Participant 4) revisits a defining moment of 11 years before. She describes this moment as though it occurred yesterday. The meaning of the event hits her full force. "My voice was gone." A voice merged with self. Indistinguishable from self. All of her self. Teresa knew her life had changed at this moment and with it, the self she had been in the past. Perhaps time collapses as Teresa returns to the defining moment. Perhaps we see the self of the 30-year-old woman become again the 19-year-old girl who faced losing the only self she had known and valued.

Meanings of time permeate Teresa's narrative. The past, present, and future take on intensified meaning, as Teresa's story unfolds. She had recounted the incident earlier in her story and in her statement above describes the surgery as a point in time. Teresa treats having thyroid cancer as a defining event that separated past and present. Her surgery becomes a benchmark of time and demarks her changed self. It marks the reality of loss of the voice that had defined her and had shaped her life. As Teresa struggles with losing her voice, she juxtaposes the event against her past and future. Her story goes beyond an account of an "unfortunate event." Rather, Teresa tells a tale of devastating loss and of regaining a revised but valued self.

For Teresa, her cancer, surgery, and lost voice merge into an overwhelming experience that forced loss of self. The past shaped the force of the event and the life-changing spiral of events that rapidly followed. Yet she had gained both a stance and skills in the past that turned her tragic narrative into the beginnings of a positive new direction.

FIGURE 6.2. Early memo on connections between losing voice and self.

tial loss had become actual loss at this point and thus formed the core of my analysis. As is typical of grounded theorists, I tried to conceptualize the larger category of loss of self and treat it in relation to the process of losing a valued self as well as analyze the concrete precipitating event. The themes of loss of self, suffering, and meanings of time in this paper certainly resonate with my earlier work. Yet the category of loss of self—voice—resounds with remarkable clarity in these data. Consistent with grounded theory strategies, I wrote my analysis before using other material. Reading my coauthors' analyses of these data; reviewing earlier work, including my own; and attempting to integrate material from the literature all came later. A few references came to mind while I was writing this draft, so I simply noted them to check later while revising the paper.

The classic grounded theory texts (Glaser, 1978; Glaser & Strauss, 1967) instruct readers to discover a fundamental social or social psychological process about which to theorize. Unlike much of my work, two fundamental processes, losing and regaining a valued self, stood out in Teresa's story.[6] After I defined the properties of the core category, loss of self, the phases of the process were readily identifiable in other codes. The subsequent analysis essentially consists of memos about phases in the process.

My construction of this analysis does not end with a theoretical rendering of loss and regaining self. It also resides in my arguments, selected excerpts, chosen words, and crafted mood. We can talk about using grounded theory strategies to construct an analytic tale. But how we write this tale is yet another story.

Losing and Regaining a Valued Self: A Constructivist Grounded Theory Analysis

"I'd never been anything but my voice." So begins my analytic story of Teresa's portrayal of experiencing a devastating event that occurred 11 years earlier when she was a 19-year-old college student. Teresa's astonishing talent as an opera singer had already set her apart from other voice students and destined her for stardom. But tragedy intervened. A rapidly growing lump in Teresa's neck turned out to be a deadly cancer that required delicate surgical excision.[7] Consider Teresa's story as she seeks to account for what happened to her voice:

> It's been theorized that the surgery was responsible for shifting some things around, so things were just going to be different from that point on. That was difficult . . . healing physically and coming to terms with the fact that things would have to be so different from then on. I wasn't even myself anymore after that. ***My voice was gone, so I was gone, and I'd never been anything but my voice.*** (emphasis mine)

Through these words, Teresa revisits the tumult of 11 years before when she experienced the reality of loss of her voice, self—a life. This earlier moment becomes an irrevocable turning point in a story sprinkled with such instantaneous turning points. Teresa describes the moment as though it had happened yesterday. Its meaning had ripped through her consciousness and had torn apart the self she had known and valued. "My voice was gone." A voice merged with self. Indistinguishable from self. All of her self.

GTM

Voice is a metaphor for self. Voice unifies body and self. Voice conveys self and expresses its passions. Before having cancer, Teresa's voice had structured her college days and shaped her future as a professional mezzo-soprano. Her life irrevocably changed the instant she realized that her voice was gone and with it, the self she had been in the past. This pivotal moment simultaneously revealed and foretold tragic loss. Such loss of self is a "searing disruption" (Charmaz, 1997) of how one knows the world and oneself (Bury, 1982; Charmaz, 1991). Perhaps time collapses as Teresa returns to the crucial event. Perhaps we catch a glimpse of the 30-year-old woman becoming again the 19-year-old girl who lost the only self she had known and valued.

At 30, Teresa's clear reflective voice amplifies the story of losing her singing voice and, therefore, her self. Her loss of voice was involuntary, uncontrollable, and irrevocable. She felt like she had lost control of her life. Teresa's cancer, surgery, and lost voice merge into an existential crisis that forced loss of self and resulted in enormous suffering (Charmaz, 1983, 1999, 2002).[8] The past shaped the force of the crisis and the life-changing spiraling events that rapidly followed and still echo through her life today. An ominous cancer lurked in the background of her life, ever present, usually quiescent, but there. Yet Teresa had gained both a stance and skills in the past that turned a tragic narrative into a tale of hope, courage, and positive growth.

Meanings of time permeate Teresa's story. She looked back at the past through the prism of the present (Mead, 1932; Ross & Buehler, 2004). As Teresa's story unfolds, the past, present, and future take on intensified meaning. Her story also teaches us about meanings of moments. Telling moments mark and symbolize tumultuous changes. Teresa had earlier recounted how her ordeal unfolded before she made the stunning statement about losing her self. The moment when Teresa learned that she might lose her voice became the defining event in her life. The news separated the present from her past. This moment marked the shattering of Teresa's self. What could life be without singing?

After Teresa's surgery, potential loss became actual loss. Trauma disrupted the rhythm of the past. As Teresa struggled with losing her voice, she juxtaposed these events against her past and future. Her story surpasses an account of an "unfortunate event." Instead Teresa told a tale of devastating loss of self and of regaining a revised but valued self. The specter of death enters this tale, although we cannot ascertain when or how because, as Teresa divulged, "I try to play things off like there's nothing wrong."

A social psychological analysis of Teresa's story illuminates the process of losing a valued self, an embodied self, and suggests ways of regaining a valued self while living with uncertainty. For analytic clarity here, my rendering of her story (1) treats losing and regaining self as two ends of a continuum of reconstructing self, (2) emphasizes the conditions under which loss of self develops, (3) describes those conditions necessary to effect *intentional* reconstruction of self, and (4) links intentionality with meanings of moments. When I use similar data to trace biographies over time, I find that these processes are seldom singular and linear. Instead people move between, through, and around these processes, depending on the vicissitudes of health and life (Charmaz, 1995).

What is loss of self? How might it be related to a disrupted self and a changed self? Which experiences contribute to suffering loss of self? How do people who suffer loss of self regain a valued self? I address these questions in this chapter and show how a grounded theory perspective guided my analysis. I concentrate here on Teresa's story but offer some comparisons with Gail's account of her gymnastics injury to clarify analytic points. Teresa and Gail speak as graduate students in a psychology class who are asked to write about an unfortunate event in their lives and subsequently answer a classmate's interview questions about this event. Thus they have shaped their written stories for an imagined audience and coconstructed their interview responses with an acquaintance with whom they could share a sustained connection.

The very methods of collecting data position these two young women as heroines of their own stories (Mathieson & Stam, 1995; Ricoeur, 1991). Interviews and autobiographical accounts place the storyteller on center stage. What we analyze is predicated on this positioning, which may have shifted or distorted their experienced locations and relationships with other people. I note this point but treat their narratives as revealing telling personal disclosures to analyze.

The context of forming the accounts, the purpose of producing the accounts, and the availability of the accounts to the instructor and class all affect Teresa and Gail's construction of their narratives. They both highlight their heightened awareness of crucial moments and their reverberating effects. Each woman's story reflects her interpretation of past events and present situations and the imagined self she wishes to present. These women may have told a tale that supports or expands the identity they had previously claimed in their class and graduate program. Versions of each woman's story likely change as time unfolds, perspectives shift, and audiences vary. Nonetheless, grounded theorists treat such data as plausible accounts from which we can begin to theorize.

What Is Loss of Self?

Defining Loss of Self

Loss of self symbolizes more than bodily losses. It means loss of the ways people know, define, and feel about themselves. Their identifying attributes are gone. The foundations of their lives have weakened or crumbled. Loss of self alters how people compare themselves with others and locate themselves in their worlds. It means losing their way of being in the world—and, moreover, in its most intense forms, losing their personal and collective worlds (Ciambrone, 2007; Charmaz, 1983, 1997; Mathieson & Stam, 1995). Chaos erupts. Communities disappear and lives irrevocably change.

Loss of self resides at the far end of a continuum of reconstruction of self, with regaining a valued self at the other end. Both are played out in a situation that ranges between certainty and uncertainty (see Figure 6.3).[9] Loss of self makes life uncertain and chaotic; regaining a valued self fosters a sense that life has become more predictable and manageable. Hence, regaining a valued self also implies that the person has reestablished a stable self-concept, although it may be based on new attributes and values.

The depth, extent, and existential meaning of loss define loss of self. Such losses are devastating, uncontrollable—overwhelming. These losses impose uncertainty, portend permanence, undermine autonomy, and cause grief and suffering. Teresa's tale of wrenching loss suggests the suffering that she endured. She lost what had made her distinctive, given her solace, and formed a way of life. When her interviewer asked about her relationship with God, Teresa revealed how losing her voice reverberated through her life.

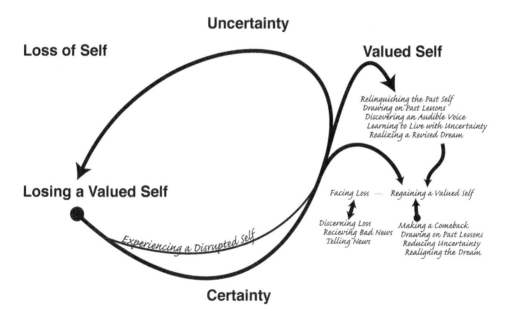

FIGURE 6.3. Effecting intentional reconstruction of self: Losing and regaining a valued self.

Singing was my prayer. That was my connection. That was my big gift. I was a fat kid with no friends for as long as I could remember, but I could sing! That was the "in" for me. When I lost that, I lost my connection with God, I lost all my friends, I lost my calling in life, I lost my passion in life, I lost my trump card . . . the thing that was gonna get me out of being that fat kid with the oppressive dad, and whatever . . . that was going to be my ticket out. I lost my ticket! So I lost my connection to God. Gone.

Loss of voice spread throughout Teresa's life as she lost relationships, her passion, and her purpose—and one identity after another. The prospect of possible loss of function can initiate loss of self. For Teresa, loss of self began with the threat of losing her voice. Her suffering was immediate. The instant the surgeon said "You may not be singing anymore after this," Teresa understood how fragile her voice and her world had become. With the force and clarity of his statement, Teresa experienced this moment as one of immediate, piercing awareness that the unsuspected catastrophe was real. Teresa recalled feeling shock and anguish overtake her during this defining traumatic moment.

I froze. I couldn't breathe, couldn't move, couldn't even blink. I felt like I had just been shot. My gut had locked up like I'd been punched in it. My mouth went dry and my fingers, which had been fumbling with a pen, were suddenly cold and numb. Apparently picking up on my shock, the surgeon smiled a little. "We're going to save your life, though. That's what counts. And you know what? The other surgeon working with me is a voice guy. We're going to do everything we can not to be too intrusive." I started to breathe a little, very little, and I felt myself trembling. I tried to say something meaningful, expressive . . . all that I could manage was, "Man . . . I was actually pretty good."

Then, all of me let loose. I was sobbing, but there was no sound; just a torrent of tears, and the hiss of crying from my open mouth, pushing through the pressure from the accursed mass.

Within seconds, the tempo of conversation had quickened, signaling the crisis and subsequent profound loss. The defining moment may come quickly, but the pain and suffering it causes feels timeless. The immediacy, force, and severity of misfortune intensify the sense of loss of self when people recognize what is happening to them. Sudden thudding awareness of immediate, extensive, and life-threatening loss is overwhelming, particularly when people are young. Critical illness is out of synchrony with the rhythm of their lives. Thoughts of dying may be unimaginable. Teresa's tumor had appeared suddenly. Not only had she been without warning, but also her two earlier

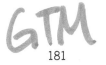

diagnoses of merely having a goiter made the threat of losing her voice all the more shocking.

> I was sure this [the surgery] was no big deal. After all, this was just a thyroidectomy, and only affecting one lobe . . . people have their thyroids taken out all the time. I was actually just taken up in the whole strangeness of suddenly being on the verge of surgery. "Wow," I thought. "My first surgery . . . weird."

Being absorbed by immediate but minor troubles, such as Teresa's initial concentration on her impending surgery, deters redefining symptoms and hence intensifies shock. In turn, shock amplifies suffering and feelings of loss of control. The sounds of sorrow alternate with the silence of numbing shock. At this point, suffering consumes the person and drains the self. The self-concept of the past crumbles in the exigencies of the present. Teresa experienced losing its very substance—a death of self.

> I was completely drained, like a ghost of my former self. I felt as though the biggest and best part of me had died in that office. Cancer wasn't as frightening to me as never being able to sing again. Singing had been my life for as long as I could remember; the one thing I could excel at, the only thing I knew. It had been my solace in all my times of distress, through every hardship . . . this would be the most grueling hardship of all, and I wouldn't be able to sing my way out of it. Literally. Worst of all, I still had to tell my mother.

After the actual loss occurs, suffering increases as the effects of loss spread (Charmaz, 1999). Loss of voice hurled Teresa out of the familiar present into a foreboding future. The music stopped. She foresaw being deprived of consolation. She foretold the end her relationship with her beloved voice teacher:

> If I couldn't sing, I was going to lose this guy. As far as I was concerned, not being able to sing would destroy not only everything that we'd worked toward that past 2½ years, but also our relationship . . . professionally, personally, you name it. And I just couldn't deal with that.

Did Teresa's suffering become silent at this moment, silenced by the daunting events? Can words express what she felt then? Could she voice her sorrow? How did this moment of realization influence her subsequent actions? Realization of overwhelming loss may flash in an instant, but its meaning may henceforth pervade one's consciousness. If an illness is episodic, such mean-

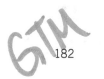

ings may linger only to ignite again when disturbing symptoms arise. By losing her valued self, Teresa suffered a psychological death that overshadowed the sudden fragility of her life.

Objective misfortune merges with subjective meaning when people experience loss of self. Nonetheless, not everyone is aware of physical changes or their implications. Not everyone views symptoms or impairment as reflecting a body in trouble (Mairs, 1986)—and therefore as symbolizing a precarious or lost self. One's imagined self may not be the person that other people see. Meanings of body and self frame responses to illness, loss of function, and disability—of those who witness such changes as well as of those who experience them. Lack of bodily control or impaired function, however, makes physical loss tangible and undermines a person's earlier images of self (Charmaz, 1995). Some people can distance themselves from their now erratic bodies, but most cannot. For them, body and self are intertwined.

In Teresa's case, body and self had merged and were expressed by the beauty and emotionality of her voice. Without her body working smoothly to sustain her voice, *she* could not function. Teresa's present and future self depended on her trained throat muscles and controlled vocal chords. Here, body and self are markedly intertwined and unified.[10] Nevertheless, this unity of body and self may not have included all of Teresa's body—but likely centered on the parts and functions that she used in singing. These bodily attributes had tempered and superseded being "a fat kid," for they gave her the tools of the trade and a "ticket" to an identity.

Loss of self increases as one's life purpose dissolves. The zeal with which Teresa had pursued realizing her dream made losing it all the more unbearable. The identity and relationships gained in the voice program had shaped who she had been and would become. Envisioning a singing career meant more than pursuing an elusive youthful fantasy. Teresa's quest for voice training transcended a fervent college pursuit. Instead, singing was her calling. Through her voice, Teresa's spirit could sing. She could make her most authentic self audible—a reality. Teresa had enacted a plan to fulfill her dream, created a path, and found the requisite training and support in her teacher.

> I wanted very much to be an opera singer, and do it well, to the best of my ability . . . the only way to do that was to be around this man [her voice teacher] 24/7 . . . .I had very monocular vision when it came to my goals in life, which contributed to me being very intimately involved with working in the studio and with my teacher . . . and which is why it was so devastating when all of this happened.

Teresa went from having a benign goiter to an "accursed mass." She plunged from being absorbed by the prospect of having her first surgery into

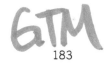

the abyss of losing her voice and therefore herself. What had looked like a minor disruption had become a devastating loss of self. If Teresa just had had a goiter, she might instead have experienced a disrupted self.

Distinguishing between Loss and Disruption of Self

The magnitude of losing a valued self becomes apparent when we compare it with experiencing a disruption of self. Here continuity of self is broken, but not irretrievably. Loss of self shares certain properties with a disrupted self but also has some significant differences. As I analyze them here, experiencing loss of self and a disrupted self both (1) result from misfortune, (2) typically cause distress, and (3) impose immediate changes in daily life. In addition, each may affect the person's sense of purpose, require sustained effort, and perhaps elicit questions about the person's prior actions or judgment. Whether and to what extent people are aware of what has happened to them affects what they say, do, and feel about it.

The immediacy of disruption of self may elicit similar feelings as arising with loss of self. Similarly, a person may feel cast adrift. As Ville (2005, p. 332) points out, following injury, "the broken body occupies the entire field of experience." Gail recalled what she felt after dislocating her elbow during gymnastics practice. "When I got home that evening . . . I felt like my life lost some of its purpose. I felt handicapped and I really felt the physical pain. . . . It was nice that a lot of the girls [teammates] came over, but I felt really horrible. I was upset, I was disappointed, and I was still a little shocked."

Feelings of disappointment and depression accompany the experience of a disrupted self. Yet loss of self reaches deeper and extends further. Loss of self is the end point on the continuum of reconstructing self. Experiencing a disrupted self resides closer to the middle of the continuum between loss and regaining a valued self, but it is not neutral. Rather the "unfortunate event" interferes with how people live their lives and delays their ability to realize valued goals.

In short, experiencing a disrupted self is temporary. The event encompasses a discernible period of time with boundaries—beginning and ending points. From the start, Gail's time projections shaped her expectations and reached beyond the time horizon enforced by her injury. She said, "The cast would heal the bone chip and the good news was that I would be casted for only 3 weeks." The uncertainties caused by the precipitating event are more specific and limited than those experienced with loss of self. The promise of realizing a valued self remains, although finding ways to achieve it may not be clear. Gail mentioned, "Of course I was upset . . . but at the same time I knew that my career wasn't over. It wasn't like what am I going to do? It was, just how do I move on?"

Loss of self means at least relative permanence, if not lasting change. Life is irrevocably altered. No possibilities of regaining the lost self exist. No alternative paths to realizing it appear. The force, intensity, and uncertainty typifying loss of self distinguish it from experiencing a disrupted self. Teresa's comment below not only suggests the magnitude of loss that occurs when people's lifelong dreams are smashed but also their acute awareness of this moment and its meaning:

> I'm not the only one walking around, thinking, as a singer, "That's my voice, and without my voice I have nothing." It's a huge step for a singer to say, "Eh . . . maybe I'll try *this* career change." That's huge. It's almost as big as religion. It may be bigger. Because for a musician to devote themselves that completely to their art and to even consider the thought of straying from that path, even for a moment . . . that moment is very pivotal for a singer. Whenever you hear about people who have degrees in music and do completely different things . . . there was a big choice that took place there. In my case, it was forced on me.

The event leading to a disrupted self can take several forms, including an unexpected setback, a distressing interruption along a life path, or a personal defeat while pursuing this path. These unfortunate events may force a time out from usual pursuits; however, such events rarely preclude a return to these pursuits. Granted, some individuals may abandon efforts to resume their former lives. But the possibility is there.

In this case, the precipitating event may be inconvenient, frustrating, and embarrassing, but it does not force reconstruction of self. Rather, this event impedes and delays actions to realize a valued self. The event strikes a dissonant chord now but will eventually pass and reside in the past, and perhaps be forgotten. Reminders of this event fade because it no longer intrudes on daily life. While experiencing the disruptive event, however, its relative significance may assume large proportions. If so, objective assessments of its impermanence, lack of dangerousness, and the like, may not allay a person's thoughts and feelings about either the unfortunate event or self. Gail said:

> On the one hand, it was just a bone chip and dislocation. I did not have to get surgery, and after 3 weeks, rehabilitation could start because my cast would come off. The coaches were optimistic that I'd be able to condition myself back to shape in a few months and still be able to compete this season. Their hope kept my hopes up, because it seemed as though they hadn't given up on me yet. On the other hand, I had been in such great shape before the injury. This was supposed to be my year. And there I was . . . handicapped. These thoughts kept running through my head.

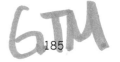

A disrupted self may be shaken. Losing a valued self is shattering. The cast permitted Gail's arm to mend, but surgery silenced Teresa's voice.

Facing Loss

Facing loss is a prerequisite for intentional reconstruction of a valued self after an unfortunate or devastating event. Typically people must understand what has happened to them, so that they can act to change its effects. In some situations, however, individuals can move forward without realizing what could happen to them in the future. Because the self is a process as well as an object to assess (Blumer, 1969; Strauss, 1959/1969), construction of self continues, although not everyone engages in intentional, focused reconstruction of self. Life goes on, time passes, things happen, and people may change without realizing it. Teresa and Gail, however, had to face what happened, and both were determined to exert control over their fates. Which conditions foster facing loss? What does it entail?

Discerning Loss

Teresa and Gail each evinced tangible, audible—and visible—signs of bodily difference from their known, "normal" bodies and from those of other people. They did not have to strain to listen to their bodies. Their bodies spoke but did not sing. Gail heard the sound of her elbow tearing apart. Teresa recalled, "Following the surgery, there was a notable inability to speak well for about a month, when my phonation was very definitively affected. Slowly, it started coming back here and there, but something had definitely changed." By saying "*there was*," Teresa distanced herself from her body and treated it as an object to observe. Her word choice might symbolize the sudden lack of unity between body and self that she felt during the experience.

An injury may occur so quickly that it collapses time into a surreal second, but simultaneously this moment stretches before the instant of impact expands and engulfs the person. Gail recounted her growing awareness of her injury:

> I was so high, but too far away from the high bar to catch it. I'm coming down fast. Even though it was so fast, I felt that moment take forever. All of a sudden I hear a crack. Or was it a tear? It sounded like the Velcro that holds the mats together ripping apart. I almost turned to see what it was. Wait. Something feels funny. Wait. Something doesn't feel right. I was on the floor kneeling down underneath the high bar. I feel my right elbow with my left hand. Something feels very, very wrong. There was no elbow anymore, my arm was contorted. I couldn't feel that bony part of my

arm. It was bent the wrong way. I panicked. *That Velcro sound was from my elbow?* Then it hits me. Look at what happened to me, in a split second. I thought about my competitive season . . . going down the drain. I thought about sitting out all those meets . . . again. I thought about the doctor. I thought about surgery. I panicked more when I thought about surgery. I remember the shock. When I felt my elbow, I said "Oh my God! Oh my God!" in panic and disbelief that something so intense could happen in a split second. Then, as it all started to sink in and the panic came over me, I kept saying, "No!! No!! No!!" first in denial and passionate, then through sobs and a feeling of defeat and frustration.

Both women were attuned to their bodies and had attended to learning from them. Both realized what the moment portended while experiencing it. Visible symptoms prompt awareness of change.[11] Gail saw her contorted arm. Teresa's "large, two-or-so-inch long bump" appeared in one day. She saw it and began her diagnostic search. As it grew, Teresa realized that she was "singing against something that was causing pressure on my vocal apparatus," although its seriousness eluded her. Gail could not ignore the look and feel of her twisted arm, nor could Teresa normalize her distorted neck and difficulty in singing.

Receiving Bad News

Receiving bad news can wreak such havoc in people's lives that it reaches into their selves and situations. Bad news catapults them into unwelcome categories and situations. Someone may, however, receive bad news without believing or accepting it. If so, and should events prove the news to be consequential, facing loss may occur months later. A person may lose the optimal time and opportunity for subsequent reconstruction of a valued self.

Time shrinks between receiving a discouraging diagnosis and accepting it when a person already feels uneasy about alarming bodily changes (Charmaz, 1991). Gail needed no diagnosis to know that she had suffered an injury. Teresa's endocrinologist had withheld crucial test results from her. Nonetheless clues had begun to accrue. A scary biopsy. "Inconclusive results." Surgery in 2 days. And then the fateful visit to the surgeon.

Note the speed with which the surgeon imparted clues that broke through Teresa's initial surprise and confusion and how he moved from "you" to "we" and thereby enlisted her cooperation. She recalled:

The surgeon seemed to have gotten very angry with something I'd said. "Damn it," he grumbled. "I hate when they do this. I hate when they make it so that I'm the one that's saying this right before surgery." For the first time, I was stunned, confused. There wasn't anything that made

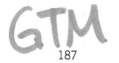

sense for me to say, so I couldn't say anything. Then, the surgeon sat down across from me at his desk. "Do you want your mother to come in?" Instantly, I declined. He asked me again, looking a bit puzzled. Again, I said no. Then he shifted a little in his seat and leaned in, resting his elbows on the desk and looking intently at me. "I don't know why your endo didn't tell you this. Your biopsy wasn't inconclusive. You have anaplastic carcinoma. That's thyroid cancer. We've got to get that thing out of there right now."

The speed, clarity, and form of imparting the news matter. Teresa and Gail each felt the immediate impact of Teresa's bad news. They went from being caught unaware to a heightened awareness of their situations. Clues about what had happened to them appeared in condensed form, one after another. These fleeting but inescapable moments locked them into the present. The surgeon's repeated question, body positioning, and intent gaze set the stage for his candid announcement of carcinoma. However unwittingly, he subsequently imparted further clues of its seriousness, and then broached the surgical risk and ended with Teresa's devastating prognosis.

He asked, "So, you're a college student . . . what's your major?" I told him it was vocal performance, and his face went white. He looked grimmer now than he had at any point in our conversation. "Look," he said very gently, "because of where this thing is and what we're going to have to do, there's a chance you won't be able to even speak the same way again. *You may not be singing anymore after this.*" (emphasis mine)

The surgeon's grim expression and blanched face attested to the truth of his pronouncement. The intrusive, expanding lump on Teresa's neck affirmed its authenticity. He cut through her sorrow and gave her hope when he predicted, "You're going to beat this. You're young, and you're going to beat this thing. And you'll get your voice back, and you'll be singing at the Met. And I want tickets, so don't forget me." But did he tell her anything more about anaplastic carcinoma?

Telling News

Receiving unsuspected bad news sets in motion a chain of spiraling events and actions.[12] Foremost among them is telling one's family and close friends and doing it quickly enough to control information. Telling reaffirms the reality of the situation—to self as well as others (Charmaz, 1991). People must look at their loss, if only taking one glimpse at a time, and hear themselves acknowledge it. Telling the news over and over again pounds the bad news into the person's consciousness.

Telling the news tests emotional fortitude because the person's shock, fear, anger, and sorrow may erupt while imparting the details (Charmaz, 1991). In addition, a teller may need to assuage the other person's grief and disappointment. Telling can recast or end a significant relationship and elicit considerable distress and dilemmas for all involved. Because Teresa viewed her mother as emotionally fragile, she reproduced similar strategies in telling her mother as she had experienced with the endocrinologist:

> I told her they might have to do a full thyroidectomy, and that the lump . . . I basically pulled the same game that the other doctor did . . . that the lump was *probably* cancer. That they didn't know exactly what it was. I left it at that, but that was enough . . . she lost it . . . I made the executive decision to moderate her amount of knowledge at that point.

Observe who takes control of this situation. Teresa assumed that control over her body, life, and decisions resided with her. She had no difficulty in withholding certain facts. What facts did she have? How did she obtain them? Teresa's strategy of information control with her mother aimed to control her mother's emotions but likely amounted to information delay.[13] Despite her mother's emotional vulnerability, Teresa knew her mother would see her through this crisis and remain in her life, no matter what happened.

> I didn't tell my voice teacher before my mother, but, for whatever reason, it was a lot harder to tell him. Where my father lacked, my voice teacher sort of picked up the slack. He was very supportive, he was about the right age to be my dad . . . he was, um . . . he understood my passion for singing, and believed in it, whereas my father, quite frankly, thought it was a pipe dream, and I ought not give money and time to a university to learn how to sing.

Such difficulties in telling news arise when the individual being told symbolizes the tie to one's actual or potential loss. Teresa's image of her teacher as an ideal father further complicated her tie to him. Losing her voice and therefore losing her teacher left Teresa without the validating counterpoint to her father's view of a singing career as a pipe dream. She would now have to contend with her father on his terms. Thus, losing her voice intensified her conflict with her father rather than muting it. She said, "I lost my identity. I lost myself. And now I didn't have a leg to stand on, like, with my dad, because I'd always fought him on being a good enough singer to make a living. Well, now he had me. So that was horrible."

The telling did not end but instead took another turn. Teresa became the object rather than the source of the telling. She received tacit identity reminders and overt identity pronouncements about whom she had become.

Everyone knew that Teresa's voice had sustained severe and lasting damage. Friends disappeared. Fellow students could see the unmistakable gash on Teresa's neck, hear her speak, and witness her struggles to regain her voice. Teresa could no longer compete much less get the coveted solos. The students' visible awareness of her new status imparted constant identity reminders of her now marginalized position (Charmaz, 2008c). The audience for sound had become an audience for sight—and dismissal. Teresa recalled how other voice students had acted, "So when this happened to *me*, it scared the crap out of everybody . . . scared the *crap* out of everybody. And I even had a couple of them tell me how tragic it was . . . like I was dead, and they were telling me about it. It was weird. But essentially, I *was* dead. To them."

Each similar incident became another identity pronouncement. The telling forced Teresa to face her loss and simultaneously allowed others to affirm her social death. If she could not resume her role as the star soprano, she no longer existed. A person may not be able to avoid such encounters and escape the ensuing identity pronouncements and reminders. While trying to get her voice back, Teresa endured hearing her teachers repeat renditions of her story as a tragic narrative for *them* to ponder.

> Having been called in by every single professor and conductor in the music school, to sit down and have a moment with me in their offices . . . just to reflect on life, and how tragic it is for this 19-year-old kid with so much promise to be taken out by cancer. I mean . . . again, being spoken to as though I was already dead.

These pronouncements and reminders portrayed Teresa as a symbol of death. She had become a ghost of her past self and an outcast from her world. Teresa cast no blame on the students because she understood their discomfort about including her. She no longer could participate in the voice program. Perhaps Teresa minimized the effects of fellow students' identity reminders and pronouncements. She could not, however, ignore the image of herself reflected in her voice teacher's tears. The most powerful identity pronouncements occur not with words but through a beloved person's telling emotions. Teresa said, "My voice teacher, who was like another father to me, greeted me in tears each time he saw me afterwards. . . . Seeing the dreams we had built together go to pieces the way they did was just too much for either of us, and we spoke very little after that."

Regaining a Valued Self

After facing loss in the concrete world, what can a person do? How can he or she reverse the present situation and the unwelcome identities inherent in it?

What does regaining a valued self entail? Each woman tried to make a comeback, reclaim her competitive edge, and thus regain the self she had valued. How did they accomplish their goals? For Gail, making a successful comeback meant doing the hard work to realize her goal. For Teresa, the path was more complicated. They each drew on lessons from the past, but Teresa also had to discover an audible new voice and live with continued uncertainty.

Making a Comeback

For people with the residuals of serious illness or injury, making a comeback means reclaiming the valued identity while still under duress (Charmaz, 1973, 1987; Corbin & Strauss, 1988). A plan to make a comeback implies that misfortune has caused the lapse of time since the person had held this identity. Making a comeback takes more than asserting identity claims. It means taking control. It takes planning and effort. It is more than a mere return after an imposed time out. These two cases indicate the ingenuity and effort required to make a comeback and therefore to effect intentional reconstruction of self.

Time constraints may determine how long a person can take to make a comeback. As this time period shrinks, the present tightens like a vise clamped between past and future selves. Gail's slowed recovery belied her earlier optimistic time estimates and, to her chagrin, the competitive season started without her. She recalled:

> I was determined to get back as fast as I could, but it was as if my body wasn't prepared to.
>
> It took another two doctor visits until I was cleared to put pressure on my right arm. By this time, it was halfway through the competitive season. I had my work cut out for me. I was *so* focused at this time. I was determined to make the fastest comeback ever.

Gail made a comeback through her systematic work to strengthen and retrain her arm. Teresa also worked hard to regain her voice, despite lack of progress and her teacher's tears.

> I just couldn't handle that, you know? I mean, I really cared about this guy, and I was just bringing him way down. And then one day, I was leaning on the piano in the studio, and he was sitting at the keyboard, and we were having this sad lesson . . . and he just looked at me and said, "Why don't you just stop coming?" And I said, "You're right." And that's the last time I went to the studio.

Teresa relinquished having a voice, her voice, *the* voice that identified her and made her unique.[14] The overriding question in her life had shifted during

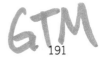

this moment. What could life be without singing? What *would* life be without singing?

Drawing on Lessons from the Past

The effort involved in making a comeback directs consciousness and orders life. What does one do when hopes of making a comeback have been dashed? The ominous present tightened like a vise after Teresa was locked out of her anticipated future.

> As soon as the voice was gone, I had to find something or I was going to die. I really felt that I was going to have to die, or kill myself . . . or hold my breath until it ended. Anything but feel like that. It was miserable and painful, and terrible. I can't explain in words how awful it was.

Teresa's wording, "*the voice*," suggests that by this time, she viewed herself as changed, now separated from that which had defined her in the past. The foreclosed future left an empty present. Although the pain of devastating loss consumed Teresa, it also spurred her to seek new directions and to reconstruct a new self.

Teresa's voice was gone, but the principles she had gained from earlier voice lessons lived on. All of Teresa's self was not gone. Parts of her former self continued. Teresa's handling of her diagnostic search showed her initiative and ability to take control over her life at an early age. Her willingness to struggle and fight poor odds had long exemplified her stance toward the world. Her father's outbursts had taught Teresa to temper her emotions and to follow her own path, despite his displeasure. Through pursuing her dream, she had learned the value of taking action, persevering, and feeling well-earned pride in her progress. Teresa had learned to control her physical tensions, keep her emotions in check, and retain her focus.

> Being in a very emotional household also contributed to the emotionality of my performance . . . .When you're emotional, you get physically tense . . . and . . . that kind of messes with what you're doing vocally . . . and that's what was happening to me. So getting away from that emotionality and reminding myself why . . . which, of course, takes logic . . . was actually very instrumental in the long run, not in quashing my emotions . . . I still listen very much to my emotions . . . but understanding that they're just a part of what needs to take place in order to help me function in a given scenario.

Throughout her ordeal with and beyond the surgery, Teresa invoked the same kind of dispassionate logic with which she had once analyzed her voice.

Not only had she relied on logic, but she also had established a partnership with the surgeon to address the problem in her now objectified body. She said:

> I remember thinking that panicking wasn't going to do any good. I remember thinking that the best thing to do at that point was to be just as methodical and professional as he had to be, and sort of remove myself from my physical self, as it were . . . to look at the problem as though I was a cohort of his, trying to analyze the problem . . . trying to take on my own role in this cancer battle we were about to embark on. It was the best possible thing I could do to, for one, maintain my sanity at that moment in time, because that's a little heavy, and two, to just get it done.

Perhaps this pragmatic stance later helped Teresa to realize that she couldn't recapture the past and led her to pursue another path.

Discovering an Audible Voice

Discovering that one can claim an audible voice derives from the convergence of individual factors and social circumstances. Life circumstances matter. When an assault on the self occurs in an otherwise stable world, possibilities exist for reconstruction of self and life. Youth and opportunity ease the challenge of taking another path. Affluent college students can change majors and pursue new fields. Taking an extra year in college while young differs from taking a year without income to retrain when middle-aged. In addition, college offers students a world with multiple possibilities to develop their untapped potentials.

Reaching a point of readiness for change allows people to relinquish their past selves.[15] Teresa had reached that point. Her voice had not allowed her to make a comeback, and she knew it. The mutual distancing between Teresa and her fellow students made it easier to leave the voice studio for an unknown future. As the voice students receded from the present into the past, she viewed them as vapid. Teresa's comparisons of the voice students with her interesting new friends kept her earlier compatriots in the past and validated the superiority of her present new world.

A long history of functioning autonomously, seeking achievement, and managing time and resources to realize goals seldom ends with critical illness. Moreover, a life-threatening crisis can refocus a person's outlook. If so, then people pinpoint their priorities, embrace life, and live intensely during a condensed period of time. By the time she left the voice studio, Teresa had a heightened awareness of time passing and quite possibly of a foreshortened life. She disclosed:

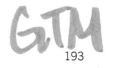

Because what if this thing comes back? I won't have done anything important if it were to come back today. I better get on with it. Yeah, it took a long time to come to terms with not being an opera singer . . . maybe two years of straight misery. Then, in my senior year of undergrad, my voice started coming back. And that was terrible.

The felt pressure to live a full life pushes the person to act. Teresa's grief over her lost self had faded without her awareness as she flourished in her new life. Getting a second chance to reclaim one's lost self is shocking, especially after one's self-concept has changed. This second chance divides the person between past and present selves and reinvokes the sorrow of loss. Reconstructing one's earlier self may seem to require giving up the gains reflected in one's new self. Getting a second chance may, however, permit a person to stand between past and present and the identities given in them. For Teresa:

That's when I started doing auditions, doing the professional opera chorus gigs . . . and still, I realized I had kind of gotten used to the idea of not being an opera singer . . . and it wasn't that bad. And I *was* kinda smart . . . and my friends who weren't musicians were a little less vapid.

Teresa found a new voice and with it a new self. Her voice had begun singing in a new key, singing a new song. Teresa's pleasure in her new life and pride in her intelligence becomes a counterpoint to her tragic narrative.

Learning to Live with Uncertainty

Living with continued uncertainty is the reality for many people with chronic and life-threatening illnesses. Teresa revealed her awareness of continued uncertainty when she compared herself to her mother-in-law, who died of cancer. She said, "The same thing could have happened to me . . . that it might still happen to me." People in Gail's position, however, experience a temporary disruption that delimits the period and content of the felt uncertainty.

Lengthy intervals between episodes of illness may quell some people's sense of uncertainty. Conversely, other people experience relentless signs of an uncertain future. Their symptoms multiply, occur with force and frequency, and defy escape. People who have suffered a serious first episode likely consider the possibility of another. If so, they may keep uncertainty in the foreground even though overt signs of illness have receded into the background. Teresa said, "There was always a bunch of 'what if-ing,' and it never really went away. With cancer, it doesn't goes away. So you always have to wonder . . . you know, if it's going to come back. Or if it never left. Or if they haven't caught it all."

Surviving against the odds adds to the "what ifs." Uncertainty hovers over one's life. The threat of recurrence remains. Identity reminders reemerge. An actual recurrence catapults the person into crisis and raises the specter of experiencing loss of self, loss of life, all over again. Uncertainty escalates. Teresa not only faced a recurrence but also alluded to what its dangerous location meant.

> The last year of my undergrad, they found another tumor, and this time it was a pituitary tumor . . . this time, it was a freakin" brain tumor. And it was inoperable, so we just sit around and watch it. It doesn't do any tricks . . . it just kind of sits there. I mean, it grows, and it shrinks, but it's not doing anything amazing. But what can you do? So that sucked. "Here we go again," is what that was. It was a little scarier, because of it being in the brain, but whatever. What can you do? Me, I turned to logic. So I ended up doing my undergrad thesis on the psychological side effects of pituitary tumors. I figured that, if I had to have this thing, I may as well get something out of it.

Uncertainty floods life when metastatic cancer persists. People's actions toward uncertainty suggest the meanings they hold of it. To talk about it at all reveals the continued significance of illness. Some people who live with uncertainty struggle to change it. They enlist collective effort to struggle against the illness and may resist thinking of death or decline. They believe that such thoughts will erode hope. This stance often occurs during the first crisis of illness and may be invoked during subsequent crises as well. Yet other people believe that they can never fully share their periods of greatest uncertainty. The experience separates them from ordinary reality and even from their beloved spouses (Frank, 1991). In her comment below, Teresa speaks to the consequent loneliness and the effects of illness and uncertainty on her husband:

> When you go through something like that, it's very lonely, very isolating, no matter what you do. I mean, even other cancer patients didn't know what it was like, because the cancer I had was so weird. Anaplastic carcinoma is a weirdo cancer that can kill you in a couple of weeks. And then the thing in my brain . . . well, that's just a lot for a new spouse to handle. So I certainly don't hold it against him . . . he was definitely standoffish.

Teresa's explanation of the inherent loneliness in having anaplastic carcinoma offers a glimpse of the kind of uncertainty she faces. The future may be foreboding. Unsettled emotions may lurk beneath the surface of her story, as frequently occurs in interviews of people whose lives have been torn apart (see also, Lillrank, 2002).

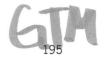

Realizing the Dream

Intentional reconstruction of self after loss takes work. It likely takes even more work when one is forced to construct a new dream. Teresa's new goal emerged during the course of her involvement in new pursuits and was a logical outcome of them. The continuity of Gail's goal before and after her injury helped her to maintain focus. For those under duress, realizing their dreams means overcoming fear and doubt.

Before their respective precipitating events, neither woman had fully realized her dream. Everyone had treated Teresa as the contender slated for stardom. Gail had to work to become a contender. Her performance before the accident, in contrast, had neither matched her expectations nor her coaches' standards for the team. Gail said, "I hadn't done as well . . . competitively and I hadn't impressed my coaches enough for them to have enough faith in me. I still had to prove myself. I needed to be in there more." For Gail, realizing her dream meant more than making a comeback to her prior performance. Instead, she had to surpass it. She had begun to make substantial progress just before her accident, but it was not enough. To be chosen for the team's starting lineup required much more. Only making the lineup would affirm Gail's competitive value and validate that she had reached her goal.

Gail worked to achieve her interrupted performance goals and previously unmet expectations. She had to deal with the disadvantages of slow healing, lost time, and lack of strength. The help, support, and empathy of her teammates spurred Gail on and a coach's proclamation, "She's going to be back," inspired her. One teammate's systematic assessments of what she had to achieve each day helped Gail manage her frustration. Yet her greatest challenge was overcoming the fear of falling again. The image of witnessing a teammate fall in a similar way that she had became etched on her mind.

With support Gail persevered and managed to overcome obstacles while grappling with fear and frustration. The effort she made and the distance she traveled gave her an enormous sense of accomplishment (see also, Galvin, 2005). She said, "During these few meets, I truly enjoyed every moment of competition. Even though I had been competitive for 13 years, never did my performance feel so significant." Paradoxically, her determined struggle to excel, despite the setback imposed by her injury, perfected her performance and placed her at the top of her game. She observed, "What had once been my weakness now became my legacy. Three years later, I continue to strive for excellence on the uneven bars, as my focus carries me closer to my dreams of athletic success than ever before."

Teresa also made great gains, perhaps not as immediately visible as Gail's but nevertheless discernible. Teresa's transition to a new life coincided with her husband's entry into her life. His view of her was not tied to her singing. He complemented her newfound intellectual interests. Teresa revealed that she now had dual sources of reference: the "more intellectual crowd" and "other cancer patients." By becoming involved in her new academic pursuits, Teresa discovered an intellect she had not realized that she possessed. As a cancer patient, she stated, "I'm proud of what I've done. . . . Feeling like, 'Okay, for a cancer patient, I'm kind of doing okay.' I'm doing stuff."

As she regained a valued self, Teresa also gained a new voice and venue as a singer. She repositioned the place of singing in her life, and now it is only part of her self-concept. Rather than seeing her current involvement in music as indicative of loss, she attributes less importance to being an opera singer. Still the shadow of cancer persists. However, Teresa will bring her experience of the past 11 years to whatever the future holds. Having endured losing her self in the surgeon's office 11 years before has given her the strength to face what lies ahead. Teresa has come full circle. She sees herself as a cancer patient who has realized new potentials and lives fully. Body and self are again unified; the devastating experience of loss has become part of her.

I can sing my own music now, so I'm a singer in an entirely new way. I've officially been in remission for over a year now, and, since my type of cancer is an angry sort, I have to go in for scans twice a year. As I see it, though, if I could get through that day in the office with that surgeon (who, by the way, I fully intend to invite to my first breakthrough gig, whatever style of music I'm singing at the time), I suppose I can get through just about anything.

Will Teresa's voice give rise to a joyous song or a melancholy refrain? Her story has not ended. The music soars and stills and yet a distant melody lingers on.

Implications

The above analysis has theoretical implications for how we view relationships between inner and outer defining attributes of self and identity and their relative visibility or invisibility. How these relationships are played out become conditions that foster either the losing or regaining of a valued self. For both these young women the relationship between visibility and invisibility became inverted. Both women had achieved visibility in their respective worlds because of their talents and skills. The illness and injury changed all that.

The evident displacement of Gail's elbow proclaimed her unmistakable injury. Simultaneously, she lost all her earlier efforts to make the team. The speed in which changes from visible performance to invisible status occur heightens loss of self. Teresa's past performance had made her recognizable

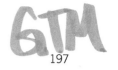

to all in her world. What had been visible and envied had become silenced and invisible. Subsequently the contrast made her disability all the more apparent and pronounced. The singer that she had been receded into the past to be replaced by the obvious scars of her surgery and the jarring sounds of her struggles to sing and to speak. In addition, the stark contrast alone between her current disabled self and her fellow music students magnified her loss. Teresa's scars and voice may not only have marked her loss of self but also symbolized it. Subsequently these symbols rendered her vulnerable to further loss as she sensed other students' stigmatizing identifications of her.

In both situations, these young women realized their loss of crucial bodily function and, by extension, their selves. They each had a heightened awareness of her body, and each predicated her self-concept on it, albeit in different ways. Hence, neither of them could ignore or minimize the losses she had sustained. Loss of self is more masked when people gradually relinquish valued pursuits or when their lives become less demanding at the same time they experience diminished physical functioning (Charmaz, 1991).

Regaining a valued self for Teresa meant leaving the world of her inspiration and her aspirations. She relinquished her hopes and her ties, both of which had been vital parts of her self. What are the conditions under which someone can relinquish such a valued part of one's life? How does a person give up those aspects of self that had uniquely defined him or her? Teresa attempted to make a comeback, but her efforts came to no avail within a time frame that she and her voice teacher could accept. Certainly a marker event can propel relinquishing the past and with it the past self. Surely the words and actions of significant people influence relinquishing a self, particularly when a person's self is already so vulnerable. Experiencing multiple moments of heightened awareness and intensified meanings of loss fosters relinquishing the past self. Teresa's voice teacher's question, "Why don't you just stop coming?" could have marked not only the end of her quest to become a mezzo-soprano but also marked a symbolic death and separation from the past. From Teresa's account, she readily agreed. If people have experienced their inability to recapture a lost self and recognize it, then they more likely accept relinquishing the past self.

Such recognition and acceptance indicates awareness of one's plight and altered self. People with a heightened awareness of loss may come to relinquish their past selves yet continue to seek to control their lives. If so, then they may make similar efforts to reestablish a new life and self that they had given to their earlier pursuits. Perhaps Teresa's awareness of her situation enabled her to reach the point of readiness to relinquish the past and move to a different future. Perhaps she gained strength from knowing that she had tried to make a comeback and had not easily given up.

The conditions that make loss so overt and overwhelming also support regaining a valued self. These two young women's sense of purpose, commit-

ment to action, and pride in achievement gave them the fortitude to perse-
vere after loss and devastation. Gail moved closer to the world in which she
aimed to achieve. She had the supportive help of teammates and coaches to
move beyond where she had been before the accident. Teresa, in contrast,
received constant messages of devaluation and difference. The students separated themselves from her as though she personified death, and the faculty
treated her as if she were dead.

The suffering caused by such loss of self cannot be denied. Yet suffering
and loss occur within a social context that may or may not support regaining
a valued self. Many poor people have lives beset by crises, and many elderly
individuals have few, if any, possibilities to reconstruct a new life and self after
serious illness. Teresa had such possibilities, and Gail apparently could afford
the needed time to return to the team and surpass her earlier performance
level. In their respective ways, both Teresa and Gail experienced an assault on
the self but not a destruction of their lives. Gail immersed herself in training,
and Teresa plunged into a new world where she found acceptance and opportunities. Not surprisingly, she found this world preferable to her former life.
Teresa emphasized the positive gains she found in this world and viewed the
voice students negatively in contrast to the people in her new life.

Quite possibly, the greater the loss, the greater the emotion work (Hochschild, 1979) in which people engage to loosen their self-concepts from the
moorings of their previous life. Perhaps Teresa's negative views of the voice
students let her relinquish what she had so greatly cherished. Teresa's hierarchy of values had shifted to fit her new life and, by contrast, the voice students
failed to measure up.[16] Forming a revised, critical view of the voice students
might be one way Teresa could neutralize loss and, simultaneously, realign
herself with new sources of identification. If so, then criticizing the voice
students likely helped solidify Teresa's belief that her life had taken a better
direction and perhaps quelled lingering regrets she might have had. By this
time, Teresa's intellectual companions and other cancer patients provided
her with new frames of reference and new measures of self. Both negative
judgments and positive measures give an individual the comparative material
to articulate a new narrative of self with fresh purposes. In sum, the person's
subsequent sense of coherence and feeling of growth allow him or her to separate self from the chaos of the past.

Notes

1. The short explanation of grounded theory in this chapter summarizes points in
   earlier writings. For more detailed portrayals of the history and logic of grounded
   theory, see Bryant and Charmaz (2007a, 2007b) and Charmaz (1983, 1990, 2000,
   2006a, 2007, 2008a, 2008b).

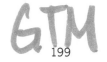

2. Curiously, Strauss's pragmatist heritage does not come across as strongly in his coauthored grounded theory manuals with Corbin as it does in his and their empirical works (Corbin & Strauss, 1988) and in his early and final works (Strauss, 1959/1969, 1961, 1993).

3. My definition of self derives from sociological social psychology in which analytic distinctions are made between concepts of self, self-concept, personal identity, and social identity. These terms may hold somewhat different meanings in psychology. In sociology, *personal identity* refers to the way an individual defines, locates, and differentiates self from others (see Hewitt, 1994), whereas *social identity* means those definitions, attributes, and social locations that others confer on the individual. Because of the fluidity and multiplicity of the self in process, the term *self-image* includes fleeting images given in experience that may or may not be congruent with the person's self-concept (Charmaz, 1991).

4. What is most significant in a study seldom is as explicit as I read these data to be. Often researchers struggle to explicate liminal processes. Grounded theory provides tools for such tasks, but ironically many grounded theorists analyze overt rather than covert processes and assumptions.

5. These properties define the loss of self that Teresa experienced and serve to define the category, "losing a valued self." I chose not to present them as formal properties because I wished to reproduce the power of the experience in the writing of it.

6. I have long argued that the quest to find a single basic social process forces a preconceived frame on the data analysis. By now, Glaser (2003) also sees this quest as derailing researchers.

7. Anaplastic carcinoma of the thyroid is a rare, fast-growing cancer that has typically metastasized by the time most patients discover the growth on their neck. Survival rates are low; fewer than 10% of those diagnosed live longer than 5 years. Health professionals describe it as an "angry" form of cancer. For more medical information about anaplastic carcinoma, see Konstantokos and Graham (2006).

8. We don't know whether Teresa was told or realized that having anaplastic carcinoma meant a struggle against death when she first received the news. Her story indicates that she realized it was a struggle against cancer but not necessarily against imminent death. Throughout Teresa's account of the unfortunate event, she emphasized loss of voice; however, she become more explicit about clinical projections of her type of cancer as the interview proceeded. Perhaps Teresa became more willing to indicate its seriousness as her rapport with the interviewer built. What she knew, when she knew it, and what meanings she attributed to it may form a silent frame around her story. She might have known the poor prognosis for some time and, of course, after learning it, she might have thought that she could beat it. Because other thyroid cancers are seldom lethal, Teresa may have had some latitude about disclosing specifics of her case. Yet the treatment she received from students and professors in the voice program suggests that they may have known which kind of cancer she had and its usual outcome.

9. Figure 6.3 diagrams the process of losing and regaining a valued self as I saw it in Teresa's data, outlines conditions for regaining a valued self, and introduces comparisons with experiencing a disrupted self.

10. Of course, the extent to which body and self are intertwined varies. A person may have long placed emphasis on other aspects of him- or herself than the functions or body parts he or she has lost. Some women who have mastectomies, for example, see themselves as much more than their missing breasts, whereas others view their femininity, sexuality—and selves—as irretrievably diminished (see, e.g., Gross & Ito, 1991).

11. For an analogous depiction of how people with mental illness define change and come to see themselves as different than other people, see Karp (1996).

12. These events and actions may include distressing medical procedures. Teresa's surgery was already scheduled, but its meaning had changed from a routine to a risky procedure that imperiled her voice.

13. Teresa's strategies resemble how professionals once controlled what patients knew about their cancer and prognosis (Quint, 1965).

14. Note that she took responsibility for *his* emotions. We don't know if this incident symbolized a culminating event or if the prospect of the changed relationship with her teacher suddenly sent her away. Was she shying away from facing yet another enormous loss head on? Was this incident the final impetus for acknowledging permanent loss of voice? We don't know. Either possibility is theoretically plausible.

15. Frail elders sometimes insist on remaining in their homes despite professionals' judgments that they cannot handle self-care. When these elders attempt to live independently but know they have failed, they become more amenable to institutional placement (Hooyman, 1988).

16. Teresa's situation is reminiscent of Festinger's (1957) treatment of cognitive dissonance. Teresa likely experienced profound dissonance as she tried to establish her new path as better than that of becoming a singer. Other individuals, such as injured athletes who are forced to seek other careers, may evince similar responses as Teresa's. Andrew Roth studied marathon runners and found that those who quit the sport describe other runners in pejorative terms. Roth heard them make derogatory statements such as, "All runners care about is their times" (personal communication, October 11, 2007).

References

Atkinson, P., Coffey, A., & Delamont, S. (2003). *Key themes in qualitative research: Continuities and change.* New York: Rowan & Littlefield.

Blumer, H. (1969). *Symbolic interactionism: Perspective and method.* Englewood Cliffs, NJ: Prentice-Hall.

Bryant, A. (2002). Re-grounding grounded theory. *Journal of Information Technology Theory and Application, 4,* 25–42.

Bryant, A. (2003). A constructive/ist response to Glaser. *FQS: Forum for Qualitative Social Research, 4*(1). Retrieved September 4, 2008, from *www.qualitative-research. net/index.php/fqs/article/view/757.*

Bryant, A., & Charmaz, K. (2007a). Grounded theory in historical perspective: An epistemological account. In A. Bryant & K. Charmaz (Eds.) *Handbook of grounded theory* (pp. 31–57). London: Sage.

Bryant, A., & Charmaz, K. (2007b). Introduction. In A. Bryant & K. Charmaz (Eds.), *Handbook of grounded theory* (pp. 1–28). London: Sage.

Bury, M. (1982). Chronic illness as biographical disruption. *Sociology of Health and Illness, 4,* 167–182.

Charmaz, K. (1973). *Time and identity: The shaping of selves of the chronically ill.* Doctoral dissertation, University of California, San Francisco.

Charmaz, K. (1983). Loss of self: A fundamental form of suffering in the chronically ill. *Sociology of Health and Illness, 5*(2), 168–195.

Charmaz, K. (1987). Struggling for a self: Identity levels of the chronically ill. In J. A. Roth & P. Conrad (Eds.), *Research in the sociology of health care: The experience and management of chronic illness* (Vol. 6, pp. 283–321). Greenwich, CT: JAI Press.

Charmaz, K. (1990). "Discovering" chronic illness: Using grounded theory. *Social Science and Medicine, 30,* 1161–1172.

Charmaz, K. (1991). *Good days, bad days: The self in chronic illness and time.* New Brunswick, NJ: Rutgers University Press.

Charmaz, K. (1994). Discoveries of self in chronic illness. In M. L. Dietz, R. Prus, & W. Shaffir (Eds.), *Doing everyday life: Ethnography as human lived experience* (pp. 226–242). Mississauga, Ontario: Copp Clark Longman.

Charmaz, K. (1995). The body, identity and self: Adapting to impairment. *Sociological Quarterly, 36,* 657–680.

Charmaz, K. (1997). Grief and loss of self. In K. Charmaz, G. Howarth, & A. Kellehear (Eds.), *The unknown country: Death in Australia, Britain and the U.S.A.* (pp. 229–241). London: Macmillan; New York: St. Martin's.

Charmaz, K. (1999). Stories of suffering: Subjects' tales and research narratives. *Qualitative Health Research, 9,* 369–382.

Charmaz, K. (2000). Constructivist and objectivist grounded theory. In N. K. Denzin & Y. Lincoln (Eds.), *Handbook of qualitative research* (2nd ed., pp. 509–535). Thousand Oaks, CA: Sage.

Charmaz, K. (2002). Stories and silences: Disclosures and self in chronic illness. *Qualitative Inquiry, 8,* 302–328.

Charmaz, K. (2006a). *Constructing grounded theory: A practical guide through qualitative analysis.* London: Sage.

Charmaz, K. (2006b). The self. In G. Ritzer (Ed.), *Encyclopedia of sociology.* Cambridge, MA: Blackwell.

Charmaz, K. (2007). Constructionism and the grounded theory method. In J. A. Holstein & J. F. Gubrium (Eds.), *Handbook of constructionist research.* (pp. 397–412). New York: Guilford Press.

Charmaz, K. (2008a). Grounded theory as an emergent method. In S. N. Hesse-Biber & P. Leavy (Eds.), *Handbook of emergent methods* (pp. 155–170). New York: Guilford Press.

Charmaz, K. (2008b). Grounded theory. In J. A. Smith (Ed.), *Qualitative psychology: A practical guide to research methods* (2nd ed., pp. 82–110). London: Sage.

Charmaz, K. (2008c). The legacy of Anselm Strauss for constructivist grounded theory. In N. K. Denzin (Ed.), *Studies in symbolic interaction* (Vol. 32, pp. 127–141). Bingley, UK: Emerald.

Charmaz, K. (2009). Recollecting good and bad days. In W. Shaffir, A. Puddephatt, & S. Kleinknecht (Eds.), *Ethnographies revisited: The stories behind the story*. New York: Routledge.

Charmaz, K., & Henwood, K. (2007). Grounded theory in psychology. In C. Willig & W. Stainton-Rogers (Eds.), *Handbook of qualitative research in psychology* (pp. 240–259). London: Sage.

Ciambrone, D. (2007). Illness and other assaults on self: The relative impact of HIV/AIDS on women's lives. *Sociology of Health and Illness, 23*(4), 517–540.

Clarke, A. E. (2003). Situational analyses: Grounded theory mapping after the postmodern turn. *Symbolic Interaction 26*(4), 553–576.

Clarke, A. E. (2005). *Situational analysis: Grounded theory after the postmodern turn*. Thousand Oaks, CA: Sage.

Clarke, A. E. (2006). Feminisms, grounded theory, and situational analysis. In S. Hesse-Biber & D. Leckenby (Eds.), *Handbook of feminist research methods* (pp. 345–370). Thousand Oaks, CA: Sage.

Corbin, J. M., & Strauss, A. (1988). *Unending care and work*. San Francisco: Jossey-Bass.

Corbin, J. M., & Strauss, A. (2008). *Basics of qualitative research: Grounded theory procedures and techniques* (3rd ed.). Thousand Oaks, CA: Sage.

Denzin, N. K., & Lincoln, Y. S. (1994). Preface. In N. K. Denzin & Y. S. Lincoln (Eds.), *Handbook of qualitative research* (pp. ix–xii). Thousand Oaks, CA: Sage.

Festinger, L. (1957). *A theory of cognitive dissonance*. Palo Alto, CA: Stanford University Press.

Frank, A. W. (1991). *At the will of the body*. Boston: Houghton Mifflin.

Galvin, R. D. (2005). Researching the disabled identity: Contextualizing the identity transformations which accompany the onset of impairment. *Sociology of Health and Illness, 27*(3), 393–413.

Gecas, V. (1982). The self-concept. *Annual Review of Sociology, 8*, 1–33.

Glaser, B. G. (1978). *Theoretical sensitivity*. Mill Valley, CA: Sociology Press.

Glaser, B. G. (1992). *Basics of grounded theory analysis*. Mill Valley, CA: Sociology Press.

Glaser, B. G. (1998). *Doing grounded theory: Issues and discussions*. Mill Valley, CA: Sociology Press.

Glaser, B. G. (2003). *The grounded theory perspective: Description's remodeling of grounded theory methodology*. Mill Valley, CA: Sociology Press.

Glaser, B. G. (2008). *Doing quantitative grounded theory*. Mill Valley, CA: Sociology Press.

Glaser, B. G., & Strauss, A. L. (1967). *The discovery of grounded theory: Strategies for qualitative research*. Chicago: Aldine.

Goffman, E. (1963). *Stigma*. Englewood Cliffs, NJ: Prentice-Hall.

Gross, A., & Ito, D. (1991). *Women talk about breast cancer*. New York: HarperCollins.

Hallberg, L. R. M. (2006). The "core category" of grounded theory: Making constant comparisons. *International Journal of Qualitative Studies on Health and Well-Being, 1*(3), 141–148.

Henwood, K., & Pidgeon, N. (2003). Grounded theory in psychological research. In P. M. Camic, J. E. Rhodes, & L. Yardley (Eds.), *Qualitative research in psychology: Expanding perspectives in methodology and design* (pp. 131–155). Washington, DC: American Psychological Association.

Hewitt, J. P. (1994). *Self and society: A symbolic interactionist social psychology.* Boston: Allyn & Bacon.

Hochschild, A. (1979). Emotion work, feeling rules, and social structure. *American Journal of Sociology, 85*, 551–575.

Hood, J. C. (2007). Orthodoxy vs. power: The defining traits of grounded theory. In A. Bryant & K. Charmaz (Eds.), *Handbook of grounded theory* (pp. 151–164). London: Sage.

Hooyman, N. (1988). *Taking care of your aging family members.* New York: Free Press.

Karp, D. (1996). *Speaking of sadness: Depression, disconnection, and the meanings of illness.* New York: Oxford University Press.

Konstantokos, A. K., & Graham, D. J. (2006). Thyroid, anaplastic carcinoma. *E-medicine from Webb MD.* Retrieved July 28, 2006, from *www.emedicine.com/med/topic2687. htmon.*

Lillrank, A. (2002). The tension between overt talk and covert emotions in illness narrative: Transition from clinician to researcher. *Culture, Medicine and Psychiatry, 26*, 111–127.

Madill, A. J., Jordan, A., & Shirley, C. (2000). Objectivity and reliability in qualitative analysis: Realist, contextualist, and radical constructionist epistemologies. *British Journal of Psychology, 91*, 1–20.

Mairs, N. (1986). *Plaintext: Essays.* Tucson, AZ: University of Arizona Press.

Mathieson, C., & Stam, H. (1995). Renegotiating identity: Cancer narratives. *Sociology of Health and Illness, 17*(3), 283–306.

Mead, G. H. (1932). *The philosophy of the present.* La Salle, IL: Open Court.

Melia, K. M. (1996). Rediscovering Glaser. *Qualitative Health Research, 6*, 368–378.

Mills, J., Bonner, A., & Francis, K. (2006a). Adopting a constructivist approach to grounded theory: Implications for research design. *International Journal of Nursing Practice, 12*(1–February), 8–13.

Mills, J., Bonner, A., & Francis, K. (2006b). The development of constructivist grounded theory. *International Journal of Qualitative Methods, 5*(1–April), 1–10.

Murphy, R. F. (1987). *The body silent.* New York: Henry Holt.

Peirce, C. S. (1958). *Collected papers.* Cambridge, MA: Harvard University Press.

Quint, J. C. (1965). Institutionalized practices of information control. *Psychiatry, 28*, 119–132.

Reich, J. A., & Brindis, C. D. (2006). Conceiving risk and responsibility: A qualitative examination of men's experiences of unintended pregnancy and abortion. *International Journal of Men's Health, 5*(2), 133–152.

Reichertz, J. (2007). Abduction: The logic of discovery of grounded theory. In A. Bryant & K. Charmaz (Eds.), *Handbook of grounded theory* (pp. 214–228). London: Sage.

Ricoeur, P. (1991). Life in quest of narrative. In D. Wood (Ed.), *On Paul Ricoeur: Narrative and interpretation.* London: Routledge.

Rosenthal, G. (2004). Biographical research. In C. Seale, G. Gobo, J. F. Gubrium, & D. Silverman (Eds.), *Qualitative research practice* (pp. 48–64). London: Sage.

Ross, M., & Buehler, R. (2004). Identity through time: Constructing personal pasts and futures. In M. B. Brewer & M. Hewstone (Eds.), *Self and social identity* (pp. 25–51). Malden, MA: Blackwell.

Scambler, G., & Scambler, S. (Eds.). (2010). *New directions in the sociology of chronic and disabling conditions: Assaults on the life-world.* London: Palgrave Macmillan.

Scott, K. W. (2004). Relating categories in grounded theory analysis: Using a conditional relationship guide and reflective coding matrix. *Qualitative Report, 9*(1), 113–126.

Strauss, A. L. (1959/1969). *Mirrors and masks.* Mill Valley, CA: Sociology Press.

Strauss, A. L. (1961). *Images of the American city.* New York: Free Press.

Strauss, A. L. (1987). *Qualitative analysis for social scientists.* New York: Cambridge University Press.

Strauss, A. L. (1993). *Continual permutations of action.* New York: Aldine de Gruyter.

Strauss, A., & Corbin, J. (1990). *Basics of qualitative research: Grounded theory procedures and techniques.* Newbury Park, CA: Sage.

Strauss, A., & Corbin, J. (1998). *Basics of qualitative research: Grounded theory procedures and techniques* (2nd ed.). Thousand Oaks, CA: Sage.

Torres, V., & Hernandez, E. (2007). The influence of ethnic identity on self-authorship: A longitudinal study of Latino/a college students. *Journal of College Student Development, 48*(5), 558–573.

Turner, R. (1976). The real self: From institution to impulse. *American Journal of Sociology, 81,* 989–1016.

Tweed, A., & Charmaz, K. (in press). Grounded theory for counseling psychologists. In A. Thompson & D. Harper (Eds.), *Qualitative research methods in mental health and psychotherapy: A guide for students and practitioners.* London: Wiley-Blackwell.

Ville, I. (2005). Biographical work and returning to employment following a spinal cord injury. *Sociology of Health and Illness, 27*(3), 324–350.

Whiting, J. B. (2008). The role of appraisal distortion, contempt, and morality in couple conflict: A grounded theory. *Journal of Marital and Family Therapy, 34*(1), 44–57.

Williamson, K. (2006). Research in constructivist frames using ethnographic techniques. *Library Trends, 55*(1), 83–101.

? ethnographic ?

A Discursive Analysis of Teresa's Protocol

Enhancing Oneself, Diminishing Others

Linda M. McMullen

My analytic location for our project is discursive psychology, which involves the application of ideas from discourse analysis to issues in psychology (Potter, 2003). Discourse analysis has been designated a method of analysis; a methodology; a perspective on social life that involves metatheoretical, theoretical, and analytic principles; and a critique of mainstream psychology (Crotty, 1998; Potter, 2003; Willig, 2003; Wood & Kroger, 2000). It is both a way of conceptualizing and analyzing language.

The numerous varieties of discourse analysis reveal its multidisciplinary origins in various branches of philosophy, sociology, linguistics, psychology, and literary theory (Wood & Kroger, 2000). From a focus on how sentences are put together (e.g., linguistics), to how conversation or talk-in-interaction is structured (e.g., conversational analysis), to how sets of statements come to constitute objects and subjects (e.g., Foucauldian discourse analysis), to how discourse can be understood in relation to social problems, structural variables (e.g., race, gender, class), and power (e.g., critical discourse analysis), this approach to thinking about and analyzing language encompasses varied (and often opposing) sets of principles (Potter, 2004; Willig, 2003; Wood & Kroger, 2000). As outlined by Wood and Kroger (2000, p. 18), the many varieties of discourse analysis differ on dimensions such as epistemological position (e.g., constructionist vs. critical realist), nature and role of theory (e.g., as explanatory tool or discursive text available for analysis; as foundational or peripheral), the sorts of data that are analyzed (e.g., researcher-generated or naturalistic), how context is understood and treated (e.g., as background and to be acknowledged or as determinative and to be analyzed), and how claims are warranted (e.g., empirically, theoretically, ideologically). As such, *discourse analysis* is a nonspecific term.

While the variation in types of discourse analysis enables the articulation of similarities and differences on these dimensions, it has also facilitated the blurring of boundaries between approaches and the opportunity for researchers to adapt particular approaches to their research questions and goals. For example, Wetherell (1998) argued for a synthesis of the more "molecular" approach of conversational analysis with the more "molar" style of poststructuralist or Foucauldian analysis. Such a combination focuses attention on how discursive resources are deployed in particular contexts in order to accomplish specific social actions as well as on the wider social and institutional frameworks that shape such deployment (Willig, 2003). Following the spirit of Wetherell (1998), I relied, in the present project, on a form of discourse analysis that has its basis in social psychology (Potter & Wetherell, 1987) and that is sometimes referred to as discourse analysis in social psychology (DASP; Wood & Kroger, 2000), and I attended to context and social consequences and to background normative conceptions (Wetherell, 1998, p. 405) in my analysis.

The foundations of DASP are typically located in Austin's (1962) speech act theory, which stressed the performative aspects of language use, and in ethnomethodology, which shifted the study of talk to a topic of research in its own right (Potter & Wetherell, 1987). The earliest work appears to be a 1985 publication by Litton and Potter, which was followed by the first major statement of the approach in Potter and Wetherell's 1987 book (Potter, 2003). As a critique of mainstream social psychology, DASP took several key constructs (e.g., attitudes, cognitions, categories, the self) and reworked them (Potter, 2004). For example, attitudes were no longer thought to be something "held" by people "about" an object or event. Rather, they were understood as discursive positions variously taken up in the interest of accomplishing specific ends in a particular context. Contradiction became, then, something expected and worthy of study, rather than a problem to be explained away. Similarly, talk was no longer understood solely in representational terms and as a route to cognitions; rather, it became a focus of research in its own right. Objects and events were understood not as giving rise to mental representations, but rather as being actively constructed through language itself. The consequence of this radical move is that many of our taken-for-granted, so-called foundational psychological concepts (e.g., prejudice, identity, or, in the present case, resilience) become something people *do* rather than something people *have* (Willig, 2003). So, unlike many other qualitative methodologies, the focus of analysis is not the person. As noted by Wood and Kroger (2000), discourse analysis does not assume that "personality traits, as conventionally defined, determine actions in a variety of different situations." (p. 10)

This approach emphasizes three core features of discourse, as outlined by Potter (2003). The first—action orientation—sees discourse as a form of social action; as such, the focus of a discursive analysis is on how participants use discursive resources (e.g., metaphors, narrative, categories) and with what effects. With this focus on performance, the goal becomes to identify the business that is being done in talk. The second feature—situation—is understood in three ways. That is, discourse is organized sequentially such that each utterance is understood (at least in part) in relation to what precedes and follows it; it is situated institutionally in the sense that it may be shaped (again, in part) by local norms; and it can be situated rhetorically in that it can be fashioned to resist attempts to undermine or counter it. The third feature—construction—refers to the notion that discourse is both constructed—that is, built from various resources, such as categories, narrative, and metaphor—and constructive—that is, versions of the world, actions, and events are built in talk.

One of the criticisms of this way of conceptualizing discourse is that DASP restricts its focus to the texts that are being analyzed and, by doing so, overlooks the influence of who the speakers are and the broader social context in which the texts are produced. This latter emphasis is in keeping with a poststructuralist (sometimes designated *Foucauldian*) approach to discourse analysis, which is distinguished from DASP in at least two other significant ways. First, discourse is assumed to construct its subjects and to make meanings available to them rather than, in DASP, being a tool that can be used by active agents, and second, discourse is considered to be implicated in experience, as opposed to invocations of experience being considered a discursive move (Willig, 2001, 2003). Although not all discourse analysts agree that these two approaches can be combined (e.g., Parker, 1997), I take up Wetherell's (1998) position that it is possible to attend both to the ways in which speakers deploy discursive resources in particular situations and to the broader social and institutional contexts that shape such deployment.

From years of empirical research with these discursive approaches and others, there now exists a number of analytic concepts and strategies that can be drawn upon in any investigation. For example, Wood and Kroger (2000) specified numerous concepts that relate to content, features, form, structure, or function, as well as many notions that derive from other discourse analytic traditions (e.g., positioning, facework, narrative, ideological dilemmas) and are used by those who situate themselves in the DASP tradition. In addition, they outlined several strategies (e.g., reframing, focusing on participants' meaning, being sensitive to multiple functions and variability) that can be employed in the process of analyzing discourse.

These concepts and strategies can be applied to a range of written, spoken, and visual materials. Although the researcher-generated interview has typically been a method of choice, there is now a move away from this method of data generation to what are deemed "naturalistic" sources of data, that is, material that exists independently of the research project. The analysis typically begins with relatively unmotivated reading(s) of the materials as a way of developing a sense of what they are doing. "Readings" can involve not only involvement with the written word, but also engagement with audio and visual materials. Following these initial readings, the analyst begins to develop a broad set of concerns or questions, often on the basis of what has struck him or her as intriguing. The analyst then searches all of what is available for analysis in order to select those parts of the materials that are considered relevant to the initially articulated concerns or questions. At this point, all potentially relevant parts are included, with the understanding that as the focus of the investigation is further refined, many of these parts will be excluded from the detailed analysis. Further work with those parts selected for in-depth and intensive analysis involves an iterative cycling between specifying and addressing the question(s) of the investigation. Questions often take the form of "How is X constructed?", "What is being done and how is it being done?", or "What are the functions and consequences of what is being done?"

While working with the selected parts, the analyst attends to context and variability and to those concepts deemed relevant to the research question(s) (e.g., content, stylistic and grammatical features, figures of speech, interpretative repertoires or systematically related sets of terms, categories, forms of argument) (Potter, 2003; Willig, 2003). Analytic strategies can include substituting terms to determine function, reframing participants' utterances in terms of the discourse analytic perspective, alerting oneself to the possibility of multiple functions, attending to similarity and difference in accounts, and focusing on participants' meaning (Wood & Kroger, 2000). The outcome is an empirically based set of claims and interpretations. That is, the analyst shows how his or her claims are warranted by referencing specific features and functions of the text. In the spirit of Wetherell (1998), interpretations are understood in terms of, and placed in a description of, background normative conceptions deemed relevant by the analyst. It is important to note that the focus of the investigation can change many times throughout the analysis, that many questions can be asked of the data, and that one's analysis is never complete.

The Process of My Analysis

I began the process of analysis by noting the kind of material with which we were working and the contexts in which this material was produced. Specifically, we had four texts available to us. Each was produced as part of a project exploring how people resiliently come to terms with misfortune; this project was conducted to enable students in a graduate course on qualitative methods in psychology to learn about interviewing. The first was a protocol written by Teresa, a 30-year-old doctoral student in psychology, in response to the following instructions: *Describe in writing a situation when something very unfortunate happened to you. Please begin your description prior to the unfortunate event. Share in detail what happened, what you felt and did, and what happened after, including how you responded and what came of this event in your life.* The second was a short synopsis written by a fellow graduate student, a male who served as the interviewer of Teresa, in which he outlines his goal for the interview, how he conceptualized the notion of resiliency, and how this conceptualization influenced his questioning. The third text was the transcript of the interview with Teresa, and the fourth was a transcript of another interview from the same project to be used for comparison purposes, if desired. I consider the data from which we worked as four texts rather than two data sets—that of Teresa and of Gail—because each of the four texts is generated in a particular context that must be taken into account in the analysis.

I read the first three texts in their entirety in a fairly undirected fashion, without making any notes. I then waited a week, read them again in their entirety, and began to jot notes in the margins. These notes were not particularly directed; some were paraphrases of parts of the text, some consisted of what I thought might be key words, some were descriptions of what I thought the speaker was doing. In subsequent readings, I began to be more directed and to draw on analytic concepts used by discourse analysts—for example, positioning of oneself and others (how and in what ways people locate themselves and others in the talk about a topic; Davies & Harré, 1990), interpretative repertoires ("recurrently used systems of terms used for characterizing and evaluating actions, events and other phenomena"; Potter & Wetherell, 1987, p. 149), patterns, and variability. I then stepped back and thought about how the original project might have come to be framed in terms of *resilience*, *coping*, and *recovery* and about the possible consequences of such framing. I then searched for a definition of *resilience*. I wondered what a common (perhaps Westernized) understanding of this word was, and how such an understanding might have influenced what and how the participants talked about the topic. A common dictionary definition was "the ability to recover quickly from illness, change, or misfortune; buoyancy" (Morris, 1970, p. 1106). I then searched for a definition of *recover*, which I found to mean "to regain a normal or usual condition or state, as of health; the getting back of something lost" (Morris, 1970, p. 1090). In thinking about the focus of the project from which the data were derived, these definitions of key words, and my initial set of notes, I began to think in terms of actual or implied contrasts: before and after; normality and unusualness; illness and health; misfortune and survival.

With the notion of contrast in mind, I engaged in several analytic maneuvers. For example, I read the interviewer's turns of talk in isolation from those of the interviewee. I read the second interview with a student we had named "Gail," not so much for the purpose of analyzing it, but with an eye to how it contrasted with the interview with Teresa. I then considered several questions: How are the three primary texts similar and different from each other? What is absent from/present in them? How are the writer/interviewee and others positioned in these accounts? At this point in the analysis, I began to think about how Teresa had positioned herself (on occasion) as a special, talented, unusual, take-charge person, and others as flawed, weak, and not there for her.

Before proceeding further, however, I decided to step back from the analysis and pose a series of questions that could be asked of the data. These questions included: How does one structure an account of "resiliently coming to terms with misfortune" (or trauma)? How is misfortune constructed in the texts? How is the psychology of resiliency constructed in the texts? How do the participants "do resilience"? Although such questions are often interrelated and are typical foci for discourse analysts, they do offer different ways of proceeding with an analysis, and I knew I had to articulate precisely what my focus would be.

At this point, I became intrigued with the notion of the instrument and of instrumentality as metaphors for Teresa's story about the loss of her singing voice (her instrument) and her response to this loss (her instrumentality). I played around with the multiple meanings of *instrument* (e.g., a device for giving controlled musical sounds; a means by which something is done; a person used and controlled by another to perform an action) and of *instrumentality* (serving as an instrument or means; agency), and I began to think of how Teresa was "doing instrumentality" and of how she was constructing others as instruments (i.e., in terms of what they did for her or what they failed to do for her).

I began, then, to extract excerpts that I thought might speak to the notion of the instrumentality of oneself and others. During this part of the analytic process, I also thought about how the contexts in which these data were generated—that is, as a written account and via an interview produced for a class project—might have influenced the data. Specifically, we were informed that in preparation for carrying out the class project from which these data were derived, students had discussed pursuing themes of social support and agency in their attempts to learn something about how people resiliently come to terms with misfortune. I wondered about the extent to which the graduate students involved in this project might want to show themselves (to each other and to their professor) as agents, and I reasoned that if "doing agency" was important, then too much talk of social support might be deemed to undermine this action.

My selection of extracts for analysis then became more focused. I chose extracts in which Teresa variously positions herself as an agent or a patient; in which she provides significant detail about her own actions and accomplishments or an absence of details about the actions of others; in which she dismisses others; in which others' support is constructed as naturally provided and to-be-expected, contingent, or not readily available; or in which she undoes such support.

It was only at this point that I did a brief search of the literature on loss, trauma, and resilience. One of the so-called pathways to resilience, self-enhancement or overly positive biases in favor of the self (Bonanno, 2004), seemed a particularly apt term for what I deemed a primary action that Teresa was performing in her talk. Because I saw her talk about others as contrasting with her talk about herself, I then searched for a word that I thought captured this contrast and eventually settled on *diminishing*.

For the purposes of illustrating how discourse analysis can be applied to the texts we have chosen for analysis, I focus, then, on what I consider to be one prominent social action that was performed by Teresa: what I label "enhancing oneself, diminishing others." I use the word *enhancing* in the sense of increasing the value or reputation of oneself, and I use *diminishing* to refer to a lessening of the presence of the other, to a construction of the other as less able to cope, and to criticizing the other.

My Analysis: Enhancing Oneself, Diminishing Others

From the material available to us, I worked up two variations of how "enhancing oneself, diminishing others" is performed discursively. The first pattern, based on two extracts from Teresa's written account, consists of enhancing oneself through detailed claims of being an accomplished, in-charge agent and diminishing others by constructing them as unable to cope or by making them peripheral to the account.

Pattern One

EXTRACT 1

1 All my friends had been fellow singers, and I knew that they couldn't bear the discomfort of
2 being around me under the circumstances; my voice teacher, who was like another father to me,
3 greeted me in tears each time he saw me afterwards . . . he was there for my surgery, and was the
4 last person I saw before my anesthesia kicked in. Seeing the dreams we had built together
5 go to pieces the way they did was just too much for either of us, and we spoke very little after
6 that.

7 Many suggested that I take a break from school, that no one would think any less of me, but I
8 was determined to move on as if nothing had happened. When I met new people, I no longer
9 introduced myself as a singer, which was strange for me. Now, I was a psychology major, and I
10 told people this as though I had always been. I suddenly had nonmusician friends, which was
11 also odd, yet strangely refreshing. I was having conversations that I never had the opportunity for
12 in my previous life; my friends now were philosophers, scientists, poets, and historians, and I
13 was learning of a life beyond the hallowed catacombs of practice rooms, voice studios, and
14 recital halls. On top of that, I took up fencing, motorcycling, rock climbing, and theater
15 acting, and seemed to do pretty well. Frankly, I just wanted to live as much as I possibly could,
16 and do everything imaginable while I was at it.

In lines 1 and 2, Teresa constructs her friends and fellow singers as distressed by what has happened to her, but also implies that they were not there to support her. The statement "I knew they couldn't bear the discomfort of being around me under the circumstances" casts them as not up to the task that was required of them. Note that there is no mention of any actions undertaken by these fellow singers. Teresa then constructs her voice teacher as an important person in her life and as one who is deeply affected by her circumstances, but with whom her relationship fades over time (lines 2–6). Although she supplies a few details about her encounters with her voice teacher, his actions are cast as invariable and passive. For example, saying that he "greeted me in tears each time he saw me afterwards" constructs him as having only one rather passive response, and the phrase "he was there for my surgery" is notable for its absence of details about his actions during this important time. A lack of agency or intervening action is also present in the statements "[s]eeing the dreams we had built together go to pieces that way" and "we spoke very little after that."

In lines 7–16, Teresa makes an abrupt shift away from others as subject to herself as subject. She introduces and prefaces this part of her account by first setting herself apart from others. The statement "Many suggested that I take a break from school, that no one would think any less of me, but I was determined to move on as if nothing had happened" casts her as taking an un-ordinary and self-directed path. She then goes on to construct herself as having fashioned a new life as "a psychology major" and as actively embracing life ("I took up fencing, motorcycling, rock climbing, and theater acting"), and she evaluates this new life and her performance of it positively (having nonmusician friends is "strangely refreshing"; she "seemed to do pretty well" at fencing, motorcycling, rock climbing, and theater acting). In addition, she claims status for herself by categorizing her new friends as "philosophers, scientists, poets, and historians." In this latter part of the extract, which is structured as a long list, nearly all sentences begin with "I" followed by an action verb. This repeated use of similar sentence structure works to emphasize her point. Other people are occasionally mentioned, but only as the generalized other—for example, "many," "new people," "nonmusician friends," "philosophers, scientists, poets, and historians." They do not figure prominently as coproducers of her new life.

Of note, then, in this extract is that Teresa's construction of others is comparatively brief and lacking in agential actions, while her construction of herself is longer, more detailed, and full of such actions. I argue, then, that she diminishes others by constructing them as sensitive and unable to cope and by supplying relatively few details about their actions, while she engages in self-enhancement by adopting a discourse of agency, independence, and self-directedness.

The second extract that illustrates this particular pattern of "enhancing oneself, diminishing others" occurs three sentences later and forms most of the last paragraph of Teresa's written account.

EXTRACT 2

1 It took an extra year to get through my undergrad work due to the change of major, during which
2 I met and married my very nonmusical, very academically inclined husband. I began
3 contemplating what to do with my bachelor's degree in psychology when, three years after my
4 surgery, my singing voice began to come back. Ridiculous timing. While holding down my nine-
5 to-five job, I bean [sic] working slowly toward getting my voice back in shape, and eventually
6 maintained my own voice studio of around sixty students, serving as my own poster child for the
7 miracles of good voice technique. I sang with two opera choruses, got back into singing at
8 weddings and church services a bit, even visited my old voice teacher a few times for a few
9 lessons. Still, I loved my newfound intellectual life, and I didn't want to give it all up and go
10 back to the grind of full-time classical singing. Besides, I had discovered that, while my voice
11 was still misbehaving (and often does, to this day), I could sing other kinds of music pretty well,
12 particularly rock and blues. I began tinkering with writing my own music, and eventually
13 acquired my own regular gigs at night clubs and live music venues. I continued in my
14 psychology work, as I do now, for I love it dearly, particularly in that it brought forth in me a part
15 of myself I never knew I had, one that seems to hold its own well enough with the more
16 intellectual crowd.

From lines 7–9 and again from lines 12–14, there is, as in the previous extract, a focus on the "I" as agent and a detailed listing of her actions (e.g., "I sang with two opera choruses, got back into singing at weddings and church services a bit"; "I began tinkering with writing my own music"; "I continued in my psychology work"). In addition, Teresa continues to construct herself as determined. For example, her use of *eventually* in line 5 and again in line 12 implies that it took time to accomplish what she did. And her accomplishments continue to be constructed as extraordinary. She not only worked toward getting her voice back in shape; she did so "[w]hile holding down [her] nine-to-five job." She not only maintained her own voice studio, but it was a voice studio "of around 60 students"—clearly no small feat. Again, Teresa also engages in positive self-evaluation (e.g., "serving as my own poster child for the miracles of good voice technique"; "I could sing other kinds of music pretty well"; "a part of myself . . . that seems to hold its own well enough with the more intellectual crowd").

This construction of oneself as exceptional, along with the positioning of oneself as agential, is woven around two very brief mentions of others. In lines 1 and 2, she states that it was during her undergraduate program that she "met and married my very nonmusical, very academically inclined husband." Then in lines 8 and 9 she states that she "even visited my old voice teacher a few times for a few lessons." In both of these instances, the other is referenced in terms of the role they occupy in Teresa's life—as husband, as teacher. No actions are attributed to them, and no mention is made of their impact in Teresa's life.

In this second extract, then, the other is again diminished by a sheer absence of detail. In contrast, Teresa enhances herself by providing a lot of detail about her actions and accomplishments, and by positioning herself as an independent agent in charge of her own life. Taken together, these first two extracts indicate a pattern of talk in which others are diminished by constructing them as unable to cope or by making them peripheral to the account, while one's own person is enhanced through detailed claims of being an accomplished, in-charge agent. Such a pattern might be understood, at least within parts of the Western world, in terms of a cultural discourse of resilience as exceptionality—that is, as thriving under adversity largely due to one's own initiative and talents and with little involvement of, or assistance from, others.

Pattern Two

The second variation in the discursive action of "enhancing oneself, diminishing others" consists of enhancing oneself by claiming to be unique, unusual, and especially talented, and diminishing others by constructing their actions as having adverse consequences for oneself. The following two extracts are from the interview between Teresa, as interviewee, and her fellow male graduate student, as interviewer. In the very brief introduction to the interview that was written by the interviewer, he states that "[a]fter conducting the interview, I realized how I had 'conceptualized' the idea of resiliency. My questions were geared towards trying to find sources of support because I believed that resilience cannot happen without a source of strength or support." I found this statement particularly interesting in light of how little of Teresa's written account was focused on others' support. The third extract begins with a comment and a directive from the interviewer (in italics):

1 *You mentioned your friends not being able to stand being around you because they knew how*

2 *much pain you were in. Describe how that manifested itself, in terms of their actions or their*

3 *relationships with you.*

4 They disappeared from my life. And I think that was on both our parts; we're talking about dear,

5 dear friends, of which I've retained one . . . I think we were so close that nothing was going to

6 drive a stake through that. But you have to remember that we're dealing with a voice studio and a

7 voice school where everything is very competitive, and everybody knows who's who and what

8 they're capable of, and voice parts having their different animosities between themselves . . .

9 there's always a queen bee. I was the freak *wunderkind* mezzo-soprano at the music school that

10 got the auditions, got the solos, got the favoritism from directors. I didn't really want things like

11 that, because it sucked. By default, people started hating me. I had graduate students come up to

12 me in the halls and threaten me . . . it was weird. But it was my calling . . . it was me, it was what I

13 had to do. To hell with the grad students. It was me, who I was . . . and everyone just kind of knew

14 I was going to be something someday.

Of note at the beginning of this extract is how the reaction of Teresa's friends is constructed. Recall that in extract 1 from her written account she stated "All my friends had been fellow singers, and I knew that they couldn't bear the discomfort of being around me under the circumstances." Such a statement has the potential to cast the friends as empathically in tune with (and perhaps overwhelmed by) Teresa's (and perhaps their own) pain over the loss of her singing voice. In lines 1 and 2 of extract 3, the interviewer recasts this statement as "You mentioned your friends not being able to stand being around you because they knew how much pain you were in." The phrase "not being able to stand being around you" can be understood in two ways: (1) that they could not tolerate Teresa's (and perhaps their own) pain, or (2) that Teresa was unbearable to be around. This statement by the interviewer is then followed by Teresa's crisp, direct, evocative statement, "They disappeared from my life." Again, in contrast to her written account in which there is no mention of any actions taken by her friends, she now constructs their actions as active avoidance. Although Teresa concedes in a qualified way that she, too, might have disappeared from their lives ("And I think that was on both our parts"), she does not elaborate on her own actions. Her use of the phrase "we're talking dear, dear friends" (lines 4 and 5) also suggests that one would expect behavior other than disappearance from them. Again, there is a brief interlude where Teresa makes reference to the one friend she has retained (lines 5 and 6). However, like the absences of detail noted in the previous two extracts, she makes no further mention of this person's contribution during her cancer treatment.

Teresa then constructs the voice studio/school as a competitive, status-conscious ("everybody knows who's who and what they're capable of"), hostile environment (lines 6–9). Doing so enables her friends' actions to be explained as normative, rather than as particular to her, and, as such, can serve a face-saving function. Although it is unclear in line 9 whether Teresa is claiming the "queen bee" status for herself, she clearly constructs herself in lines 9 and 10 as unusual, talented, and special, and as getting what presumably every voice student would want. Her use of the German "*wunderkind*" rather than the English "child prodigy" (line 9) also serves as a way of setting herself apart. She goes on to claim not to "really want things like that," and constructs others' responses to her talent and special recognition as out of her control ("by default"). She continues to position herself as a "patient" (i.e., as someone who is seen to suffer the consequences of external forces or internal compulsions) as opposed to as an "agent" (as she did in the previous two extracts) by constructing her talent as her "calling," by using "Dummy it" (i.e., a pronoun whose referent is unspecified; Penelope, 1990) rather than "I" as the subject, and by employing the modal element "had to" as a way of denying her agency (lines 12 and 13). In contrast, her fellow students (even those who were more senior than she) are constructed as jealous and spiteful (". . . people started hating me. I had graduate students come up to me in the halls and threaten me . . ."), and as not worth worrying about ("To hell with the grad students").

I am arguing, then, that in this extract Teresa diminishes others by constructing them as unavailable, competitive, and jealous and by dismissing their significance, while she enhances herself by claiming to be unusual, unique, and destined for fame. Of note is that this extract marks a shift away from the positioning of others as passive or inconsequential, and herself as active and agential, as was the case in the first two extracts. However, this pattern of talk that casts others as nonsupportive, or even vengeful, in circumstances and situations over which one has no control can, again, make the achievement of actions that we, in the Western world, label "resilience" all the more noteworthy. It also highlights a conception of social support as necessary and expected for this achievement.

EXTRACT 4

1 of course, my voice teacher would just openly cry in front of me. I just couldn't handle that,
2 you know? I mean, I really cared about this guy, and I was just bringing him way down. And
3 then one day, I was leaning on the piano in the studio, and he was sitting at the keyboard, and
4 we were having this sad lesson . . . and he just looked at me and said, "Why don't you just stop
5 coming?" And I said, "You're right." And that's the last time I went to the studio. It was like
6 that. It was like that. Plus, I was in every top choir in the school . . . and this was a school with
7 a pretty hard-core choral program . . . recordings, international tours, the works. I was a
8 member of the elite chamber choir, the youngest member, so it was a big deal. This thing was
9 like lighting [*sic*] when it hit. So I became like this weird kind of ghost, like a pariah . . . the
10 untouchable one that everybody talked about.
11 *Do you have any resentment for your teacher?*

12 No . . . well, a little bit, a little bit. Because, even though I expected us to drift apart because
13 of this, I harbored this secret hope that there was more to it than just the singing . . . that we
14 could find common ground as people.

In the first five lines of this extract, Teresa constructs an account of her relationship with her voice teacher in which she positions her voice teacher and herself as both agent and patient. Her voice teacher "would just cry openly" in front of her, but did take the initiative to end their professional relationship—an ending that was perhaps necessary, inevitable, and known but unspoken, as is suggested in the use of *just* in line 4. Similarly, Teresa positions herself as having an impact on her teacher ("I was just bringing him way down"), as well as the one who agrees with (rather than initiates) the recognition of the inevitability of ending the relationship.

The repetition of "It was like that" (lines 5 and 6) suggests a significance to this evaluative phrase, but because *it* and *that* are vague referents, the meaning is unclear. In the absence of access to the audiotape, it is not possible to determine which of at least two possible ways of interpreting this phrase is more justifiable: (1) that one can be cut loose from a voice studio rather precipitously; or (2) that voice studios are governed by norms. In either case, however, a lack of control is implied.

Beginning in line 6 and continuing through line 10, we see, once again, the pattern of a quick shift away from talk about others to talk about herself, and, once again, Teresa engages in self-enhancement by claims of having significant talent ("I was in every top choir in the school"), by constructing the school as being only for the very serious and talented singer ("a pretty hard-core choral program . . . recordings, international tours, the works"), and by allusions to the child prodigy ("I was a member of the elite chamber choir, the youngest member"). This positioning of herself as extraordinarily talented serves to emphasize the significance of her having had thyroid cancer and having (at least temporarily) lost her singing voice, which she summarizes as "so it was a big deal."

Comparing her cancer to lightning (line 9) carries the connotation that it was quick, precise, potentially devastating, unpredictable, and uncontrollable. Equally provocative is Teresa's construction of her social significance and status after have been stricken with cancer: It is like she is dead, a social outcast whose circumstances are so unusual as to generate significant conversation (lines 9 and 10). Here, again, Teresa constructs herself as a patient (rather than an agent), as someone to whom others do things, as suffering the consequences of external forces, but also as being special and in the limelight.

The interviewer's query (in italics) brings the focus back to Teresa's relationship with her voice teacher, a move that can be understood as in keeping with the interviewer's admission that he "believed that resilience cannot happen without a source of strength or support" (see Introduction to the interview transcript), and that he had interpreted Teresa's written account as evidence that people in her life were not supportive. His query prompts a self-repair by Teresa ("No . . . well, a little bit, a little bit"), which signals a trouble source for her. A self-protective move ("Because, even though I expected us to drift apart because of this") is followed by her admission that she "harbored this secret hope that there was more to it than just the singing . . . that we could find common ground as people." In this sequence, others are diminished by being constructed as disappointing her. Again, the discourse being drawn upon by Teresa in this extract disrupts the notion of social support as being necessary for the achievement of what might be deemed "resilience."

Summary

To summarize, then, I have focused on two discursive patterns that I interpret as "enhancing oneself, diminishing others." I have also highlighted how agent and patient positions are flexibly taken up by Teresa as she employs these two patterns. Of possible note is that I worked up the first pattern from extracts chosen from Teresa's written account and the second pattern from extracts chosen from the interview. In citing this distinction, I am not drawing the conclusion that each pattern was exclusive to a particular context. Rather, I think it illustrates that discursive context can matter. The written account of "a situation when something *very* unfortunate happened to you" was not a form of talk-in-interaction in real time. It did, of course, have an audience, as the students knew that their fellow students would have access to these accounts, but it was not a real time coconstruction by speakers. In this account, Teresa said little about the people in her life, other than the medical professionals with whom she interacted during the course of the diagnosis, and, as I have illustrated through analyzing the two extracts included here, she positioned herself, at some points in the latter part of her account, as an independent agent in charge of her life. It is possible to argue that producing a written account affords the writer considerable control. He or she can structure the account in innumerable ways and can edit as he or she sees fit. What is said can be carefully crafted to produce particular effects, and parts of the account can be reworked, embellished, or censored. As mentioned previously, it is possible that enhancing oneself and diminishing others is one discursive strategy that is pulled for by the way in which the instructions for the written account were worded—that is, focused on "you" and "your," and by the audience (i.e., one's fellow students and professor).

The interview, on the other hand, which is the context from which I derived the second discursive pattern, is talk-in-interaction, an event that is dynamically coconstructed by the participants. It is a context that has the potential to afford the participants less control than a written account. That is, the interviewer and the interviewee can take the conversation in various directions, and those directions can be taken up or resisted. As noted previously, following the interview the interviewer wrote that his "questions were geared towards trying to find sources of support," and that he "wanted to look at . . . betrayal" because throughout Teresa's story, there were people whom he thought were not supportive of her. And, it is in this context that we see a discursive pattern in which Teresa occasionally positions herself as being subject to external forces—that is, to others' responses to her exceptional talent and to the consequences of her cancer, and occasionally includes persons other than medical professionals as more central to her account.

What might be said about the social consequences of engaging in such variations in talk? One source of data for specifying these consequences is the brief written account produced by the interviewer subsequent to the interview. In this account, he praises the interviewee as "smart," "strong and courageous." As noted previously, he states that "my questions were geared towards trying to find sources of support because I believed that resilience cannot happen without a source of strength or support." This latter statement seems to suggest that, from the interviewer's perspective, Teresa's written account defied his expectation that support is necessarily implicated in talk about what is thought to constitute "resilience" and "recovery." Possible social consequences of these discursive patterns are, then, admiration, sympathy, and a questioning of the completeness of the account.

Another source of data for specifying these consequences is the theoretical and empirical literature on loss, trauma, and resilience. As reported by Bonanno (2004), engaging in self-enhancement can evoke negative impressions on the part of others, but can also, in the context of highly aversive events, elicit positive evaluations. That is, it can be seen as evidence of high self-esteem and good adjustment in the face of serious adversity. As such, it is an instantiation of a cultural imperative to show that one can not only cope with adversity, but can thrive from it. However, in combination with a diminishing of others, it is possible that such evaluations can co-occur with other consequences, such as disbelief, criticism for failing to acknowledge what others have offered, or compassion for one not getting what one needs. That is, doing self-enhancement can have different meanings and different consequences when done in combination with different forms of diminishing others.

Contextualizing My Analysis

This contribution illustrates how discourse analysis can be conducted, what can be produced from the analysis, how claims are justified, and how the analysis is contextualized and interpreted. Although the analysis is in keeping with what I typically do, there is much about this project that departs from how I would normally proceed. First, I would not normally frame a project in terms such as *resilience, recovery,* or *coping.* Such terms are typically eschewed by discourse analysts because they imply that what is being got at is something inside the person, for example, a trait, an attribute, or an ability. Discourse analysts (particularly those who work within the tradition of DASP) claim instead that what we are showing are the performative capacities of language—that is, what speakers *do* with language. If I were to do a project on misfortune, I would frame it very openly as, perhaps, how people talk about misfortune or what they do when they are asked to talk about misfortune, along with focusing on the cultural discourses upon which the speakers draw. If terms such as *resilience, recovery,* or *coping* became part of the discussions about the project, I would query them as taken-for-granted concepts and note how they are used by participants, by members of my research team, by me, and in the culture at large.

Second, I would typically work from data produced by more than one person. Although this project was based on data generated from more than one context, which is particularly important in the search for variability in discourse analysis, and by more than one person (i.e., Teresa, the interviewer, and Gail [the comparative written account]), the focus was on Teresa's written account and interview. Although such a focus is certainly not prohibited in discourse analysis, it runs the risk of limiting the range of discursive patterns that are available for analysis and has the potential to communicate that the focus of the analysis is the person. In discourse analysis, the unit of analysis is *not* the person; rather, it is the extracts of discourse. Third, I would likely use the data to produce several analyses. That is, I would use the present analysis as a way of directing my gaze to other discursive patterns that have become clearer to me, perhaps because these patterns are in contrast to those that I have already worked up in detail. Asking several questions of the same data set speaks again to the central place that variability occupies in discourse analysis.

In further contextualizing my analysis, I want to highlight that, in relying on a particular form of discourse analysis that focuses on the performative aspects of language and on how culturally and historically available discourses are drawn upon, I have neglected features of other forms of analysis with rich theoretical groundings. For example, what some writers refer to as Foucauldian discourse analysis is based in conceptions of technologies of power and of the self—that is, the means and techniques used to govern, regulate, or enhance human conduct—and in the notion of subject positions, which invokes not only the idea that discourses afford positions from which a person speaks, but that these positions are moral locations (Arribas-Ayllon & Walkerdine, 2008). In addressing questions such as "What characterizes the discursive worlds people inhabit and what are their implications for possible ways-of-being?" (Willig, 2004, p. 162), this type of discourse analysis draws attention to the power of discourse to construct the human subject and to how human subjects act upon themselves and others within a particular moral order. Although I incorporated the notions of subject positioning and of culturally and historically available discourses into my analysis of the protocols used in this project, I did not engage in a historical inquiry of the genealogy of, for example, discourses of exceptionality or social support and did not attend in an in-depth fashion to relations of power as enacted either through institutional or self-regulatory practices.

By grounding my analysis in a constructionist epistemology, I have also not relied on recent attempts to combine relativist and realist positions as they relate to discourse analysis. Often referred to as a critical realist approach to the analysis of discourse, this stance affords materiality and material practices the same ontological status as discursive practices. In this approach, features of human existence such as physicality, embodiment, economic or social conditions, and institutional power are said to provide the context from which the use of certain discourses and engagement in ways-of-being are enabled or constrained (Sims-Schouten, Riley, & Willig, 2007). Rather than ignoring these features or considering them only in terms of how they are constructed in various versions of reality, they can be analyzed, for example, through a review of literature, documents, or policies that are relevant to one's research questions and via careful observations of relevant social and physical environments (see Sims-Schouten, Riley, & Willig, 2007, for an illustration). Taking such an approach in the present project would have required the generation of additional forms of data and a focus on questions related to, for example, embodiment and illness, or institutions of power, such as the medical system, the family, or voice schools.

I have also not engaged with the texts of this project or with the topic in ways that would fit with what Parker (2005) has labeled "radical research." For example, in addition to not employing Foucauldian notions about how knowledge is produced, I have not relied on resources such as feminist or Marxist theory as a means by which to consider questions of gender, race, and class, and have not fully developed how notions such as contradiction or resistance are evidenced in the texts; nor have I shown how the culturally and historically available discourses to which I allude function ideologically. While it is possible to do radical research with existing texts, Parker (2005) also advocated for a type of discourse-analytic interviewing that enlists the persons one is interviewing as coresearchers. In the present project, this way of generating data would have involved, for example, enrolling Emily as a discourse analyst of her own and the interviewer's language, highlighting points of contradiction in the interview and engaging Emily with them, encouraging her to refuse assumptions and common sense, making the analysis visible to her, and discussing and deciding what the coresearchers make of each other's take on the analysis.

Conclusion

My focus for this project is on the variations in how one social action—what I label "enhancing oneself, diminishing others"—is performed. I could have chosen other social actions performed by Teresa, but I found this one most compelling. I understand my analysis not as evidence that Teresa is a "self-enhancer," and that this trait serves as a pathway to resilience, as might be the understanding in much of the literature on loss, trauma, and resilience (e.g., see Bonanno, 2004). Rather, I see the variations in how this action is performed as serving specific ends, as drawing on specific culturally and historically available discourses, and as having a variety of social consequences in the particular contexts in which the data for this project were generated.

References

Arribas-Ayllon, M., & Walkerdine, V. (2008). Foucauldian discourse analysis. In C. Willig & W. Stainton-Rogers (Eds.), *The Sage handbook of qualitative research in psychology* (pp. 91–108). London: Sage.

Austin, J. (1962). *How to do things with words.* Oxford, UK: Clarendon Press.

Bonanno, G. A. (2004). Loss, trauma, and human resilience: Have we underestimated the human capacity to thrive after extremely aversive events? *American Psychologist, 59,* 20–28.

Crotty, M. (1998). *The foundations of social research: Meaning and perspective in the research process.* London: Sage.

Davies, B., & Harré, R. (1990). Positioning: The discursive production of selves. *Journal for the Theory of Social Behaviour, 20,* 43–63.

Litton, I., & Potter, J. (1985). Social representations in the ordinary explanation of a "riot." *European Journal of Social Psychology, 15,* 371–388.

Morris, W. (Ed.). (1970). *The American heritage dictionary of the English language.* New York: American Heritage & Houghton Mifflin.

Parker, I. (1997). Discursive psychology. In D. Fox & I. Prilletensky (Eds.), *Critical psychology: An introduction.* London: Sage.

Parker, I. (2005). *Qualitative psychology: Introducing radical research.* Berkshire, UK: Open University Press.

Penelope, J. (1990). *Speaking freely.* New York: Pergamon.

Potter, J. (2003). Discourse analysis and discursive psychology. In P. M. Camic, J. E. Rhodes, & L. Yardley (Eds.), *Qualitative research in psychology: Expanding perspectives in methodology and design* (pp. 73–94). Washington, DC: American Psychological Association.

Potter, J. (2004). Discourse analysis as a way of analysing naturally occurring talk. In D. Silverman (Ed.), *Qualitative research: Theory, method and practice* (pp. 200–221). London: Sage.

Potter, J., & Wetherell, M. (1987). *Discourse and social psychology: Beyond attitudes and behaviour.* London: Sage.

Sims-Schouten, W., Riley, S. C. E., & Willig, C. (2007). Critical realism in disourse analysis: A presentation of a systematic method of analysis using women's talk of motherhood, childcare and female employment as an example. *Theory and Psychology, 17*, 101–124.

Wetherell, M. (1998). Positioning and interpretative repertoires: Conversation analysis and post-structuralism in dialogue. *Discourse and Society, 9*, 387–412.

Willig, C. (2001). *Introducing qualitative research in psychology: Adventures in theory and method.* Buckingham, UK: Open University Press.

Willig, C. (2003). Discourse analysis. In J.A. Smith (Ed.), *Qualitative psychology: A practical guide to research methods* (pp. 159–183). London: Sage.

Willig, C. (2004). Discourse analysis and health psychology. In M. Murray (Ed.), *Critical health psychology* (pp. 155–169). Hampshire, UK: Palgrave Macmillan.

Wood, L. A., & Kroger, R. O. (2000). *Doing discourse analysis: Methods for studying action in talk and text.* Thousand Oaks, CA: Sage.

Additional Examples of Discourse Analysis

Clarke, V., Kitzinger, C., & Potter, J. (2004). "Kids are just cruel anyway": Lesbian and gay parents' talk about homophobic bullying. *British Journal of Social Psychology, 43*, 531–550.

Edley, N., & Wetherell, M. (2001). Jekyll and Hyde: Men's constructions of feminism and feminists. *Feminism and Psychology, 11*, 439–457.

Liebert, R., & Gavey, N. (2009). "There are always two sides to these things": Managing the dilemma of serious side effects from SSRIs. *Social Science and Medicine, 68*, 1882–1891.

McMullen, L. M., & Herman, J. (2009). Women's accounts of their decision to quit taking antidepressants. *Qualitative Health Psychology, 19*, 1569–1579.

Potter, J., & Hepburn, A. (2003). "I'm a bit concerned": Early actions and psychological constructions in a child protection helpline. *Research on Language and Social Interaction, 36*, 197–240.

Wetherell, M., & Edley, N. (1999). Negotiating hegemonic masculinity: Imaginary positions and psycho-discursive practices. *Feminism and Psychology, 9*, 335–356.

CHAPTER 8

Narrative Research

Constructing, Deconstructing, and Reconstructing Story

Ruthellen Josselson

T he link between life and story in psychology has traditions going back to Freud, Murray (1938), and Allport (1937). Theodore Sarbin (1986) was probably the first to coin the phrase "narrative psychology," although psychologists for many years had been doing "case study" research. While there are today many definitions of narrative research, it shares a fuzzy border with other forms of qualitative research and is distinguished by a focus on narrated texts that represent either a whole life story or aspects of it. Narrative research is, in Clifford Geertz's phrase, a "mixed genre" in the sense of integrating systematic analysis of narrated experience with literary deconstruction and hermeneutic analysis of meaning.

Narrative research takes as a premise that people live and/or understand their lives in storied forms, connecting events in the manner of a plot that has beginning, middle, and end points (Sarbin, 1986). These stories are played out in the context of other stories that may include societies, cultures, families, or other intersecting plotlines in a person's life. The stories that people tell about their lives represent their meaning making; how they connect and integrate the chaos of internal and momentary experience and how they select what to tell and how they link bits of their experience are all aspects of how they structure the flow of experience and understand their lives. Narratives organize time (Ricoeur, 1988) and are performed for particular audiences.

Most generally, narrative research is an interpretive enterprise consisting of the joint subjectivities of researcher and participants subjected to a conceptual framework brought to bear on textual material (either oral or written) by the researcher.[1] It aims to explore and conceptualize human experience as it is represented in textual form. Grounded in hermeneutics, phenomenology, ethnography, and literary analysis, narrative research eschews methodological orthodoxy in favor of doing what is necessary to capture the lived experience of people in terms of their own meaning making and to theorize about it in insightful ways.

Narrative research epistemologically respects the relativity and multiplicity of truth and relies on the foundational work of such philosophers as Ricoeur, Heidegger, Husserl, Dilthey, Wittgenstein, Bakhtin, Lyotard, MacIntyre, and Gadamer. While narrative researchers differ in their view of the possibility of objectively conceived "reality," most agree with Donald Spence's (1982) distinction between narrative and historical truth. Narrative truth involves a constructed account of experience, not a factual record of what "really" happened. The focus is on how events are understood and organized.

Within psychology, Jerome Bruner (1990) has championed the legitimization of what he calls "narrative modes of knowing," which privilege the particulars of lived experience. Meaning is not inherent in an act or experience, but is constructed through social discourse. Meaning is generated by the linkages the participant makes between aspects of the life he or she is living and by the explicit linkages the researcher makes between this understanding and interpretation, which is meaning constructed at another level of analysis.

While I ground my thinking in the work of such writers as Bakhtin, Ricoeur, Bruner, and Geertz, other narrative researchers, depending on their primary academic discipline, have been strongly influenced by such thinkers as Dewey, Labov, and Rosaldo. Narrative researchers work in symbolic interactionist, feminist, and psychoanalytic traditions, among others. What is common to all is approaching the problem of the analysis of lived experience, represented in words rather than numbers, for the benefit of social science understanding.

Narrative inquiry works with detailed stories drawn in some way from participants, stories that reveal how people view and understand their lives. Generally, narratives are obtained through interviewing people around the topic of interest, but narrative research may also involve the analysis of written documents. Narratives are understood contextually, as influenced by the circumstances under which they were obtained, with consideration given to the intended audience and the motives the narrator may have had for constructing the narrative in a particular way.

Narrative analysis emphasizes content and its meanings, which are sometimes revealed in structural forms. The narrative telling is not mimetic; it is not an exact representation of what happened, but a particular construction of events created in a particular setting, for a particular audience, for particular purposes, to create a certain point of view (Mishler, 2004). Therefore, we pay a lot of attention to the context (both relational and social) in which the narrative is constructed. In addition, the principles of reflexivity require that the researcher regard findings as relative to his or her standpoint as an observer.

Readings of narrative materials can be conducted along two major dimensions: holistic versus categorical approaches and content versus form (Lieblich et al., 1998). In a holistic analysis, the life story, as represented in the narrative, is considered as a whole and sections of the text are interpreted with respect to the other parts. A categorical analysis abstracts sections or words belonging to a category, using coding strategies, and compares these to similar texts from other narratives. Maxwell (1996) refers to this distinction as one between contextualization and categorization. The dimension of *content versus form* refers to readings that concentrate on either *what* is told or *how* it is told.

Narrative analysis is conducted within two hermeneutic traditions detailed by Ricoeur: a hermeneutics of faith, which aims to restore meaning to a text, and a hermeneutics of suspicion, which attempts to decode meanings that are disguised (Josselson, 2004). Thus, a narrative analysis may both re-present the participant's narrative and also take interpretive authority for going beyond, in carefully documented ways, its literal and conscious meanings (Chase, 1996; Hollway & Jefferson, 2000).

Narrative researchers read texts for personal, social, and historical conditions that mediate the story. Analysis is aimed at discovering both the themes that unify the story and the disparate voices that carry, comment on, and disrupt the main themes.

Narrative research relies on thematic analysis, discourse analysis, and the other frameworks that my colleagues detail in the other chapters. What is perhaps unique to narrative research is that it endeavors to explore the whole account rather than fragmenting it into discursive units or thematic categories. It is not the parts that are significant in human life, but how the parts are integrated to create a whole—which is meaning. Fundamental to this approach is Schleiermacher's idea of the "hermeneutic circle," in which an understanding of the whole illuminates the parts, which in turn create the whole. Narrative inquiry approaches recognize that narrators are constructing ordered accounts from the chaos of internal experience and that these accounts will likely be multivocal and dialogical in that aspects of self will appear in conversation with or juxtaposed against other aspects. There is never a single self-representation.

Many practitioners and theorists of narrative research draw on the work of the philosophical anthropologist Mikhail Bakhtin (1981) and his ideas of the dialogical, multivocal self as expressed in novelistic form. In Bakhtin's conception, the self is construed as always in relationship to some other, "whether that other be another person, other parts of the self, or the individual's society or culture" (1986, p. 36). It is also a dynamic, unfinished self, with potentialities that point to the future. Following Bakhtin's lead, narrative analysis does not regard a person as fixed in any representation of his or her words and cannot claim any finality as to what a story means, since any story has potential for revision in future stories.

The construction of the story reflects the current internal world of the narrator as well as aspects of the social world in which he or she lives. Rather than just identifying and describing themes, narrative analysis endeavors to understand the themes in relation to one another as a dynamic whole. The self is regarded as multiple, as different voices in dialogue with one another. The narrative is conceived as a multiplicity of "I" positions (Hermans & Kempen, 1993) where each "I" is an author with its own story to tell in relation to the other "I's." Some of these selves may be strongly developed, whereas others may be suppressed or even dissociated. Bakhtin emphasizes the dynamics of inconsistency and tension that resist closure.

Narrative analysis focuses, then, on patterned relationships in the flow of events and experience within a multivoiced self that is in mutually constitutive interaction with its social world. It tries to maintain a view of how the person integrates multiple psychic realities.

The process of analysis is one of piecing together data, making the invisible apparent, deciding what is significant and insignificant, and linking seemingly unrelated facets of experience together. Analysis is a creative process of organizing data so that the analytic scheme will emerge. Texts are read multiple times in a hermeneutic circle, considering how the whole illuminates the parts, and how the parts in turn offer a fuller and more complex picture of the whole, which then leads to a better understanding of the parts, etc.

Narrative researchers focus first on the voices *within* each narrative, attending to the layering of voices (subject positions), their interaction, and the continuities, ambiguities, and disjunctions expressed. The researcher pays attention to both the content of the narration ("the told") and the structure of the narration ("the telling"). Narrative analysts may also pay attention to what is unsaid or unsayable (Rogers et al., 1999) by looking at the structure of the narrative discourse and markers of omissions. After each participant's story is understood as well as possible, cross-case analysis may be performed to discover patterns across individual narrative interview texts or to explore what may create differences between people in their narrated experiences.

There is, mercifully, no dogma or orthodoxy yet about how to conduct narrative research. The aim is to elicit stories around a theme in as unobtrusive a manner possible, attending to the context of the relationship between interviewer and interviewee, and then to analyze these stories in the framework of the questions that the researcher brings to them, giving due consideration to the linguistic and cultural contexts that shaped the account, both immediate and in terms of the larger culture.

Narrative Analysis

Analysis from the stance of the hermeneutic circle involves gaining an overall sense of meaning and then examining the parts in relation to it—which will involve changing our understanding of the whole until we arrive at a holistic understanding that best encompasses the meanings of the parts. In order to approach such a text, we would engage in the following operations:

1. We do an overall reading of the interview to get a sense of how the narrative is structured and the general theme or themes. Then we return to each specific part to develop its meaning, and then consider the more global meanings in light of the deepened meaning of the parts.
2. We do multiple readings to identify different "voices" of the self and to create a view of how these selves are in dialogue with one another.
3. These iterative readings continue until we develop a "good Gestalt" that encompasses contradictions. The different themes make sensible patterns and enter into a coherent unity.
4. The work also enters into conversation with the larger theoretical literature so that the researcher can remain sensitive to nuances of meanings expressed and the different contexts into which the meanings may enter.

Always we attempt to be aware of our own presuppositions—how the interviewer and the interpreter are shaping the text as a coconstructed situation. Finally, we hope that the interpretation brings forth something new—something not apparent in the surface of the text.

The Current Project

This research project was framed within a context of understanding something about processes of psychological resilience, and my reading of this interview would perhaps offer a critique of the concept of resilience. The word resilience derives from the Latin *resilire,* to spring back, rebound. It is defined as an ability to recover from or adjust to misfortune or change, but has some implication of returning to an original state. This life narrative, the story of a woman whose whole sense of self was bound to being a singer but who lost, through cancer, her ability to sing well enough to become a lead opera singer, can be construed, however, more as a narrative of transformation. The process of identity formation, in this narrative, is intertwined with a narrative of tragedy that redirected her location of herself in the world. In terms of narrative form, derived from literary theory, it is structured both as a tragedy and a romance, the tragedy inhering in the emphasis on all that was lost, the romance in the overcoming of this massive loss and creating something new, a story in which the essence of the journey is the struggle itself.

We must first consider the relational context of this interview. It occurred as part of a class assignment, and the interviewer was a classmate of the interviewee, a man of about the same age. We don't know what their prior relationship may have been like, but the interviewer is clearly a novice who is awkwardly pursuing his own agenda in the interview. This agenda seems to be to discover the interpersonal support system that he is convinced is crucial to overcoming adversity and engendering resilience, but Teresa, the interviewee, staunchly resists this framing. The interviewer's rigidity here may have led her to an even greater emphasis on her individual, internal, intrapsychic modes of coping than she might have offered under other interviewing circumstances—and her refusal to comply with his direction suggests something about her capacity to hold to her own definitions in the face of external pressure, something that was also apparent in her construction of her identity as a singer in opposition to her father.

We must also reflexively consider the interpretive context. I read the transcript as a person who is a psychodynamically oriented clinical psychologist, actively engaged as a therapist, so I am accustomed to hearing accounts of personal tragedy and loss and am attuned to affect and to psychological mechanisms of coping. I am also a researcher of identity, so the issues of identity in this narrative leap out at me. I am not a cancer survivor but, through colleagues, have some familiarity with wellness groups. Still, my personal reaction to this narrative is to be very moved, amazed by, and admiring of this woman's courage and fortitude—and also to feel worried about her current physical state, perhaps more worried than she allows herself to be.

Overall Characteristics of the Narrative

Theresa's narrative of coping with the loss of her voice focuses almost exclusively on *internal* reworkings of her experience of self. Her narrative is one of personal agency and a determination to overcome adversity. Her stories illustrate internal rather than interpersonal realities. Other people in her life are painted, in relation to her loss, as disappointing, emotionally unreliable, betraying, or abandoning—though adequately available to care for her physically when she is in need.

We have here two narratives that are interesting to compare—one written and one oral. The primary thematic and emplotted contents are similar, but the written narrative has more evocative language and more quoted direct speech of others. Not surprisingly, there is more complexity and more hesitation in the interview. In its bare bones, Teresa's story is one of having lost everything—everything that anchored her in her world, coming to terms with this, and then reintegrating herself. Teresa emphasizes her sense of aloneness with the diagnosis, treatment, and aftermath. Psychologically, she stresses her reliance on cognitive modes of coping, eschewing or distancing herself from her emotions.

Teresa's evocative language communicates the depth of her sense of loss. "I was a ghost of my former self," she says in her written narrative, "Cancer wasn't as frightening to me as never been being able to sing again. Singing had been my life for as long as I could remember: the one thing I could excel at, the only thing I knew. It had been my solace in all my times of distress, through every hardship." So she lost not only her identity, but her customary means of coping. But, she says in her written narrative, "I was determined to move on as if nothing had happened." This, then, is a marker of one of Teresa's main internal dialogues: her feeling that she had lost everything ("I had never been anything but my voice") and her wish to move on as though "nothing had happened."

There are some definite differences between the written and the oral narratives that we don't have enough information to explain. In the written narrative, Teresa focuses on the details of the day when she first learns that she might lose her singing voice through a surgery to remove an aggressive thyroid tumor. She structures her story as one of shock, loss of nearly all aspects of self, reconstruction of herself as a student of psychology, and also as "a singer in an entirely new way" who sings in a variety of venues and writes her own music—but to whom being an opera singer is no longer so important. In the oral narrative, told in person to a fellow student, the current sense of herself in relation to singing is much less clear than in the written narrative, and she stresses more her identity as a psychologist, but still describes little of how she got there.

Both of these tellings, however, can be read as narratives of transformation and integration. In the oral narrative, she details the nature of the meaning of the loss. The interviewer, clumsily, tries to direct and structure the story, and this makes it difficult to analyze its formal and organizational properties. At the same time, there are many hints about important aspects of her experience that are not explored in the interview.

Theresa presents herself as someone who is attentive to the ways in which she defines herself, even enacting this in relation to the interviewer, whose efforts to reframe her experience into his own categories she doggedly resists. This idea of defining herself underlies the central motif of her story. In losing her voice, she tells us, she lost all of her identity. As she constructs her world, she experiences herself as a compound of a physical self, an emotional self, and a logical self. Before her cancer, her physical self, expressed in singing and in perfecting herself as a singer, was paramount. Once she learned that there was a tumor on her thyroid, she tried to "sort of remove myself from my physical self" in order to be able to cope and plan, but she was uncertain what there was of her besides her physical self as manifested in her voice. Having lost her singing voice, she tells us, "My voice was gone, so I was gone, and I'd never been anything but my voice." Her relationship with God, with her peers—everything had been predicated on her singing, even her capacity to soothe herself following disappointments. After her surgery, which took away her capacity to sing, her former fellow music students treated her as though she were dead, and this is how she felt about herself.

One important focus of Teresa's narrative was her experienced loss of the person who had been most important in her life—her voice teacher, who had been a kind of idealized father to her. After her diagnosis, she says, "It was harder for me to even conceive of telling him, because our relationship hinged solely on the fact that I was a singer. My mother would have been there for me. But as far as my voice teacher? If I couldn't sing, I was going to lose this guy. As far as I was concerned, not being able to sing would destroy not only everything that we'd worked toward that past 2½ years, but also our relationship . . . professionally, personally, you name it. And I just couldn't deal with that." The loss of this relationship becomes a kind of metaphor for the sense of total loss, her recognition that, before the loss of her voice, she had "monocular vision"—a whole life predicated on being special as a singer. The cancer, then, was not just on her thyroid, but on her very identity. And singing had always been the solution to any other problem she may have had, her form of self-soothing. This was a situation that she could not sing herself through.

Thus, we have the outlines of the Gestalt, the general narrative thread of Teresa's story. She lost the central anchor of her existence—of her identity and of her most important relationship—and yet she found the internal capacity to come to terms with herself and to reinvent herself, deliberately and intentionally, with new goals and new ways of being with others and in the world. We then look for the primary subthemes: Teresa's explication of how she went about coping with the loss and creating a new life.

Procedure to Identify Themes

I read the narrative several times, marking passages I thought were significant in relation to both coping with loss (the tragic narrative) and engendering a new life (the romance narrative). I paid particular attention to statements about self experience ("I statements") and her descriptions of others
in relation to herself. I then grouped these passages into broad categories
that became "emotion and logic," "identity," and "self with others." Once I
had these grouped passages, I then reread the passages within each category
examining their interrelationship and looking for shifts in "voice" or locations of the self that spoke different experiences with regard to each category.
Then, as I go to write my findings, I see that the categories are themselves
intertwined, one affecting the other in complex ways, so much so that I can't
really discuss them separately without blurred boundaries. This reassures me
that I have done my work reasonably well: Categories that are too separate are
artificial. Human life is of a piece, multilayered, contradictory, and multiva-
lent, to be sure, but the strands are always interconnected.

Emotion and Logic

A central theme that marks Teresa's coping is the tension between her intense
emotions and her preference to live through logic and reason, with a cool
head. Asked to explain her response to learning that, after the surgery, she
might not be able to sing again, Teresa expresses a kind of dissociative state.
She says she sort of removed herself from her physical self: "I reverted completely to logic at that point." In the written narrative, she eloquently expresses
the intensity of the emotions she was removing herself from, emotions that
were utterly disabling: "I froze. I couldn't breathe, couldn't move, couldn't
even blink. I felt like I had just been shot. My gut had locked up like I'd been
punched in it. My mouth went dry and my fingers, which had been fumbling
with a pen, were suddenly cold and numb. . . . Then, all of me let loose. I was
sobbing, but there was no sound; just a torrent of tears, and the hiss of crying from my open mouth, pushing through the pressure from the accursed
mass." In this state, overwhelmed with anguish and despair, Teresa is without
sound, without self. As she continues the narrative, she says that, in response
to the surgeon's attempt at reassurance, "Slowly, I came back to myself." Her
"self," then, is a self that can think and give voice to her experience. But, a few
sentences later she says, "I felt as though the biggest and best part of me had
died in that office. . . . Singing had been my life for as long a I could remember, the one thing I could excel at, the only thing I knew." Thus, Teresa also
defines her sense of self—and her sense of loss—in her capacity to sing.

As the narrative progresses, Teresa moves far beyond this disabling affect
and relies on her reasoning and planning to create a new sense of identity,

ultimately redefining herself in terms of her turn to psychology and recasting of herself as an intellectual self. She also finds ways to sing and express herself musically that are not part of becoming an opera singer. She subsumes this progression toward new career goals under an effort to use logic and reason to lead her to a new path.

Teresa locates her coping capacity largely in her effort to "move on as if nothing had happened," detailing one aspect of her self-experience. She begins to introduce herself to new people as a psychology major rather than as a singer, which was "odd," but, she says, "strangely refreshing." She uses this new identity to distance herself from her loss and takes up new activities, such as rock climbing and fencing, in order to "live as much as I possibly could." But, there is yet another part of Teresa that sees the limits of this effort. She says, in the written narrative, that the frequent readmissions to the hospital reminded her that she was "fool[ing] myself into thinking I was normal again."

Teresa's capacity for putting her emotions aside (but not completely) also becomes salient at the end of her oral narrative, where she indicates that this is not indeed a narrative of happy endings. She is not cancer free by any means and lives with a brain tumor that threatens her very existence. This, on the heels of a pituitary tumor. Her attitude to this, unspoken, seems to be a kind of emotional denial or a characterological stoicism. She will carry on as though it is not there. Thus, for Teresa, a central psychological dilemma is managing the affective aspects of her situation that accompany her experience of herself as ill. The despair, the out-of-control expression of feeling (very much a part of her warded-off self), is largely placed into others—her parents, for example. She locates her grief in the tears of her voice teacher. And here is where my own worry about her may be reflexively relevant. She speaks without much affect of the recurrence of cancer, of her brain tumor that waxes and wanes, but I find myself deeply troubled on her behalf. Perhaps I am experiencing part of what she does with others—avoiding her own feelings by perceiving or injecting them in to those close to her.

Teresa talks about "getting away from emotionality" and also about listening to her emotions and "tempering" them. She very much fears "going completely off kilter and looking like a moron" or becoming "completely pathetic under the weight of your emotions." We also learn that she disliked the "emotionality" of her household, marked by her father's outbursts, so even before the thyroid cancer, the construction of experience as divided between emotion and reason—and the discomfort with emotion—marked Teresa's psychological organization.

Teresa relates that she was able to rely on skills she had learned as a singer to manage her emotions, a passage in which she juxtaposes physical control and emotionality. She says:

I was very emotional . . . and of course, being in a very emotional household also contributed to the emotionality of my performance. When I
got to college and entered the voice studio, I was told to restrict that
emotion and to focus more on the physicality of what I was doing, on
releasing tension. When you're emotional, you get physically tense. And
when you get physically tense, that kind of messes with what you're doing
vocally . . . and that's what was happening to me. So getting away from
that emotionality and reminding myself why . . . which, of course, takes
logic . . . was actually very instrumental in the long run, not in quashing
my emotions . . . I still listen very much to my emotions . . . but understanding that they're just a part of what needs to take place in order to
help me function in a given scenario.

As a singer, she had learned to "restrict" her emotions, and this is what
she called into play in dealing with her losses. Her development as a singer
involved becoming very attentive to the relation between her emotions, her
physical state, and her capacity to control her voice. "I still listen very much
to my emotions—but understanding that they're just a part of what needs to
take place in order to help me function in a given scenario," she says, thus
proclaiming executive control for the rational side of herself.

From a psychological point of view, we are unable to determine what of
Teresa's management of her emotions is a product of conscious control (as she
proclaims it to be) and what represents unconscious defenses. But the issue of
how she experiences the interplay between reason and feeling represents the
intersection of important parts of herself, and from this we can perhaps learn
something about what it means to cope with and transcend such a loss.

Teresa's psychological framing of coping with her personal tragedy is
largely in terms of the balance between reason and feeling, between determination and helplessness. At least in this context, of being interviewed by a
classmate in a psychology graduate program, her narrative privileges rationality and determination. She is more expressive of her emotional states in
the written narrative, a context that is more neutral in relational terms in the
sense that she does not have to detail her feelings (or sense of helplessness
and vulnerability) in the physical presence of another person.

Still, she discloses in the oral narrative that when she is sick, she is "sick
with a vengeance" and that her treatments sometimes lead to "weaknesses
that are pretty bad." There are markers in the interview of her emotional
states that she experiences as out of control or incompatible with her view of
herself. She also indicates that her emotional expression is often trying for
others. The subtext is one of suffering and torment that is largely downplayed
as she, in her life, strives to "play things off like there's nothing wrong."

Thus, as we assemble these pieces of Teresa's narrative related to her
experience of logic and emotion, we see that she is aware of intense, possibly

disabling feeling but has found a way to keep these emotions at bay so that she can reason her way to a new life. This raises some psychologically interesting questions about the role of suppression, denial, and dissociation in successful coping. Teresa says that she tries to act "like there's *nothing* wrong" and that she tried to "move on as though *nothing* happened." I am captured here by her use of the word *nothing*. How could it be that there is *nothing* wrong or that *nothing* happened when she is narrating a story of losing everything? These are extreme statements. How are these two states of experience (*total loss* and *nothing happened*) held psychologically?

Identity

In terms of identity, we listen to the alternate selves available to Teresa. We learn, in the oral narrative, that being a singer disavowed the other identity offered to her—that of the "fat kid with no friends . . . the fat kid with the oppressive dad." Singing gave her "a ticket out" of both of these imposed identities. And there was another self that she is somewhat relieved to have left behind—the "*wunderkind*" at the music school who got the solos and the favoritism—and also had to cope with the envy of others who, now that she was no longer a "threat" to them, simply lost interest in her. Thus, she experienced herself as having the awful choice of being the envied one or being erased. At least, after she could no longer sing, she no longer had to cope with the envy. But looking at herself through the eyes of her peers and teachers, she experienced herself as "dead," as no longer existing. The dominant self-image, repeated in both tellings, is that of a ghost, being a member of the living dead who was frightening to others, including to other cancer survivors. At best, if she was noticed at all, she became "the untouchable one that everybody talked about." Teresa, then, was without a reference group of any kind, quite alone in terms of being understood.

Teresa found herself confronting the task of creating a new self and a new life, but the (combined) narrative tells little about how she actually did this. At first, she tried to resume her vocal training in hopes of carrying on, suffering through the dissuasion of her professors until, in a moving scene, even her primary, much-loved voice teacher suggests that it is over for her. "I had to find something or I was going to die. I really felt that I was going to have to die, or kill myself . . . or hold my breath until it ended." I find this locution about holding her breath until she died to be very important and very telling. Breath is the major focus of a singer, and it is with breath that she thinks of controlling whether and how she lives—or dies. She speaks then of discovering that she was smart and of valuing an intellectual life with new friends—and this leads her to a new path. But she doesn't define it as completely new, rather as "a part of myself I never knew I had." Thus, Teresa is able to link her new sense of identity to her prior self. Still, she mentions "2 years of straight misery" as she came to terms with not being an opera singer. She also got married somewhere in the midst of her adjustment, but we know little about her decision to marry at this time. She also speaks of having "a sick passion to fight odds. . . . I gotta go do more stuff. I gotta go be a fencer, go rock climbing, get a Phd. I have to keep going, like I'm obsessed with it."

Why she chose psychology—and what other options she may have considered—is not clear from the narrative, although she mentions having done a paper in her psychology class on the psychological effects of pituitary tumors, a project that may have allowed her some reflective distance on her experience and given her an opportunity to apply her intellectualizing defenses against disabling affect. Writing this paper, she says, was another aspect of her "turn to logic." That she does not elaborate her interest in psychology or speak about its current meaning to her may reflect what she thinks is already apparent to the interviewer—given that they are both students in a graduate psychology class.

Teresa also alludes to, but does not elaborate, another significant choice point in the story of her identity formation. This was the moment where her voice comes back, just as she had managed to grieve its loss. She returned to singing, but "I realized I had kind of gotten used to the idea of not being an opera singer . . . and it wasn't that bad. And I *was* kinda smart . . . and my friends who weren't musicians were a little less vapid." And here her husband enters the story and takes a role. He never knew her as a singer; he is very academic. So something about the way in which he held her new identity helped her resist the impulse to try to resume her previous one. (He also got her involved in fencing.) But there is also a story of the integration of her singer self into her current one—"becoming a musician again in a new way." She is still performing, at clubs and in opera choruses, but "being an opera singer . . . doesn't seem so important to me any more." She writes her own music and had created her own voice studio with 60 students. So her identity as a singer/musician is not lost; rather, it has a different place in the pattern of her life, one that is not well detailed in the narrative, perhaps because the interviewer did not pursue this line of inquiry. But this belongs to the aspect of Teresa's narrative that cannot be finalized. Her musical self is still very much present, and it remains unclear how she will express it as her life unfolds.

Relations with Others

While the interviewer began the interview certain that others were central as sources of support for Teresa, we find instead that others played a more complex role in shoring up or assaulting her identity definitions, of carrying warded off emotions, and of providing or dismantling a social context in which she can function. It is telling that Teresa, in her initial written narration, chooses to dramatize a part of the interaction with the surgeon who tells her that the lump in her throat is thyroid cancer. She details how, before telling her this, he asked if she wanted her mother to come in, and she declines. Thus, in narrating the scene this way, Teresa stresses her sense that she will go it alone, will cope alone. After describing her shock and terror, Teresa then says, "Worst of all, I still had to tell my mother." In the oral narrative, Teresa returns to the scene of telling her mother who, she had feared, would "freak out." That Teresa anticipated the most intense and least controlled response from her mother suggests that she may experience her most painful emotions located in others.

Similarly, she describes her former teachers in her voice program speaking to her "as though I was already dead . . . everybody kept looking at me like I was already death warmed over." We hear in these words echoes of how Teresa regarded herself at times, or at some levels of herself, as dead, as a ghost. Thus, there appears to be some fluidity in the way her feelings about herself and her trauma move their location between being clearly her own and being expressed by others.

We are acquainted with the other people in her relational world primarily through their reactions to her loss of her voice and her ongoing illnesses. (This is, in part, a result of the interviewer's line of questioning.) As she speaks of the role of others' actions in relation to her ordeal, we see that other people are variously resented for being solicitous of and upset by her illness (her mother, her voice teacher, her father) and resented for not being solicitous or concerned enough (her fellow voice students, her father). This pattern may suggest that she locates expressions of her rage about her vulnerability in her intimate relationships.

We know little of the nature of Teresa's ongoing relationships with her family, husband, or friends, but she certainly maintains relationships, at least superficially. In her interpersonal world, no one seems to her to be willing or able to join her fully in her pain and in her struggles—although people do try to help her manage. She ambivalently and distantly acknowledges her father's effort to soothe her by buying her "stuff" after her surgery before he became "his old belligerent self again." Although she was rueful about the extent of her mother's emotional pain in response to her illness, she appreciated her mother's serving as the "master hub" of managing the physical and logistical aspects of her recovery—of doing "what needs to be done." Ultimately, Teresa does forgive her voice teacher for distancing himself from her.

She recognizes how difficult it was for her husband to have to cope with her cancer so early in their relationship. "I wanted to be seen as strong. But whenever I was falling all over myself because of the radiation, he didn't know how to deal with it. He would just kind of look at me and say, 'Come on, get up.' And I couldn't get up. So then he thought that I was trying to milk this whole thing for attention. He didn't think it was that bad, I guess, because I tended to downplay things." Teresa, then, has still not found a comfortable way to be both strong and in need with the others who care about her.

Summary

A narrative reading of these texts, written and oral, then, would focus, I think, on the central tensions in regard to her coping with what was framed by the opening question as a "very unfortunate" event. One major tension involves her experience of thinking and feeling and how she has balanced or interwoven the two. A second involves the intersection of her late adolescent developmental task of forming an identity with the loss of a dream that had defined her identity throughout her life. And a third relates to her experience of self with others. All are intertwined as she makes use of others in the shifting balance between her thinking and feeling selves. Her successful quest for identity represents the triumph of her rational self and is itself shored up by others. Overall, we might come to critique the concept of resilience and wonder about processes of transformation in response to trauma and loss. Teresa does not return to a previous level of functioning, although she briefly tried to do so. Instead, her response to her loss is a narrative of rebirth and reintegration. Essentially, this is a narrative of existential aloneness, of coping with repeated threats of death and loss of function, and of using will and logic to guide her passion to overcome these threats and to live a meaningful life.

The Narrative Research Project

How one would use an analysis of this interview in a research project would depend very much on the nature of the research question. An actual narrative research project would begin with a review of the literature, on resilience, perhaps, and point to unclear areas that might be explored and better understood through a narrative investigation. Without such a guide, I here offer a reading that has tried to distill the central intentional meanings of the narrator and to suggest some thematic interactions that may lie beneath the surface of the narration (Josselson, 2004). I have also read this narrative as a romance in which resilience inheres in the journey of struggle rather than in an outcome. "I want to be seen as strong," Teresa says, and this is the essence of the narrative that she creates. The source of her strength seems primarily located in her capacity for emotional stoicism. Her focus on personal agency connects to other work on resilience, but her relative deemphasis on relationships and support systems offers a counternarrative to the one that has become more or less canonical.

The aim of narrative research is not to generalize—one cannot offer generalizations based on small samples that are not gathered to be representative. Instead, narrative research offers the possibility of exploring nuances and interrelationships among aspects of experience that the reader might apply to better understand other related situations. Narrative research explicates layers of meaning and the intersection of internal psychological mechanisms. Thus, Teresa allows us a window into the complexities of coping with tragic loss of function. This analysis offers a view of aspects of herself in dialogue with one another rather than attempting to categorize her (Josselson, 1995). We also see how other people are recruited internally to represent aspects of herself that are difficult to bear, a reading that goes far beyond the usual conceptualizations of "social support."

An interview such as this one might be used as a pilot interview in narrative research to generate potential research questions. Indeed, it raises important questions about how feeling and thinking are balanced in the face of traumatic loss, of how others are used in the service of internal disruption following loss, and how life stage timing of loss may have impact on the possibilities for transformation of identity. Any or all of these avenues could be pursued in further interviews with other participants as conceptualizations develop.

If this were part of a narrative research project on resilience, it might be read in the context of the large psychological literature on resilience (see Bonnano, 2004) or hardiness (Maddi & Khoshaba, 1994) to argue for a form of development following loss that goes beyond return to healthy functioning and to demonstrate a particular pathway to transformation following loss. Does Teresa demonstrate an individual example of, and can she teach us something about, what has been conceptualized as "posttraumatic growth" (Tedeschi & Calhoun, 2004; Park, Edmondson, Fenster, & Blank, 2008)? Narrative research is conducted in conversation with the theoretical and conceptual literature, either to critique existing concepts or to extend and deepen them.

Teresa's narrative also raises important questions about defense mechanisms in coping. The extremity of her denial of loss (*nothing* happened) in certain ego states raises questions about her ability to know and not to know at the same time. This is a complex psychological process that may be crucial to her capacity to move on, and one that could be investigated more fully in interviews with others.

If this were a study of identity formation in the context of loss, then the study might raise questions about the intersection of adolescent development and trauma and its effect on identity. Were Teresa older, her choices about how to reconstitute herself might have been more limited, and a closer investigation of the ways in which the available identity possibilities appeared to her might extend our understanding of identity formation itself. If this were the intent of the study, the interview might also have been conducted somewhat differently, focusing more on how she made the choice to enter psychology and to marry the man she chose.

Alternatively, one might create from this text a commentary on the role of inducing or experiencing one's own feelings in others (via projective identification and projection; see Josselson, 2007) as a way of coping with loss and develop further Teresa's experience of others who seem to feel her disowned anger or disruptive and chaotic distress. Aspects of the narrative reading I presented could be organized more fully along these lines.

In summary, a narrative reading of the text goes beyond identification of themes and attempts to analyze their intersection in light of some conceptual ideas that illuminate processes more generally. The aim is to illuminate human experience as it is presented in textual form in order to reveal layered meanings that people assign to aspects of their lives. Narrative research is thus a fundamentally hermeneutic enterprise, concerned with the science of meanings, using as its data base the contextualized stories that people tell to mark and understand their actions, to construct an identity, and to distinguish themselves from others. Our hope in narrative research is that the painstaking work of combing through a narrative for its various levels of meaning will bring forth some new understanding that will benefit our wider scholarly fields.

Note

1. For a general introduction to narrative research and exploration of contemporary issues, see Clandinnin (2007); Polkinghorne (1988); Sarbin (1986); and Andrews, Squire, and Tamboukou (2008). For further explanation of the conduct of narrative research, see Josselson, Lieblich, and McAdams (2003) and Lieblich, Tuval-Mashiach, and Zilber (1998). For examples of narrative research studies, see the 11 volumes of *The Narrative Study of Lives* series (6 published by Sage Publications, edited by Josselson and Lieblich (1993, 1995, 1999; Josselson, 1996; Lieblich & Josselson, 1994, 1997), and 5 published by APA Books, edited by Josselson, Lieblich, and McAdams, 2003, 2007; Leiblich, McAdams, & Josselson, 2004; McAdams, Josselson, & Leiblich, 2001; McAdams, Josselson, & Leiblich, 2006); Rosenwald and Ochberg (1992); and Andrews (2007).

References

Allport, G. (1937). *Personality: A psychological interpretation.* New York: Holt.
Andrews, M., Squire, C., & Tamboukou, M. (2008). *Doing narrative research.* Thousand Oaks, CA: Sage.
Bakhtin, M. M. (1981). *The dialogic imagination.* Austin: University of Texas Press.
Bakhtin, M. M. (1986). *Speech genres and other late essays.* Austin: University of Texas Press.
Bonanno, G. A. (2004). Loss, trauma, and human resilience: Have we underestimated

the human capacity to thrive after extremely adverse events? *American Psychologist, 59,* 20–28.

Bruner, J. (1990). *Acts of meaning.* Cambridge, MA: Harvard University Press.

Chase, S. E. (1996). Personal vulnerability and interpretive authority in narrative research. In R. Josselson (Ed.), *Ethics and process in the narrative study of lives* (pp. 45–59). Thousand Oaks, CA: Sage.

Clandinnin, J. (Ed.). (2007). *The handbook of narrative inquiry.* Thousand Oaks, CA: Sage.

Hermans, H., & Kempen, H. (1993). *The dialogical self: Meaning as movement.* New York: Academic Press.

Hollway, W., & Jefferson, T. (2000). *Doing qualitative research differently.* London: Sage.

Josselson, R. (1995). "Imagining the real": Empathy, narrative and the dialogic self. In R. Josselson & A. Lieblich (Eds.), *The narrative study of lives* (Vol. 3, pp. 27–44). Thousand Oaks, CA: Sage.

Josselson, R. (Ed.). (1996). *Ethics and process in the narrative study of lives* (Vol. 4). Thousand Oaks, CA: Sage.

Josselson, R. (2004). The hermeneutics of faith and the hermeneutics of suspicion. *Narrative Inquiry, 14*(1), 1–29.

Josselson, R. (2007). *Playing Pygmalion: How people create one another.* New York: Jason Aronson.

Josselson, R., & Lieblich, A. (Eds.). (1993). *The narrative study of lives* (Vol. 1). Newbury Park, CA: Sage.

Josselson, R., & Lieblich, A. (Eds.). (1995). *The narrative study of lives: Interpreting experience* (Vol. 3). Thousand Oaks, CA: Sage.

Josselson, R., & Lieblich, A. (Eds.). (1999). *Making meaning of narratives: The narrative study of lives* (Vol. 6). Thousand Oaks, CA: Sage.

Josselson, R., Lieblich, A., & McAdams, D. P. (Eds.). (2003). *Up close and personal: The teaching and learning of narrative research.* Washington, DC: American Psychological Association.

Josselson, R., Lieblich, A., & McAdams, D. P. (Eds.). (2007). *The meaning of others: Narrative studies of relationships.* Washington, DC: American Psychological Association Books.

Lieblich, A., & Josselson, R. (Eds.). (1994). *The narrative study of lives: Exploring identity and gender* (Vol. 2). Thousand Oaks, CA: Sage.

Lieblich, A., & Josselson, R. (Eds.). (1997). *The narrative study of lives* (Vol. 5). Thousand Oaks, CA: Sage.

Lieblich, A., McAdams, D. P., & Josselson, R. (Eds.). (2004). *Healing plots: The narrative basis of psychotherapy.* Washington, DC: American Psychological Association Books.

Lieblich, A., Tuval-Mashiach, R., & Zilber, T. (1998). *Narrative research: Reading, analysis and interpretation.* Thousand Oak, CA: Sage.

Maddi, S. R., & Khoshaba, D. M. (1994). Hardiness and mental health. *Journal of Personality Assessment, 63,* 265–274.

Maxwell, J. A. (1996). *Qualitative research design: An interactive approach.* Thousand Oaks, CA: Sage.

McAdams, D. P., Josselson, R., & Lieblich, A. (Eds.). (2001). *Turns in the road: Narrative studies of lives in transition.* Washington, DC: American Psychological Association Books.

McAdams, D. P., Josselson, R., & Lieblich, A. (Eds.). (2006). *Identity and story: Creating self in narrative.* Washington, DC: American Psychological Association Books.

Mishler, E. (2004). Historians of the self: Restorying lives, revising identities. *Research in Human Development, 1,* 1–2, 101–121.

Murray, H. (1938). *Explorations in personality.* New York: Oxford University Press.

Park, C. L., Edmondson, D., Fenster, J. R., & Blank, T. O. (2008). Meaning making and psychological adjustment following cancer: The mediating roles of growth, life meaning, and restored just-world beliefs. *Journal of Consulting and Clinical Psychology, 76*(5), 863–875.

Polkinghorne, D. (1988). *Narrative knowing and the human sciences.* Albany, NY: State University of New York.

Ricoeur, P. (1988). *Time and narrative* (Vol. 3, K. Blamey & D. Pellauer, Trans). Chicago: University of Chicago Press.

Rogers, A. G., Casey, M. E., Ekert, J., Holland, J., Nakkula, V., & Sheinberg, N. (1999). An interpretive poetics of languages of the unsayable. In. R. Josselson & A. Lieblich (Eds.), *Making meaning of narratives: The narrative study of lives* (pp. 77–106). Thousand Oaks, CA: Sage.

Rosenwald, G. C., & Ochberg, R. L. (Eds.). (1992). *Storied lives: The cultural politics of self-understanding.* New Haven, CT: Yale University Press.

Sarbin, T. R. (1986). *Narrative psychology: The storied nature of human conduct.* New York: Praeger.

Spence, D. (1982). *Narrative truth and historical truth.* New York: Norton.

Tedeschi, R. G., & Calhoun, L. G. (2004). Posttraumatic growth: Conceptual foundations and empirical evidence. *Psychological Inquiry, 15*(1), 1–18.

CHAPTER 9

Intuitive Inquiry

Exploring the Mirroring Discourse of Disease

Rosemarie Anderson

> I was learning of a life beyond the hallowed catacombs
> of practice rooms, voice studios, and recital halls.
> > —TERESA, Interview Transcript

> I was angry . . . in many ways nondirectional anger . . .
> at myself, for being defective, having the seizures.
> > —RENO, Interview Transcript

Overview

The impulse to conduct an intuitive inquiry begins like a spark in the dark of winter because this impulse to explore a topic claims the researcher's imagination, often in an unconscious and uncanny way. She cannot stop thinking about the topic. Almost everything seems to remind her of the topic in some way. A yearning begins to understand the topic fully. This yearning to understand is Eros, love in pure form, because the intuitive inquirer wants to know her beloved topic fully. The researcher examines the fine points of a research account in a manner akin to a lover exploring a beloved's hand. Details matter. Secrets matter. The ordinary is extraordinary. The particular is favored. Everything related to the topic has meaning and significance, drawing her closer to understanding. She yearns to know more. Named or unnamed, conscious or unconscious, an intuitive inquiry has begun. What matters to the researcher may be an ordinary experience latent with symbolic meaning; a transformative, anomalous, or peak experience; or a social or interpersonal phenomenon that invites inquiry for reasons that only the researcher may apprehend, albeit vaguely, at the start.

As a research method, intuitive inquiry contains five iterative cycles that form a complete hermeneutical circle of interpretation (Anderson, 2000, 2004a, 2004b, in press). Within the five cycles, analysis and interpretation pivot around the researcher's intuition, which discerns both understandings explicit in the data and those that suggest enhanced potential in human experience toward which the data point. Imaginal processes, creative expression, and a variety of intuitive styles are encouraged in all five cycles in order to (1) move the research process forward when stymied, (2) discern understandings both explicit and implicit in the data, and (3) cultivate deeper and speculative insights suggested in the data about the potential "farther reaches of human nature" (Maslow, 1971). This interpretive and interactive dynamic of intuitive inquiry tends to transform both the researcher's understanding of the topic studied and his or her personal life—sometimes profoundly so. Procedurally, this transformation of the researcher's understanding of the topic is "contained" by the five interpretive cycles. Each cycle contains both intuitive and analytic activities that invite the researcher's psyche to roam freely within the boundaries set by the cycle. The researcher's psyche roams freely but not aimlessly.

In a manner unique among research methods, both qualitative and quantitative, intuitive inquirers tend to "break set" with established theory and scholarship. Often synchronistic with events in the media and attracting public attention, intuitive inquirers explore topics that require attention by the culture at large, as though they are called to envision anew and seek solutions for dilemmas in which we as humans find ourselves embroiled. Consciously or unconsciously, from a psychoanalytic or Jungian perspective, what may seem like one researcher's dedication to a narrow topic may be the tip of an iceberg of a call from the culture at large for change.[1]

Methodologically, intuitive inquiry has been informed directly by the Biblical hermeneutics of Friedrich Schleiermacher (1819/1977), the philosophical hermeneutics of Hans-Georg Gadamer (e.g., Bruns, 1992; Gadamer, 1998; Packer & Addison, 1989), phenomenological and heuristic research as developed by Clark Moustakas (1990, 1994), and a wide spectrum of feminist scholarship in psychology and theology. My first version of intuitive inquiry incorporated intuitive and compassionate ways of knowing in the selection of a research topic, data analysis, and presentation of findings in what might be described as an in-depth qualitative research method (Anderson, 1998). Later, I developed a hermeneutical process of iterative cycles of interpretation to give a "soft" structure to the intuitive process that lends both intellectual precision and freedom of expression to the method (Anderson, 2000). The version of intuitive inquiry presented in this chapter and elsewhere (Anderson, 2004a; Anderson, 2004b; Esbjörn-Hargens & Anderson, 2005; Anderson, in press) represents a refined integration of this hermeneutical process and my experience in supervising studies using intuitive inquiry in the past 12 years. Elsewhere (Anderson, in press) I provide an in-depth presentation of intuitive inquiry along with research examples and experiential exercises of each of the five cycles. For more information about the historical development of intuitive inquiry, see my autobiographical statement in Chapter 2 of this volume.

In this chapter, I present intuitive inquiry as a distinct method of analysis. Of course, too, the intuitive and imaginal procedures of intuitive inquiry may support and enhance research praxis more generally. This chapter invites readers to explore intuitive inquiry as a unique method *and* to integrate and adapt its procedures with other analytical approaches to research and scholarship. Supported by accounts from eminent scientists and artists who have openly claimed the value of intuition to their scientific discoveries and innovations (e.g., Root-Bernstein & Root-Bernstein, 1999), intuition is commonly acknowledged as a way of knowing related to scientific insight. In a sense, the human sciences are catching up with this wider cultural discourse in the arts and literature regarding the role of intuition within the wide spectrum of human knowing.

Initially, in the mid-1990s, I developed intuitive inquiry in response to the challenges posed by my dissertation students who studied topics in the field of transpersonal psychology. "Right body size" for women (Coleman, 2000), the healing presence of a psychotherapist (Phelon, 2001), grief and other deep emotions in response to nature (Dufrechou, 2002), true joy in union with God in mystical Christianity (Carlock, 2003), storytelling and compassionate connection (Hoffman, 2003), and the dialectics of embodiment among contemporary female mystics (Esbjörn, 2003) were among early topics studied. In last several years, intuitive inquiry has spread beyond transpersonal and humanistic psychology circles. Intuitive inquiry and elements of intuitive inquiry are being used in studies in a wide variety of fields, including creative arts, ecopsychology, health and wellness, education, mainstream psychology, and nursing science. Therefore, I write and speak about the potential for integrating intuition within research praxis and intuitive inquiry per se with confidence and nuance. When research analysis is infused with the imaginal and intuitive, science is imbued with a renewed ethical and compassionate dimension. Our times press with individual, communal, and global needs that invite fresh solutions. Let us begin.

What Is Intuition?

In Latin, *intuitus* refers to the direct perception of knowledge. Jeremy Hayward (1997) defines intuition as "the direct perception of things as they are" (p. ix). Intuitions often bypass the ordinary five human senses and analytical reason. Marie-Louise von Franz (1971) described intuition as "a kind of sense perception via the unconscious or a subliminal sense perception" (p. 37). In contemporary neuropsychological research, intuition is usually described as primarily related to right-brain processes that mediate the perception of imagery, gestalts, and patterns, as differentiated from left-brain processes that mediate linear thinking, logic, reason, and analysis (e.g., Taylor, 2006). Carl Jung (1933) presents intuition as an "irrational" function—not because intuition is unreliable but because intuitive insights often elude our attempts to understand their character or origins. Intuitions often feel palpable as distinct perceptions into the nature of things; sometimes we can discern their triggers and how they support or even confound life decisions. But, more often, the occurrence of an intuition seems elusive, unrepeatable by will, and understandable conceptually only after a period of reflection and discernment.

In a phenomenological investigation of the intuitive experience, Claire Petitmengin-Peugeot (1999) described four "interior gestures" that were strikingly similar from interview to interview, despite the differences in the content of intuitive insight: (1) the gesture of letting go, slowing down, and of interior self-collection; (2) the gesture of connection with a person, object, problem, or situation; (3) the gesture of listening with senses and awareness open and attentive; and (4) the intuition itself. The intuition surges forth in many forms, as "an image, a kinesthetic feeling, a sound or word, even a taste or an odor, most of the time in several simultaneous or successive sensorial forms" (p. 69). Petitimengin-Peugeot concludes:

> This study confirms our hypothesis at the starting point: intuition does correspond to an experience, that is, a set of interior gestures which involve the entire being. Even if intuition keeps an unpredictable, capricious character, it is possible to encourage its appearing, and to accompany its unfolding, by a very meticulous interior preparation. This preparation does not consist in learning, in progressively accumulating knowledge. It consists in emptying out, in giving up our habits of representation, of categorization, and of

abstraction. This casting off enables us to find spontaneity, the real immediacy of our relation to the world. (p. 76)

Elsewhere (Anderson, in press) I present a typology of five intuitive modes of expression based on how I currently understand intuitive ways of knowing. Behaviors typical to one mode may readily blend with other modes in everyday experience. This typology has been enriched by the earlier writings of Roberto Assagioli (1990), Arthur Diekman (1982), Peter Goldberg (1983), Carl Jung (1933), Arthur Koestler (1990), and Frances Vaughan (1979) and is summarized below:

1. *Unconscious, symbolic, and imaginal processes.* Unconscious, symbolic, and imaginal processes have been explored in depth in visionary experiences (e.g., Hildegard von Bingen, 1954; Chicago, 1985; Cirker, 1982; Luna & Amaringo, 1991), Jungian and archetypal psychology (e.g., Burneko, 1997; Edinger, 1972, 1975; Jung, 1959, 1972), and more recently in imaginal psychology (e.g., Romanyshyn, 2002, 2007). Typically in these fields, researchers and scholars tend to live active symbolic lives in which dreams, imaginal processes, somatic experiences, and visionary experiences are commonplace. In my own case, my understanding of these processes has been deepened primarily through listening to and sitting with indigenous teachers from eastern Europe and Tibet.

2. *Psychic or parapsychological experiences.* Despite their common occurrence for many people, psychic and parapsychological phenomena typically are generally unacknowledged as sources of scientific insights. Such direct and unmediated experiences include telepathy, clairvoyance, and precognitive experiences that take place at a distance (in space or time). These experiences are aspects of what have been called exceptional human experiences (EHEs) by researchers Rhea White (1997) and William Braud (2002, 2003).

3. *Sensory modes of intuition.* In addition to the five senses of sight, hearing, smell, taste, and touch, kinesthesia (sense of movement in space), proprioception (sense of orientation in space), and a "visceral sense" arising from sense receptors in the organs and tissues of the body may serve as intuitive channels, conveying subtle forms of information often unavailable to the thinking mind. Awareness of visceral, kinesthetic, and proprioceptive sensations can be enhanced through focused attention and specialized training, such as the focusing method developed by Eugene Gendlin (1978, 1991, 1992, 1997), authentic movement developed by body practitioners Mary Whitehouse, Janet Adler, and Joan Chodorow (e.g., Adler, 2002; Pallaro, 1999), embodied writing (Anderson, 2001, 2002a, 2002b), and many other embodied and meditative practices.

4. *Empathic identification.* Through compassionate knowing or empathic identification, writers, actors, psychotherapists, and scientists inhabit the lived world of another person or object of study. In a seamless display of gesture and timbre of voice, a fine actor convinces an audience that Macbeth is present. Psychotherapists attend to the life of their clients, seeing the world through the clients' eyes in order to help them see possibilities they cannot imagine for themselves. Similarly, geneticist Barbara McClintock spoke about looking through a microscope at corn fungus and viewing the chromosomes as though she were "down there and these were my friends (as cited in Keller, 1983, p. 117). An extensive discussion of empathic identification as used by great artists and scientists can be found in *Sparks of Genius* by Root-Bernstein and Root-Bernstein (1999).

5. *Through our wounds.* Having conducted and supervised doctoral research for over 30 years, I am often aware that a researcher's intuitive style tends to settle along the fault lines or wounds in the researcher's personality in a manner akin to the concept of the wounded healer in religious, spiritual, and shamanic circles. Catholic priest and contemplative Henri Nouwen (1990) and Buddhist Roshi Joan Halifax (1983) characterize human wounds as sites of both suffering and hospitality to the sacred.

In *The Wounded Researcher,* Robert Romanyshyn (2007) strikes a similar theme. For Romanyshyn, "re-search" is soul work or spiritual work because in relinquishing one's claims upon the work and the narrow perspectives with which one began, "re-search" takes on a lively character all its own. The past that claims the researcher speaks through us to the future in language transformed by the act of searching again. The researcher begins to ask, "Who's doing this work after all?", begging the question even of authorship. Romanyshyn articulates this process precisely:

> The work that the researcher is called to do makes sense of the researcher as much as he or she makes sense of it. Indeed, before we understand the work we do, it stands under us. Research as a vocation, then, puts one in service to those unfinished stories that weigh down upon us individually and collectively as the wait and weight of history. As a vocation, research is what the work indicates. It is re-search, a searching again of what has already made its claim upon us and is making its claim upon the future. (p. 113)

Highly intuitive people are often intuitive from an early age, but everyone can learn intuitive ways of knowing and expand the intuitive skills they already have. See Anderson and Braud (in press) and Root-Bernstein and Root-Bernstein (1999) for suggestions on how to integrate intuitive, imaginal, and meditative practices into research practice.

Five Cycles of Interpretation

Intuitive inquiry is a hermeneutical research process requiring five iterative cycles of analysis and interpretation. In Cycle 1, the researcher clarifies the research topic via a creative process that is described in depth below. In Cycle 2, the intuitive inquirer reflects upon her or his own pre-understanding of the topic in light of relevant texts and findings found in literature and prepares a list of preliminary interpretative lenses. These Cycle 2 lenses describe the researcher's understanding of the topic *prior* to data collection and analysis. In Cycle 3, the researcher gathers original or archival data and presents the data in a descriptive form that represents the "voices" in the texts and invites readers to come to their own conclusions about the data. In Cycle 4, the researcher presents a set of interpretive lenses, which have been transformed in light of personal engagement with the data gathered in Cycle 3, and provides a lens-by-lens comparison of the Cycle 2 and Cycle 4 lenses. In Cycle 5, the researcher presents an integration of the Cycle 4 lenses with the empirical and theoretical literature relevant to the topic and theoretical refinements and discusses the implications. Reflecting the transformative and imaginative dimensions of the method, presentation of the five cycles should be written in the researcher's distinctive voice in a manner that engages readers both professionally and personally.

All five cycles of intuitive inquiry are embedded with analytic *and* intuitive processes that support and "contain" the ongoing investigation. Aligned with Petitmengin-Peugeot's (1999) phenomenological study that presents intuition as an unfolding process with distinct interior gestures, my own experience with intuition suggests that intuitive insights are encouraged by environments and often structured conditions that support these interior gestures over time. The five cycles of intuitive inquiry are illustrated in Figure 9.1. Based on my own experience in conducting and supervising intuitive inquiries, the size of the ovals for each cycle indicates the amount of time and effort each cycle typically requires, relative to the others.

This chapter is part of a book, together with the work of four other qualitative researchers, which emphasizes our individual analyses of an interview with a young woman, called Teresa, who is recovering from anaplastic throat cancer. Each of us begins with an overview of our respective analytic approaches. I provide a brief overview the five cycles of intuitive inquiry below. (See Anderson, in press, for a thorough presentation of the five cycles, experiential exercises for each cycle, and discussion of other aspects of intuitive inquiry.) Following this overview, I present my analysis of the Teresa texts as Cycle 1 of intuitive inquiry. Subsequently, my analysis of the Teresa texts is followed by an analysis of an additional interview of a man, called Reno, who is recovering from epileptic seizures, to illustrate all five cycles of intuitive inquiry.

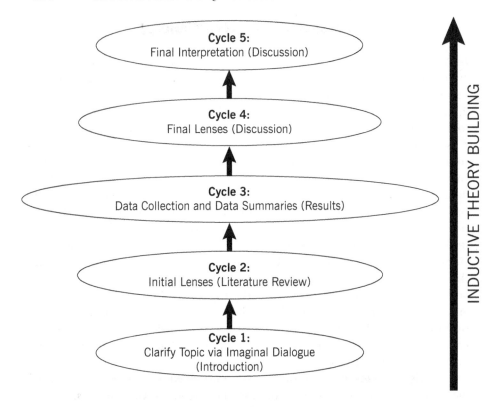

FIGURE 9.1. Intuitive inquiry: Five cycles of interpretation.

Cycle 1: Clarifying the Research Topic

The purpose of Cycle 1 of intuitive inquiry is to clarify the research topic. Since most intuitive inquirers choose topics relevant to their personal lives, it is important for them to understand the motives for their choice and their pre-understandings of the topic. To clarify and refine a topic, the intuitive inquirer selects a text or image that repeatedly attracts or claims his attention in relationship to his research topic and interests. Sometimes the relationship of the chosen text or image to a topic is ambiguous at the start. Texts and images selected for Cycle 1 may include photographs, paintings, sketches, symbols, sculptures, song lyrics, movies, poems, sacred texts or scripture, interview transcripts, recorded dreams, and/or accounts of a meaningful transformative experience. Theoretically, a statistical analysis, graph, or figure based on statistical analysis might be suitable as a "text" for Cycle 1, though no intuitive inquirer has done so yet.

Once the text, broadly defined, is identified, the researcher enters Cycle 1 interpretation via daily engagement with the text and records the insights.

Researchers should spend at least 20 minutes a day (or approximately 40 minutes every other day) reading, listening, or viewing the identified text. Thoughts, ideas, daydreams, conversations, impressions, visions, and intuitions occurring during sessions and at other times are recorded in a non-invasive manner so as not to disrupt the stream of consciousness that often accompanies intuition. Notebooks, handheld voice recorders, and art supplies should be readily available to support recording of thoughts, memories, images, and impressions. This process of engagement with the selected text should be continued until the creative tension between the intuitive inquirer and the text or image feels resolved and complete.

By repeatedly engaging with a potential text in this dialectic process, impressions and insights converge into a focused research topic. A suitable topic for intuitive inquiry is

1. *Compelling.* For a research topic to sustain the researcher's interest and energy, it should inspire his or her motivations and intellectual passions.

2. *Manageable.* A topic can vary in scope and depth, depending on the time given for a project.

3. *Clear.* Good research topics can be expressed easily in one sentence. The more a researcher understands a research topic, the simpler the basic statement of intent becomes.

4. *Focused.* A simple and focused topic with significant implications for human experience is preferable to a diffuse, ambiguously defined topic.

5. *Concrete.* The research topic should be directly related to specific behaviors, experiences, or phenomena.

6. *Researchable.* Some topics are too grand or do not (yet) lend themselves to scientific inquiry.

7. *Promising.* A topic is promising when it signifies an experience of something that is still unknown or appears to beg understanding. Since the topics pursued in intuitive inquiry tend to be at the growing tip of cultural understanding, it is often the case that only the researcher him- or herself can evaluate the potential importance of a given topic at the start of the inquiry.

Cycle 2: Preliminary Interpretive Lenses

In Cycle 2, the intuitive inquirer reflects upon the topic in light of texts found in the extant literature about the topic and prepares a list of preliminary interpretive lenses. These Cycle 2 lenses describe the researcher's understanding of the research topic *prior* to data collection. To articulate these lenses, the researcher again engages the topic through imaginal dialogues with texts that help him or her discern the values, assumptions, and understanding he or she brings to the topic from the start. This imaginal dialogue of Cycle 2 is similar to the imaginal dialogue in Cycle 1; however, in Cycle 2, the researcher's reflections and notes become more conceptual and intellectual in relationship to the topic. Usually, selecting appropriate texts for Cycle 2 takes place at the same time as the researcher reviews the theoretical and research literature on the topic. Cycle 2 texts are different texts than those used in Cycle 1. However, the meaning of texts in Cycle 2 is again broadly defined and may include empirical findings, theoretical writings, historical or archival records, literary or musical texts, symbol and images, etc. Later, by comparing Cycle 2's preliminary lenses with Cycle 4's interpretive lenses, readers of intuitive inquiries can evaluate the course of change and transformation in the researcher's understanding of the topic.

Structurally, Cycle 2 involves a three-part process. First, the intuitive inquirer becomes familiar with the empirical findings and the theoretical, historical, and literary texts relevant to the topic. Empirical literature may include quantitative and qualitative findings. Second, the researcher identifies from among the literature and research on the topic a unique set of texts for his or her Cycle 2 imaginal dialogue. Third, based on ongoing imaginal dialogue with these Cycle 2 texts, the researcher prepares a list of preliminary Cycle 2 lenses that express his or her understanding of the topic prior to data collection. This generation of preliminary lenses is often quick and free-flowing, feeling more like brainstorming or creative imagination than a formal process. At a certain point, the researcher feels that he or she has integrated the Cycle 2 texts sufficiently and sits down at the desk with pen and paper or keyboard and "roughs" them out, often in a single sitting. Through a process of combining, reorganizing, and identifying emerging patterns, the list of preliminary lenses usually shortens to less than a dozen. Ordinarily, 10–12 preliminary lenses seem sufficient to "capture" the nuance and range in content and structure of most research topics.

In intuitive inquiry, the articulation of Cycle 2 interpretive lenses completes the forward arc of the hermeneutical circle during which the intuitive inquirer seeks to identify the topic clearly and express his or her pre-understanding of it. With data collection in Cycle 3, the return arc of the hermeneutical circle begins and the researcher's focus shifts to understanding the topic in light of the experiences of others. Once data collection begins, there is no turning back to reclaim the researcher's pre-understanding of the topic because the forward movement implicit in data collection propels the intuitive inquirer into a different mode of engagement and perception. The primary mode of activity in the forward arc of Cycles 1 and 2 tends to be inward and reflective. In contrast, the primary mode of activity in the return arc of Cycles 3, 4, and 5 is more outwardly engaged in order to reimagine and reinterpret one's own understanding in light of the understanding and experiences of others. For a more complete description of this process, see Anderson (in press).

Cycle 3: Collecting Data and Preparing Descriptive Reports

In Cycle 3, the researcher (a) identifies the best source(s) of data for the research topic, (b) develops criteria for the selection of data from among these sources, (c) collects data, and (d) prepares descriptive analyses of data that represent the "voices" of the participants or other narrators in the data. Data interpretation does not begin until Cycle 4.

While researchers may be tempted to choose data that are conveniently available, rarely does any study profit from such an approach—far less the in-depth, intuitive processes invited by intuitive inquiry. Therefore, choose the data sources that best suit your unique and focused interests in the topic of study. Follow your enthusiasm and intuition. Notice what attracts your attention again and again. Choose inviting or challenging data sources, even if you do not always know why those sources attract or repel. Empirical research on intuition (e.g., Bastick, 1982; Petitmengin-Peugeot, 1999) has consistently shown that intuitive processes tend to convey an impression of certainty even when the intuitive insight proves later to be incorrect. Therefore, intuitive inquirers might consider selecting data sources that intentionally challenge their Cycle 2 lenses.

To date, most researchers using intuitive inquiry have collected original empirical data in the form of interviews or stories from research participants who meet specific criteria as informants relevant to the topic of study (e.g., Coleman, 2000; Dufrechou, 2002; Esbjörn, 2003; Manos, 2007; Perry, 2009; Phelon, 2001, 2004; Rickards, 2006; Shepperd, 2006; Unthank, 2007). However, in a study of true joy among Christian mystics, Susan Carlock (2003) chose an additional set of writings from historical mystics for Cycle 3, rather than collect data from contemporary Christian mystics, because of the spiritual depth of the historical mystical sources. In addition to interviews, Rickards (2006) made use of extensive historical narratives about, and journal accounts by, female espionage agents during World War II. Several researchers have incorporated embodied writing accounts (Anderson, 2001, 2002a, 2002b) from participants (Dufrechou, 2002; Medrano-Marra, 2007; Netzer, 2008; Shepperd, 2006) or encouraged artistic expression (Hill, 2005; Hoffman, 2003; Manos, 2007; Rickards, 2006).

To date, data analysis procedures used in Cycle 3 have included the following:

♦ Edited interview transcripts (Esbjörn, 2003; Esbjörn-Hargens & Anderson, 2005)

♦ Portraits of participants (Coleman, 2000; Rickards, 2006) incorporating procedures developed within heuristic research by Moustakas (1990)

♦ Historical portraits (Carlock, 2003)

♦ Descriptive portraits of the artists accompanied by illustrative examples of their art (Manos, 2007)

- Aspects of discourse analysis developed by Potter and Wetherell (1995) plus interviewee stories (Unthank, 2007)
- Descriptive thematic content analysis of interviews (Brandt, 2007; Perry, 2009)
- A series of embodied writing accounts by participants directly related to the topic (Dufrechou, 2002; Shepperd, 2006)
- Participants' stories accompanied by excerpts of their embodied writing (Medrano-Marra, 2007; Netzer, 2008)
- Grounded theory analysis (McCormick, 2010)

These descriptive presentations allow readers to review the data prior to the researcher's interpretation of data in Cycle 4 and come to their own conclusions. When I am teaching intuitive inquiry, a metaphor that seems to communicate the descriptive presentation of data in Cycle 3 is that of hovering low like a hummingbird, over the data and relaying what you see from that vantage point. (See Anderson, in press, for an extended discussion of data collection options for Cycle 3.)

Cycle 4: Transforming and Revising Interpretive Lenses

In Cycle 4, the researcher presents a final set of interpretive lenses, which have been transformed by personal engagement with the data gathered in Cycle 3, and provides a detailed comparison of the Cycle 2 and Cycle 4 lenses. Cycle 2 lenses are modified, removed, rewritten, expanded, etc., reflecting the researcher's more developed and nuanced understanding of the topic at the conclusion of the study.

In intuitive inquiry, the two-fold articulation of lenses in Cycle 2 and again in Cycle 4 mitigates against circularity. The degree of change between Cycle 2 and Cycle 4 lenses is, in part, a measure of the researcher's willingness to be influenced by data and to modify his or her understanding of a topic. Some changes are likely to be major, others minor. In Cycle 4, the researcher prepares a *lens-by-lens* comparison of the Cycle 2 and Cycle 4 lenses in order to make the changes obvious to the reader. By comparing Cycle 2 and Cycle 4 lenses, the reader of an intuitive inquiry report can evaluate what changed in the researcher's understanding of the research topic during the course of the study. The new, change, and seed lenses proposed by Vipassana Esbjörn (2003) provide a reader-friendly way to make both substantive and subtle changes obvious to the reader in Cycle 4.

Throughout an intuitive inquiry, the most important feature of interpreting data is intuitive breakthroughs, those illuminating moments when the data begin to shape themselves before the researcher. Generally speaking, feelings of confusion and bewilderment are indications that a researcher is encountering what he or she does not know and yet seeks to understand. When the researcher begins to see patterns in the data, interpretation in the form of Cycle 4 lenses has begun. Since the generation of Cycle 4 lenses is an interpretive task, the act of taking personal responsibility for one's own reflexivity and interpretation may challenge a researcher's beliefs about the purely objective nature of science.

My own process of generating Cycle 4 lenses involves intuitive and analytic processes based on a visual scanning for patterns. I work with a paper and pencil, drawing small and large circles—representing themes or stray ideas—then shifting the patterns and modifying the relationships and size of the circles, rather like a mobile Venn diagram. I know other researchers who work in a more narrative or auditory style, as though talking to themselves. Again and again, they bring ideas together in an array of interrelated themes, narratives, sequences, or irreducible features of the experience studied. Sometimes, intuitive inquirers start dreaming or daydreaming about final lenses or envisioning them as symbols or images. It is important to document insights along the way. This interpretive process may go on for several days or weeks, with rest or incubation periods between work sessions.

Cycle 5: Integration of Findings and Theory Building

In Cycle 5, the intuitive inquirer presents an integration of the Cycle 4 lenses, the empirical and theoretical literature reviewed at the start of the study, and theoretical refinements and speculations based on findings. Situated in the analytic, hermeneutical process of Cycles 1 through 4, in Cycle 5 the intuitive inquirer presents a final interpretation of findings and theoretical speculations related to the topic of study. As in all research reports, at the end of the study the researcher returns to the literature review prior to data collection and reevaluates prior research in light of the study's findings. In other words, the researcher must determine what is significant about his or her study and what is not, including what he or she feels is still undisclosed about the topic. In a sense, the researcher stands back from the entire research process and takes into consideration all aspects of the study anew, as though drawing a larger hermeneutical circle around the hermeneutical circle prescribed by the forward and return arcs of the study.

Similar to various forms of grounded theory (e.g., See Charmaz, Chapter 6 this volume; Strauss & Corbin, 1990), one of the most promising aspects of intuitive inquiry is its potential for inductive theory building. As a practical matter, intuitive inquirers must maintain a big-picture perspective throughout the course of a study, so inductive theory building is intrinsically embedded in the method. Reductive processes do not fit the method, and researchers usually find themselves "out-maneuvered" by their own spontaneity and intuitions. To date, two intuitive inquirers (Phelon, 2001; Unthank, 2007) have actively engaged the method's potential to generate theory inductively, based on the development of their understanding of the topic in the five cycles. At the conclusion of her study, Cortney Phelon (2001, 2004) developed a theoretical model for understanding the embodied healing presence of a psychotherapist along with recommendations for the training of clinicians. Katherine Unthank (2007) began her study of trauma survival with an implicit theory based on years of clinical practice as a therapist specializing in trauma recovery. By her own account, her study "brought her face to face with her own embodied shame and with survival habits of security in having [perceived] control" (p. 226). At the end of the study, she concluded that the deep structure of trauma survival is a learned functional neurosis of shame fused with guilt, which generates a world of perceived safety at the expense of being chronically at fault for what happened or what might happen differently. (See Anderson, in press, for additional information about the theory-building potential of intuitive inquiry.)

Analyses of Teresa and Reno Interviews

Cycle 1: Clarifying the Research Topic: Reverse Mirroring Discourse of Disease

To meet the needs of this collaborative project, I made several adjustments to the usual procedures for intuitive inquiry's five cycles described above. First, the choice of analyzing Teresa's interview was made by the group and not by me alone. Typically, in intuitive inquiry, the researcher chooses a topic based on his or her own interests and passions and then selects a text for Cycle 1 that evokes his or her intuitive understanding of the topic. However, in this case, the group decided to analyze Teresa's interview because the introductory description of the "unfortunate event" by Teresa, the interviewer's introductory notes, and the interview transcript provided richer qualitative descriptions than any of the other data available to us. I agreed with the group and hoped that my interest and enthusiasm would eventually be "hooked" by Teresa's interview texts in a manner that invites intuition. Second, the extensive analysis of identifying themes, described above, is a more elaborate intuitive and analytical process than is typically conducted in Cycle 1 of intuitive inquiry, aligning it more with the descriptive presentation of data in Cycle 3 and with the interpretation of findings in Cycle 4 of intuitive inquiry. Usually, in Cycle 1, the intuitive inquirer engages in imaginal dialogues with a text related to a topic solely to clarify and refine the topic. However, since I began this Cycle 1 *without* a statement of topic, extensive engagement with the Teresa texts was required in order to formulate an initial topic statement. Furthermore, my analysis of the Teresa texts below also invites readers to compare my analysis with that of the four other qualitative researchers analyzing these texts in this book.

As it turned out, after several readings, I found the contents of Teresa texts compelling. I started to muse and even dream about Teresa's experience while deeply immersed in the analysis, so this departure from the procedures for intuitive inquiry was successful in this instance. What engaged my enthusiasm arose out of my personal history. First, I have been an Episcopal priest since 1987, so Teresa's experience of encountering adversity, a life-threatening diagnosis, surgery, a protracted recovery period, and the possibility for a recurrence of cancer are well placed within my professional experience. Second, in the last 10 years, I have created an experientially based style of writing, called embodied writing, that expresses the lived experience of the body (Anderson, 2001, 2002a, 2002b), and I developed a scale for measuring body awareness, the Body Intelligence Scale (Anderson, 2006). Third, I have experienced the transformative dimensions of life-threatening circumstances in my own life. Fourth, my mother died of anaplastic cancer of the uterus 23 years ago; therefore, I know the aggressive course of this disease from firsthand experience. All of these factors invited me into Teresa's story in an empathic and visceral way. My experience of Teresa's experience lies somewhere in the imaginal realm between hers and mine—not mine, not hers, but something other between the two. These "flights" into intersubjectivity (e.g., Wilber, 2000, 2006) and reflectivity gave me intuitive insights that I may not have considered otherwise.

I used the Teresa interview and introductory notes as the texts for Cycle 1, engaging in the imaginal dialogues with these texts as prescribed for this cycle of intuitive inquiry (Anderson, in press). Since the purpose of Cycle 1 is to clarify and refine the topic, I entered my analysis of these texts with an open mind and heart to see what would attract my interest. Even though the interview and notes focused on the description of an unfortunate event that might suggest a variety of research topics, such as resilience, trauma, coping strategies in adversity, etc., I sought to articulate a precise topic that evolved out of my own analysis of the Teresa texts in Cycle 1. Procedurally, my analysis took a straightforward form. First, I read the Teresa texts several times. Second, once I had an overall intellectual grasp and felt sense of the texts, I highlighted the parts of the texts that interested me or aroused my curiosity. I then used these 77 highlighted texts as meaning units, most of them full sentences or full paragraphs in length, and copied and compiled them verbatim. Examples of meaning units are given below as examples of themes. Third, I sorted the 77 meaning units into thematic categories using a descriptive procedure for thematic content analysis (TCA; Anderson, 2007).

Using these procedures, I sorted the meaning units three times, reconfiguring and renaming themes for related meaning units each time. For the first two of these analyses, I sorted meanings units and provisional themes using the cut, copy, and paste edit functions in Microsoft Word. By the end of the second sort, the emerging themes and patterns between the themes were too complex for this process because I could not visually scan them all at one time on my computer screen. So I reverted to mechanical means, literally cutting out meaning units from printed copies and arranging them on large sheets of paper with themes provisionally inscribed at the top of various assortments of meaning unites. I placed these sheets on a large picnic table in my home and, from time to time over the next few days, I mused about the themes and rearranged the placement of meaning units until patterns emerged among the themes. Throughout this entire process I maintained an imaginal dialogue with the texts and experienced breakthrough insights during these dialogues, signaling to me that my intuitive process was working well. As I was finalizing this process, I reread the interview transcript and introductory notes to check whether or not I had overlooked any important dimensions of Teresa's experience in my initial highlighting for relevant meaning units. After about a week, I felt satisfied with the naming and arrangement of themes and able to state a clear research topic, the goal of Cycle 1.

Intuitively Derived Thematic Content Analysis of the Teresa Texts

My intuitive analysis of the Teresa texts resulted in five primary themes, recurring throughout the texts, namely:

1. Pragmatic and dispassionate use of denial, logic, and reason as a coping strategy
2. Emotional "shutdown" of feelings and bodily sensations of numbness
3. Personal transformation from "fat girl with no friends" to a transformed self with accompanying emotions of anger, relief, and gratitude
4. Intense feelings expressed by others
5. Angry feedback from physical body in the form of anaplastic cancer, a rare and aggressive type of cancer

The presentation of my analysis below presents Themes 1–5, along with examples of meaning units for each theme, copied verbatim from the Teresa texts. Themes 1, 3, and 4 overlap with some of the analyses of my four colleagues in this book. Themes 1–5 below are more analytically descriptive than interpretive of the Teresa texts because each theme is directly substantiated by quotes (i.e., meaning units) extracted from the Teresa texts. This descriptive presentation of themes is typical of the presentation of findings in Cycle 3 of intuitive inquiry. After presentation of the five themes, I present an overarching theme, which combines Themes 1, 2, and 5 and suggests a reverse mirroring between denial and numbing of bodily sensations and anaplastic cancer, an "angry" cancer. My subsequent articulation of the overarching theme of reverse mirroring is distinctly interpretive and more representative of the final lenses that present the researcher's understanding of the topic in Cycle 4.

Theme 1: Pragmatic and Dispassionate Use of Reason and Logic as a Coping Strategy. As evidenced throughout the Teresa texts, Teresa is an astute young woman. She is articulate about her emotional and intellectual processes. She provides considerable detail about the events surrounding her diagnosis and recovery, despite the 11 years that have passed since their occurrence. Her vocabulary and syntax reflect her graduate level of education at the time of the interview.

Teresa even speaks with nuance and awareness about her own use of logic and reason to minimize painful feelings and how these inclinations originated in experiences within her family-of-origin dynamics. Her descriptions are candid and forthcoming and are not reflective of extensive questioning by the interviewer. Specifically, in describing her conversation with her surgeon and dealing with others' reactions to her diagnosis, Teresa employs a dispassionate form of logic that allows her to distance herself from what might otherwise be emotionally overwhelming. Three meaning units follow as examples of this theme:

> I began to understand things in a very logical, philosophical way, and I took to logic because passion hurt too much.

> I reverted completely to logic at that point. I do that. In moments of stress, or anxiety, or tension, or grief . . . you name it. Um . . . I don't try to avoid the emotion, but I do try to temper it . . . by at least maintaining some degree of practical reasoning and logic as the basis of what I'm thinking and doing, just so I don't go completely off kilter and start looking like a moron.

> I took it all in very methodically, as though we were talking about someone else entirely that he'd be cutting into the next morning.

Theme 2: Emotional "Shutdown" of Feelings and Physical Sensations of Numbness. Teresa seems to have an uncanny ability to distance herself from feelings and bodily sensations. While acknowledging that the interview took place when she was 30 and the events she describes mostly took place 11 years earlier, Teresa presents a pattern of blocking, shutting down, or "freezing" in the face of strong emotions. When Teresa's surgeon informs her that she needs surgery immediately, her body becomes "cool and numb." The tumor on her throat felt like an inert object, having no sensation. Teresa also admires her voice teacher's technique of treating the body as a physical "apparatus" and attributes the success of his technique to the control of somatic emotionality in the act of singing. Teresa's admiration of his technique and her youthful success as an aspiring soprano, may in some ways, have been a result of her ability to shut down emotional sensations originating in the body—a proclivity that may have originated in the highly charged emotional environment of her family of origin. This pattern of minimizing or blocking physical sensations is the somatic correlate to the emotional coping strategies of denial and dispassionate logic in Theme 1. Four meaning units follow as examples of this theme:

> [The lump] wasn't there the day before, I was positive of that. I touched it, and it didn't hurt. I poked it, even thumped it . . . it was hard as a rock, and I didn't feel a thing.

> I froze. I couldn't breathe, couldn't move, couldn't even blink. I felt like I had just been shot. My gut had locked up like I'd been punched in it. My mouth went dry and my fingers, which had been fumbling with a pen, were suddenly cold and numb.

> When I got to college and entered the voice studio, I was told to restrict that emotion and to focus more on the physicality of what I was doing, on releasing tension. When you're emotional, you get physically tense. And when you get physically tense, that kind of messes with what you're doing vocally . . . and that's what was happening to me. So getting away from that emotionality and reminding myself why . . . which, of course, takes logic . . . was actually very instrumental in the long run, not in quashing my emotions . . . I still listen very much to my emotions . . . but understanding that they're just a part of what needs to take place in order to help me function in a given scenario.

> But this particular [voice] teacher really does have something. And the proof's in the pudding; his students do phenomenal things, and his technique is very scientifically based . . . it's not just this artsy intuition that you see so much in the field. Of course, you need to be an artist, but, if you look beyond that, you have a body and an apparatus, and a means by which it physically operates. . . .

Theme 3: Personal Transformation from "Fat Girl with No Friends" to a Transformed Self with Accompanying Emotions of Anger, Relief, and Gratitude. Through determination and courage, Teresa progressed forward in her life. Reading her texts again and again, I came to admire this young woman who took on the challenge of her cancer diagnosis, the consequent surgeries, and the creation of a new life "beyond the hallowed catacombs of practice rooms." At 19, she loses her voice to radical surgery on her throat. She fights the odds of the typical course of anaplastic cancer as a heroic journey to the other side, another life. This lonely young woman with only a voice as an identity transforms in time into a more emotionally congruent person, expressing strong feelings about her new college major, a new relationship with a man (and later her husband) outside the musical world of her past, a new form of singing in which she sings rock and blues rather than classical music, and a renewed sense of congruency and gratitude about her life. Teresa's response to cancer and surgery became a catalyst for a transformation.

For me, an interesting aspect of Teresa's postsurgery life is her participation in fencing, motorcycling, and rock climbing. All of these sports require extreme attention to outer and inner bodily sensations. One cannot be a novice fencer, motorcyclist, or rock climber without paying attention to what is happening inside and around one's physical body. That a "fat girl with no friends" who used to "numb out" in the face of emotions and bodily sensations would engage in these sports is surprising. Teresa's exploration of these sports is extreme, but then Teresa is strong-minded. Teresa's courage is a raw form of spirituality, grounded in the nitty-gritty of taking life on just as it is. Four meaning units follow as examples of this theme:

Singing was my prayer. That was my connection. That was my big gift. I was a fat kid with no friends for as long as I could remember, but I could sing! That was the "in" for me. When I lost that, I lost my connection with God, I lost all my friends, I lost my calling in life, I lost my passion in life, I lost my trump card . . . the thing that was gonna get me out of being that fat kid with the oppressive dad, and whatever . . . that was going to be my ticket out. I lost my ticket!

You're not gonna stop me. I have a sick passion to fight odds . . . I take pride in it, because . . . I don't know why.

Many suggested that I take a break from school, [that] no one would think any less of me, but I was determined to move on as if nothing had happened. When I met new people, I no longer introduced myself as a singer, which was strange for me.

Still, I loved my newfound intellectual life, and I didn't want to give it all up and go back to the grind of full-time classical singing. Besides, I had discovered that, while my voice was still misbehaving (and often does, to this day), I could sing other kinds of music pretty well, particularly rock and blues. I began tinkering with writing my own music, and eventually acquired my own regular gigs at night clubs and live music venues. I continued in my psychology work, as I do now, for I love it dearly, particularly in that it brought forth in me a part of myself I never knew I had, one that seems to hold its own well enough with the more intellectual crowd. The intensive opera chorus work still makes me an opera singer, but that doesn't seem so important to me anymore. I can sing my own music now, so I'm a singer in an entirely new way.

Theme 4: Intense Emotions Expressed by Others. Throughout the Teresa texts, Teresa describes many peoples' strong emotional reactions to her cancer diagnosis. Some of this emotional feedback was highly congruent to her and her situation. For example, her surgeon's responsiveness to her was amazingly sensitive and personal, particularly in light of his professional role. The range of the emotional responses may have helped Teresa understand ways of responding emotionally that were different from what she had experienced in her family of origin. In any case, being at the center of so much emotional tension, both inner and outer, gave her an emotional workout that she could not easily ignore and hopefully could integrate intrapsychically. Five meaning units follow as examples of this theme:

At this point, the surgeon seemed to have gotten very angry with something I'd said. "Damn it," he grumbled. "I hate when they do this. I hate when they make it so that I'm the one that's saying this right before surgery."

I knew [mom] was going to freak out, she was going to pull over, start crying, get worried, call a bunch of people, make them worry too. I thought, "Crap . . . why don't I just go through the surgery and not tell her?" And, in a sense, I did. I told her some things . . . not everything. I didn't tell her what kind of cancer it was . . . she's a med tech, so she knows things.

So for a little while, after the surgery and during my first round of radiation treatments, [my father] was very open, and was lavishing gifts on me . . . buying me lots of things. I got a new TV, I got new furniture . . . I got a new apartment! I mean, I got stuff! That's just the way he operates. He wanted to demonstrate his affection and his concern by buying me things, and, well . . . a 19-year-old college student is certainly going to take advantage of that, no doubt.

[M]y voice teacher, who was like another father to me, greeted me in tears each time he saw me afterwards . . . he was there for my surgery, and was the last person I saw before my anesthesia kicked in. Seeing the dreams we had built together go to pieces the way they did was just too much for either of us, and we spoke very little after that.

The cancer stuff is not something a guy . . . needs to have to deal with in his first year of marriage, I think. Our relationship has been very egalitarian. . . . That only becomes a problem when I get sick. I mean, we have our differences, but they're differences that we have equally. . . . But with cancer, and my radiation . . . there was no parallel for him. And I think that he tried very hard to see me as strong . . . I wanted to be seen as strong. But whenever I was falling all over myself because of the radiation, he didn't know how to deal with it. He would just kind of look at me and say, "Come on, get up." And I couldn't get up.

Theme 5: Anaplastic Cancer Portrayed as an Angry Cancer. Anaplastic cancer is a fast-growing cancer that spreads rapidly and can metastasize before the affected individual is aware of a tumor. Health care professionals commonly describe anaplastic cancer as an "angry" or "aggressive" cancer because the prognosis is poor, and death frequently occurs within months of diagnosis. Teresa also used these terms to describe her cancer. Five meaning units follow as examples of this theme:

. . . my sort of cancer is an angry sort.

I don't know why your endo didn't tell you this. Your biopsy wasn't inconclusive. You have anaplastic carcinoma. That's thyroid cancer. We've got to get that thing out of there right now.

There are different kinds of thyroid cancer. What I have is a faster type. If you're going to have a cancer, make sure it's thyroid cancer. It's great, because you can get rid of it . . . the survival rate is best. . . . The thing about my type, anaplastic carcinoma, is that it's an extremely fast-growing type. The cells are so advanced that it can grow overnight . . . my tumor *did* grow overnight, and the spreading took place in less than a week. It's the fastest growing of all the thyroid cancers, and there's something like a 15%, maybe 20% percent survival rate in the first couple of months. It seems like most everybody who gets this thing dies from it.

This thing grew overnight, while I was sleeping. Boom . . . tumor. Just like that.

Besides, when you go through something like that, it's very lonely, very isolating, no matter what you do. I mean, even other cancer patients didn't know what it was like, because the cancer I had was so weird. Anaplastic carcinoma is a weirdo cancer that can kill you in a couple of weeks.

Overarching Theme: Reverse Mirroring between Teresa's Use of Dispassionate Logic, Numbing of Feelings, and Bodily Sensation and the "Angry" Character of Her Cancer. Themes 1, 2, and 5, taken together, reveal a pattern of reverse mirroring within Teresa's descriptions of dispassionate logic, numbing of feelings and bodily sensations, *and* the "angry" character of her anaplastic cancer. On the one hand, Teresa describes coping strategies that distance her from feelings and bodily sensations, reflecting a discourse of denial. On the other hand, she describes her cancer as angry. Considering the two together reveals an overarching theme: Teresa's descriptions of her fast-growing anaplastic cancer (Theme 5) mirrors *in reverse* her descriptions of shutting down feeling and of somatic numbness in response to strong emotions (Theme 2) and the use of dispassionate logic as a means of coping (Theme 1). The simplest and most parsimonious explanation for the reverse mirroring in Teresa's discourse is to suggest that the anger Teresa may have felt in response to her diagnosis was projected on or "voiced" by her descriptions of her cancer symptoms, in the same way that important people in Teresa's life gave voice and mirrored back to her emotions that she might have understandably felt herself. If these are projected descriptions, there is no reason to assume that Teresa would be consciously aware of them. This overarching theme of reverse mirroring is embedded in the Teresa texts and does not intimate causation. Causation cannot be inferred from retrospective, self-report data.

With the help of an unusually sympathetic surgeon and the support of her family and especially her mother, Teresa rallies. She responds decisively and gets the surgeries and treatments essential for her recovery. I cannot help but wonder if her decisive, no-nonsense response to her diagnosis was as much a part of her recovery as were the surgeries and treatments. Her ability to act decisively in response to a life-threatening diagnosis of anaplastic cancer was proactive and, in some sense, the opposite of her self-described pattern of dispassionate logic and the shutting down of feelings and bodily sensation. Perhaps her ability to distance herself from feelings and bodily sensations helped her to accept the necessity of the surgery and treatments. Teresa also describes herself in ways that seem to me as more emotionally resolved and accepting as she moved forward through treatment and recovery.

Conclusion of Cycle 1: Statement of Research Topic

As a result of Cycle 1, the topic for this intuitive inquiry explores the possibility of reverse mirroring between psychological and behavioral dispositions and descriptions of disease. At the start of my analysis of the Teresa texts in Cycle 1, I had no idea that this research topic would emerge at the outcome of this cycle.

Cycle 2: Researcher's Preliminary Lenses about the Topic

Since I did not come to study this topic statement out of my own personal interests, my analysis of the Teresa texts in Cycle 1 was open-ended and exploratory. That said, I have beliefs and life experience that influence my understanding of the course of personal change, especially in the contexts of life and death struggles. As I conducted the Cycle 1 analysis of the Teresa texts, my pre-understandings of life-threatening events became clear to me. I witnessed how I encountered both my own attitudes and beliefs and the attitudes and beliefs arising from the texts themselves. In addition to noting what I observed in the texts themselves, I noted what I learned about myself in interacting with them over time. My preliminary Cycle 2 lenses for this topic are the following:

1. Somatic, emotional, psychological, and spiritual states of awareness may represent a fluid continuum rather than separate experiential states.

2. Personal metaphors and self-descriptions may represent distinctive ways of being, such as personality characteristics and coping strategies.

3. Personal metaphors and self-descriptions may morph in the context of challenges and crises, helping us cope and change.

4. Bodily processes and the ways in which we understand and describe them inform personal change in inchoate or instrumental ways whether or not we are aware of any underlying dynamics.

5. Certain diseases, such as anaplastic cancer, can be ravaging to the human body in ways that are difficult to grasp outside of firsthand experience. Perhaps all diseases, especially those that convey the prospect of death, impart a "footprint" that may be incomprehensible outside of firsthand experience.

Typically, the articulation of Cycle 2 preliminary lenses is challenging for intuitive inquirers, even excruciatingly so, because intuitive inquirers must closely scrutinize the assumptions and values they bring to the topic, a process that is likely to change their own assumptions and values concerning the topic per se. In this case, while I had not mused at length about the relationship between disease and recovery, the topic of reverse mirroring between coping strategies and the character of disease is nonetheless consonant with some of my personal attitudes and beliefs listed above.

Cycle 3: Collecting and Analyzing Additional Data

Cycle 3 of an intuitive inquiry involves the collection of original data and a descriptive presentation of them. If I were to continue this study, I would interview several dozen adults who present various types of serious and life-threatening illnesses and analyze the interviews for patterns among self-reported personal habits, coping strategies, change dynamics, and disease symptoms. To illustrate how Cycles 3, 4, and 5 might proceed, I obtained and analyzed one additional interview. I acquired this interview transcript and permission to use it from the interviewee, and from Katherine Unthank (2007), who had conducted an intuitive inquiry concerning posttrauma survival. I asked Unthank to choose a participant who had both experienced trauma and been diagnosed with a serious or life-threatening disease. Unthank chose an interview of a 57-year-old man called Reno who had experienced epileptic seizures since age 11. He began having manic episodes in his 20s and was later diagnosed with temporal lobe epilepsy. By his own account, Reno's life story was full of trauma. Throughout his childhood and adulthood, there were repeated episodes of violence and abuse, as noted in the identified themes below. At the time of the interview, Reno was in his 50s and finally receiving proper medical care for his symptoms and finding meaning in his life struggles.

I analyzed the Reno interview as I had analyzed the Teresa texts, using the procedures for an intuitively derived TCA described above. However, the analysis of the Reno interview ended up to be a simpler process for several reasons. First, the interview was about half the length of the Teresa texts, so half as much data. Second, the events described were less complex. And, more important, knowing the topic of the study allowed me to more easily identify relevant meaning units and themes, while still allowing for emergent meaning units and themes that diverged from my statement of the topic.

My intuitive analysis of the Reno interview resulted in four primary themes, recurring throughout the texts, namely:

1. Childhood trauma and onset of epileptic seizures
2. Adult incidences of trauma
3. Periodic seizures and episodes of mania, leading to diagnosis of bipolar disorder and temporal lobe epilepsy
4. Anger at self, grief, and search for meaning

Theme 1: Childhood Trauma and Onset of Epileptic Seizures. Reno described many traumatic episodes in his childhood, such as those described in the three meaning units that follow as examples of this theme:

And I've had a number of traumas in my life. I guess the earliest was at 6 or 7. And then one about 8. Another one 11. Uh (*big sigh*) and then (*pause*) in my mid 30s and early 40s there were several more traumas. Uh, first trauma was more emotional than anything else. Uh, age 6 or 7, playing with some other kids and tossing a cart, a crate back and forth, and I got hit in the mouth and busted my new teeth coming, growing in at the time. I ran home to my Mom (*pause*) with my mouth all bloody and she said "Don't come running home to me" turned and walked away. And that left me in a bit of shock (*eyes filled with tears*). And, uh, beginning not to trust her judgment, to say the least.

Uh, just about the time I turned 8 I was in the Cub Scout pack, and we were touring the jail and my father was the cop giving the tour. I decided to walk in a cell just to see what it was like for a prisoner. (*Pause*) My father backed up and the door slammed shut on me. I just froze and I wasn't able to do anything. And I was very subdued after that. Uh, a long, long time. Yeah, I got out, but I mean the door slammed shut and then I had to push it open, but I was traumatized till I got out.[2]

Uh, at age 11 I was diagnosed with epilepsy. I've been seizure free for 16 years now . . . they started about age 10 or 11. Uh, I didn't realize it until years later but it was likely due to being hit in the head with a belt . . . by my mother. Uh, I didn't make the relationship then because it was like 6 months, 8 months after before I started having any symptoms. But, uh, later in my mid- to late 20s, down at UCLA, they, uh, located a lesion in my head. Gee, just where the belt buckle hit me.

Theme 2: Adult Incidences of Trauma. Reno described many traumatic episodes throughout his 20s, 30s, 40s, and even into his 50s, including beatings, arrests, and imprisonments. Three meaning units that follow are examples of this theme:

I guess sometime during this process I had another blackout period and I found myself in the jail. With this one abusive officer who liked to kick people. Uh, so to teach me a lesson they strap me to this and take turns kicking me. Uh, they wound up breaking my left shoulder. I'm out of it again, I wake up in a hospital bed, and they'd operated on my shoulder. They put in six pins and a plate to put my shoulder together. And then they just drive me back to the board and care and literally kicked me out the back of it.

I made the mistake of getting off the bicycle, approaching the police car, and they came swinging the night clubs at me. I matched the description of someone they'd heard. . . . And so they arrested me for assaulting an officer. And then hung me in the back of the patrol, patrol car by my arm. . . . And they left me continually hanging in the car for maybe 6 hours or so.

A few minutes later another cop comes running up to me, hits me in the face, drives me to my knees. . . . I'm never allowed to speak to tell them my version of what's happening. Uh, I get arrested. I have a seizure at the police station. So I'm charged with assaulting an officer again. Uh, this is when they put me in solitary.

Theme 3: Periodic Seizures and Episodes of Mania, Leading to Diagnosis of Bipolar Disorder and Temporal Lobe Epilepsy. Reno's behaviors led to diagnoses of bipolar disorder and eventually temporal lobe epilepsy. Four meaning units follow as examples of this theme:

And I found myself carrying books downstairs, no idea why I was doing it. By the time I got downstairs, I said "This is ridiculous." I carried the books back upstairs. And then I felt compelled to carry the books downstairs. And this happened, like, seven, eight, nine times. . . . And I just feel like something's out of whack. I don't know what, but I can't control this. I've got to carry these books downstairs. Why am I doing that? It's ridiculous.

Uh (*pause*) it still took, oh, 2 months for them to dismiss the charges. And they sent me to a locked board and care for a month or two, I forget. Near. By this time they had diagnosed me as bipolar. Uh, I'm in the board and care for . . . (*sigh*).

But, uh, I was having basically a combination of seizures and, uh, manic episodes again. Didn't quite understand what the heck was going on. Uh, and my roommate called the police. Gave up on them coming. Got on my bicycle so I was riding to the hospital where I called my doctor. He told me to come on up. And one of the cops who'd just seen me ride up there says I was too . . . I was behaving weirdly. Uh I'd had a seizure the previous day, previous night.

That was at the time diagnosed as temporal lobe epilepsy, uh, complex seizures, and I think now it's a combination of the two.

Theme 4: Anger at Self, Grief, and Search for Meaning. Primarily in his late 40s and 50s, Reno's life began to calm down. Under regular and proper medical care, his epileptic seizures and manic episodes decreased in frequency. Reno also began to reflect on his life experiences, grieve some of the traumatic experiences, and move toward psychospiritual recovery and normal life. Four meaning units that follow are examples of this theme:

And just why have I got to carry this burden? And, uh, there was shame, there was guilt, there was grief. Uh, basically I was feeling sorry for myself.

Uh, I was angry. Uh, in many ways nondirectional anger, anger at my self. . . . Yeah, for being defective, having the seizures.

I mean in the jail I was put in humiliating circumstances being strapped to a bed, and I could feel things that humiliate me—well, you can't be humiliated probably without your consent—and I did not consent to it. I did not blame myself for it. I blame the screwed-up policies and procedures more than anything else. Might have been a little bit here and there but effectively not blame.

In the midst of all the trauma that is going on . . . I don't, didn't realize it at the time but it was a search for meaning. How can I turn all these negative things that happened to me to a positive?

Cycle 4: Combining the Teresa and Reno Analyses: The Mirroring Discourse of Disease

In the analysis of the Reno interview, I did not find reverse mirroring, but I did find direct mirroring in Reno's descriptions of trauma and abuse, bipolar symptomology, and epileptic seizures. All of these behaviors and symptoms can be described as forms of hyperactivity or reactivity. The intensity of his trauma, anger, and violence are mirrored by the intensity of his seizures and mania. My analysis of the Reno texts suggests a direct mirroring discourse of disease that "surrounds" the illness itself, rather than the reverse mirroring discourse that characterized Teresa's descriptions of personal dispositions, habits of coping, and the fast-growing nature of her cancer.

Viewed together, my analyses of the Teresa and Reno texts signal a modification of the statement of topic for this study, as presented above. Therefore, the research topic is now an exploration of a mirroring discourse between descriptions of psychological and behavioral characteristics and somatic descriptions of disease symptoms. As indicated earlier, to explore this topic fully, I would conduct several dozen additional interviews with people presenting various types of serious and life-threatening diseases.

As noted earlier regarding the Teresa texts, the simplest and most parsimonious explanation for the mirroring discourse found in the analysis of the Teresa and Reno texts is to suggest that both of them described their illnesses and symptoms in a manner similar to the way they generally portray their life stories and identities. In other words, the mirroring discourse patterns are correlated phenomena. Teresa's descriptions of her throat cancer may have "carried" the voice of angry emotions about the illness, and Reno's seizures and mania may be part and parcel of his patterns of hyperactivity and reactivity. I do not want readers, especially Teresa and Reno, to think that their thoughts, coping strategies, or personal habits caused their respective illnesses. The Teresa and Reno data in this study are self-reported, retrospective texts. Only pre- and postdisease data involving proper control groups could suggest causation in these or other cases.

Cycle 5: Integration of Findings and Literature Review

The preliminary findings of Cycle 4 align with some research findings regarding the value of using mental imagery in the treatment of some diseases. For example, in the early 1970s, Carl Simonton and Stephanie Matthews-Simonton conducted exploratory studies on the use of imagery and the treatment of cancer (Simonton, Matthews-Simonton, & Creighton, 1978). Because of ethical requirements not to deny potentially helpful treatment to seriously ill participants, the Simontons' early studies did not involve time-phased control groups. Nonetheless, the results were impressive. Of the original 159 highly selected patients diagnosed to have medically incurable cancer and given 1 year to live, 63 patients were alive 2 years after diagnosis. Controlled studies with delayed treatment or conventional control groups have been conducted by Achterberg (1984), Achterberg and Lawlis (1979), Spiegel (1991), Spiegel, Bloom, Kraemer, and Gottheil (1989), and others have replicated and extended the Simontons' findings, demonstrating the effectiveness of imagery in the treatment of cancer. Imagery has also been demonstrated to be effective in the treatment of a variety of other disease symptoms, including chronic pain, smoking cessation, weight management, eating disorders, cardiovascular disorders, among others (e.g., Sheikh, 2003).

While the efficacy of mental imagery in the treatment of disease symptoms requires further study, the possibility remains that mental images may allay certain disease symptoms for some regardless of the initial causes of the presenting symptoms. Of course, the origins of diseases, especially serious diseases, are multifaceted. However, regarding treatment, if future research identifies a mirroring discourse of disease in a large number of individuals, such findings may suggest a wide number of therapeutic interventions within an individual's disease-related discourse. Applying various therapeutic modalities, it may be possible to reduce disease symptoms or the psychological tension produced by them by dissembling specific patterns of mirroring embedded in a person's psychological, behavioral, and somatic self-descriptions.

While I was thinking about the possibility of such therapeutic interventions, I remembered watching my maternal grandmother, Selma, pull out yarns from old knitted garments in order to reuse the yarns to knit another garment. She would cut the garments along a knitted row at a convenient point and begin to pull and separate out long woolen threads from the interlocking knit. In pondering what this particular recollection may have to have to do with therapeutic interventions within a disease discourse, I had a hunch that some diseases for some people are a result of complex, interwoven patterns, rather like a knitted garment. Whatever the causes of an illness, it may be possible to unravel an unlocking pattern by pulling out individual "yarns" from any convenient point in the "knit." Since I came to this research topic through the collaborative project in this book and not via a search of related empirical studies, I do not know if others may have suggested such a possibility already. My hunch is but a hunch and subject to additional investigation but nevertheless a hopeful way to conclude.

Coda

I write these closing remarks on intuitive inquiry as the darkness of winter again draws near. My analyses of the Teresa and Reno texts seem sufficient for the season and I need to rest and wonder anew. If I were called to continue this study further, I trust that I would again begin to muse about the mirroring discourse of disease derived from my analyses and that new ponderings and insights would arise. I would probably find myself drawn to read all the empirical and theoretical literature on imagery and healing and related phenomena that I could find. However, I would not force this decision but allow my intuition to guide me. As readers and researchers, I invite you also to consider and muse on whether continuing this intuitive inquiry belongs to you. If your imagination begins to soar with ideas and possibilities, it might. Exploring the topic of a disease discourse that mirrors the illness itself has exciting, clinical applications if proven to be valid. I am—and you might—be curious about the phenomenon of whether or not therapeutic interventions can be made within a illness discourse itself. Perhaps I will continue this intuitive inquiry and collect and examine the additional interviews necessary to explore this topic in depth—or better yet, perhaps you will.

Notes

1. Aside from personal engagement and transformation of the researcher, intuitive inquiry and transpersonal research approaches, in general, overturn a number of conventional assumptions about research, suggesting that research can be a full psychological and cultural process that incorporates, records, and honors many forms of data in addition to physical sense data. For a more comprehensive discussion of the ways in which intuitive inquiry and transpersonal approaches to research challenge the assumptions of mainstream science, see Braud and Anderson (1998) and Anderson and Braud (in press).

2. In a personal communication (January 6, 2010), Reno indicated that the experience of being locked in a jail cell by this father at age 8 has probably led him to "always second guess [himself], coming up with reasons not to do something or alternative courses of action."

Recommended Readings

Anderson, R. (2004a). Intuitive inquiry [Guest editor]. *The Humanistic Psychologist,* *32*(4).

This issue of *The Humanistic Psychologist* explores the intuitive inquiry approach to human science research. Following my introduction, four intuitive inquiries based on doctoral dissertations are presented by Cortney Phelon, Jay Dufrechou, Sharon Hoffman, and Vipassana Esbjörn-Hargens.

Anderson, R. (in press). Intuitive inquiry: The ways of the heart in human science research. In R. Anderson & W. Braud, *Transforming self and others through research: Transpersonal research methods and skills for the human sciences and humanities.* Albany, NY: State University of New York Press.

This chapter provides a comprehensive presentation of intuitive inquiry. Many extended examples of intuitive inquiries are given, along with experiential exercises to illustrate the five cycles and other aspects of intuitive inquiry. Examples of exercises include: What Is Your Intuitive Style?, Identifying Your Intended Audience, and Visionary Trajectories Based on This Study.

Esbjörn-Hargens, V., & Anderson, R. (2005). Intuitive inquiry: An exploration of embodiment among contemporary female mystics. In C. T. Fischer (Ed.), *Qualitative research methods for psychology: Instructive case studies* (pp. 301–330). Philadelphia: Academic Press.

Based on dissertation research by Esbjörn (2003), this chapter provides research examples illustrating the five cycles of intuitive inquiry. A comparison of Cycle 2 and Cycle 4 lenses is provided, along with examples of new, change, and seed lenses, which allow readers to see changes in the researcher's understanding of the topic over the course of the study. Resonance validity and efficacy validity, modes of validity somewhat unique to intuitive inquiry, are also introduced.

Rosemarie Anderson's website, *www.rosemarieanderson.com,* provides access to articles and updates on intuitive inquiry, embodied writing, thematic content analysis (TCA), and transpersonal approaches to research.

References

Achterberg, J. (1984). Imagery and medicine: Psychophysiological speculations. *Journal of Mental Imagery, 8,* 1–13.

Achterberg, J., & Lawlis, G. F. (1979). A canonical analysis of blood chemistry variable related to psychological measures of cancer patients. *Multivariate Experimental Clinical Research, 4,* 1–10.

Adler, J. (2002). *Offerings from the conscious body: The discipline of authentic movement.* Rochester, VT: Inner Traditions.

Anderson, R. (1998). Intuitive inquiry: A transpersonal approach. In W. Braud & R.

Anderson, *Transpersonal research methods for the social sciences: Honoring human experience* (pp. 69–94). Thousand Oaks, CA: Sage.

Anderson, R. (2000). Intuitive inquiry: Interpreting objective and subjective data. *ReVision: Journal of Consciousness and Transformation, 22*(4), 31–39.

Anderson, R. (2001). Embodied writing and reflections on embodiment. *Journal of Transpersonal Psychology, 33*(2), 83–96.

Anderson, R. (2002a). Embodied writing: Presencing the body in somatic research: Part I. What is embodied writing? *Somatics: Magazine/Journal of the Mind/Body Arts and Sciences, 13*(4), 40–44.

Anderson, R. (2002b). Embodied writing: Presencing the body in somatic research: Part II. Research applications. *Somatics: Magazine/Journal of the Mind/Body Arts and Sciences, 14*(1), 40–44.

Anderson, R. (2004a). Intuitive inquiry [Guest editor]. *The Humanistic Psychologist, 32*(4).

Anderson, R. (2004b). Intuitive inquiry: An epistemology of the heart for scientific inquiry. *The Humanistic Psychologist, 32*(4), 307–341.

Anderson, R. (2006). Defining and measuring body intelligence: Introducing the Body Intelligence Scale. *The Humanistic Psychologist, 34*(4), 357–367.

Anderson, R. (2007). *Thematic Content Analysis (TCA): Descriptive presentation of qualitative data* [Electronic version]. Retrieved May 25, 2008, from *www.wellknowingconsulting.org/publications/article.*

Anderson, R. (in press). Intuitive inquiry: The ways of the heart in human science research. In R. Anderson & W. Braud, *Transforming self and others through research: Transpersonal research methods and skills for the human sciences and humanities.* Albany: State University of New York Press.

Anderson, R., & Braud, W. (in press). *Transforming self and others through research: Transpersonal research methods and skills for the human sciences and humanities.* Albany: State University of New York Press.

Assagioli, R. (1990). *Psychosynthesis: A manual of principles and techniques.* Wellingborough, UK: Crucible.

Bastick, T. (1982). *Intuition: How we think and act.* New York: Wiley.

Brandt, P. L. (2007). *Nonmedical support of women during childbirth: The spiritual meaning of birth for doulas.* Retrieved June 21, 2010, from ProQuest Digital Dissertations. (AAT 3274206)

Braud, W. (2002). Psi favorable conditions. In V. W. Ram Mohan (Ed.), *New frontiers of human science* (pp. 95–118). Jefferson, NC: McFarland.

Braud, W. (2003). Nonordinary and transcendent experiences: Transpersonal aspects of consciousness. *Journal of the American Society for Psychical Research, 97*(1–2), 1–26.

Braud, W., & Anderson, R. (1998). *Transpersonal research methods for the social sciences: Honoring human experience.* Thousand Oaks, CA: Sage.

Bruns, G. L. (1992). *Hermeneutics ancient and modern.* New Haven, CT: Yale University Press.

Burneko, G. (1997). Wheels within wheels, building the earth: Intuition, integral consciousness, and the pattern that connects. In R. Davis-Floyd & P. S. Arvidson (Eds.), *Intuition: The inside story* (pp. 81–100). New York: Routledge.

Carlock, S. E. (2003). *The quest for true joy in union with God in mystical Christianity: An intuitive inquiry study.* Retrieved June 21, 2010, from ProQuest Digital Dissertations. (AAT 3129583)

Chicago, J. (1985). *The birth project.* New York: Doubleday.

Cirker, B. (Ed.). (1982). *The Book of Kells: Selected plates in full color.* New York: Dover.

Coleman, B. (2000). *Women, weight and embodiment: An intuitive inquiry into women's psycho-spiritual process of healing obesity.* Retrieved June 21, 2010, from ProQuest Digital Dissertations. (AAT 9969177)

Diekman, A. (1982). *The observing self: Mysticism and psychotherapy.* Boston: Beacon Press.

Dufrechou, J. P. (2002). *Coming home to nature through the body: An intuitive inquiry into experiences of grief, weeping and other deep emotions in response to nature.* Retrieved June 21, 2010, from ProQuest Digital Dissertations. (AAT 3047959)

Edinger, E. F. (1972). *Ego and archetype: Individuation and the religious function of the psyche.* Boston: Shambhala.

Edinger, E. F. (1975). *The creation of consciousness: Jung's myths for modern man.* Toronto, Ontario, Canada: Inner City Books.

Esbjörn, V. C. (2003). *Spirited flesh: An intuitive inquiry exploring the body in contemporary female mystics.* Retrieved June 21, 2010, from ProQuest Digital Dissertations. (AAT 3095409)

Esbjörn-Hargens, V., & Anderson, R. (2005). Intuitive inquiry: An exploration of embodiment among contemporary female mystics. In C. T. Fischer (Ed.), *Qualitative research methods for psychology: Instructive case studies* (pp. 301–330). Philadelphia: Academic Press.

Gadamer, H.-G. (1998). *Praise of theory: Speeches and essays* (Chris Dawson, Trans.). New Haven, CT: Yale University Press.

Gendlin, E. T. (1978). *Focusing.* New York: Everest House.

Gendlin, E. T. (1991). Thinking beyond patterns: Body, language, and situations. In B. den Ouden & M. Moen (Eds.), *The presence of feeling in thought* (pp. 25–151). New York: Peter Lang.

Gendlin, E. T. (1992). The primacy of the body, not the primacy of perception. *Man and World, 25*(3–4), 341–353.

Gendlin, E. T. (1997). *Experiencing and the creation of meaning: A philosophical and psychological approach to the subjective.* Evanston, IL: Northwestern University Press. (Originally published in 1962)

Goldberg, P. (1983). *The intuitive edge: Understanding and developing intuition.* Los Angeles: Jeremy P. Tarcher.

Halifax, J. (1983). *Shaman: The wounded healer.* New York: Crossroads.

Hayward, J. (1997). Foreword. In R. Davis-Floyd & P. S. Arvidson (Eds.), *Intuition: The inside story* (pp. ix–x). New York: Routledge.

Hill, A. G. M. (2005). *Joy revisited: An exploratory study of the experience of joy through the memories of the women of one Native American Indian community.* Retrieved June 21, 2010, from ProQuest Digital Dissertations. (AAT 3200238)

Hoffman, S. L. (2003). *Living stories: An intuitive inquiry into storytelling as a collaborative art form to effect compassionate connection.* Retrieved June 21, 2010, from ProQuest Digital Dissertations. (AAT 3095413)

Jung, C. (1933). *Psychological types*. New York: Harcourt.

Jung, C. G. (1959). *The basic writings of C. G. Jung* (V. S. DeLaszlo, Ed.). New York: Random House.

Jung. C. G. (1972). *The collected works of C. G. Jung* (2nd ed., H. Read, M. Fordham, & G. Adler, Eds., R. F. Hull, Trans.). Bollingen Series. Princeton, NJ: Princeton University Press.

Keller, E. F. (1983). *A feeling for the organism: The life and work of Barbara McClintock*. New York: Freeman.

Koestler, A. (1990). *The act of creation*. New York: Penguin Books.

Luna, L. E., & Amaringo, P. (1991). *Ayahuasca visions: The religious iconography of a Peruvian shaman*. Berkeley, CA: North Atlantic Books.

Manos, C. (2007). *Female artists and nature: An intuitive inquiry into transpersonal aspects of creativity in the natural environment*. Retrieved June 21, 2010, from ProQuest Digital Dissertations. (AAT 3270987)

Maslow, A. H. (1971). *The farther reaches of human nature*. New York: Viking.

McCormick, L. (2010). *The personal self, no-self, self continuum: An intuitive inquiry and grounded theory study of the experience of no-self as integrated stages of consciousness toward enlightenment*. Retrieved June 21, 2010, from ProQuest Digital Dissertations. (AAT 3397100)

Medrano-Marra, M. (2007). *Empowering Dominican women: The divine feminine in Taino spirituality*. Retrieved June 21, 2010, from ProQuest Digital Dissertations. (AAT 3270985)

Moustakas, C. (1990). *Heuristic research: Design, methodology, and applications*. Newbury Park, CA: Sage.

Moustakas, C. (1994). *Phenomenological research methods*. Thousand Oaks, CA: Sage.

Netzer, D. (2008). *Mystical poetry and imagination: Inspiring transpersonal awareness of spiritual freedom*. Retrieved June 21, 2010, from ProQuest Digital Dissertations. (AAT 3316128)

Nouwen, H. (1990). *The wounded healer: Ministry in contemporary society*. New York: Doubleday.

Packer, M. J., & Addison, R. B. (Eds.). (1989). *Entering the circle: Hermeneutic investigation in psychology*. Albany: State University of New York Press.

Pallaro, P. (Ed.) (1999). *Authentic movement: Essays by Mary Starks Whitehouse, Janet Adler, and Joan Chodorow*. Philadelphia: Jessica Kingsley.

Perry, A. (2009). *Does a unitive mystical experience affect authenticity?: An intuitive inquiry of ordinary Protestants*. Retrieved June 21, 2010, from ProQuest Digital Dissertations. (AAT 3344550)

Petitmengin-Peugeot, C. (1999). The intuitive experience. *Journal of Consciousness Studies, 6*, 43–77.

Phelon, C. R. (2001). *Healing presence: An intuitive inquiry into the presence of the psychotherapist*. Retrieved June 21, 2010, from ProQuest Digital Dissertations. (AAT 3011298)

Phelon, C. R. (2004). Healing presence in the therapist: An intuitive inquiry. *The Humanistic Psychologist, 32*(4), 342–356.

Potter, J., & Wetherell, M. (1995). Discourse analysis. In J. A. Smith, R. Harre, & L. van Langenhove (Eds.), *Rethinking methods in psychology* (pp. 80–92). Thousand Oaks, CA: Sage.

Rickards, D. E. (2006). *Illuminating feminine cultural shadow with women espionage agents and the Dark Goddess.* Retrieved June 21, 2010, from from ProQuest Digital Dissertations. (AAT 3286605)

Romanyshyn, R. D. (2002). *Ways of the heart: Essays toward an imaginal psychology.* Pittsburg, PA: Trivium.

Romanyshyn, R. D. (2007). *The wounded researcher: Research with soul in mind.* New Orleans, LA: Spring Journal Books.

Root-Bernstein, R., & Root-Bernstein, M. (1999). *Sparks of genius: The thirteen thinking tools of the world's most creative people.* New York: Houghton Mifflin.

Schleiermacher, F. (1977). *Hermeneutics. The handwritten manuscripts* (H. Kimmerle, Ed., D. Luke & J. Forstman, Trans.). Missoula, MT: Scholars Press. (Original work published 1819)

Sheikh, A. A. (Ed.). (2003). *Healing images: The role of imagination in health.* Amityville, NY: Baywood.

Shepperd, A. E. (2006). *The experience of feeling deeply moved: An intuitive inquiry.* Retrieved June 21, 2010, from ProQuest Digital Dissertations. (AAT 3221764).

Simonton, O. C., Matthews-Simonton, S., & Creighton, J. (1978). *Getting well again: A step-by-step, self-help guide to overcoming cancer for patients and their families.* Los Angeles: J. P. Tarcher.

Spiegel, D. (1991). Mind matters: Effects of group support on cancer patients. *Journal of NIH Research, 3,* 61–63.

Spiegel, D., Bloom, J. R., Kraemer, H. C., & Gottheil, E. (1989, October 14). Effect of psychosocial treatment on survival of patients with metastatic breast cancer. *The Lancet,* 888–891.

Strauss, A., & Corbin, J. (1990). *Basics of qualitative research: Grounded theory procedures and techniques.* Newbury, CA: Sage.

Taylor, J. B. (2006). *My stroke of insight.* New York: Viking.

Unthank, K. W. (2007). *"Shame on you": Exploring the deep structure of posttrauma survival.* Retrieved June 21, 2010, from ProQuest Digital Dissertations. (AAT 3221764)

Vaughan, F. (1979). *Awakening intuition.* New York: Anchor Books.

von Bingen, H. (1954). *Wisse die wege: Scivias [Know the ways].* Salzburg, Austria: Otto Müller Verlag.

von Franz, M.-L. (1971). The inferior function: Part I. In M.-L. von Franz & J. Hillman, *Jung's typology* (pp. 1–72). New York: Spring.

White, R. A. (1997). Dissociation, narrative, and exceptional human experience. In S. Krippner & S. Powers (Eds.), *Broken images, broken selves: Dissociative narratives in clinical practice* (pp. 88–121). Washington, DC: Brunner/Mazel.

Wilber, K. (2000). *Integral psychology: Consciousness, spirit, psychology, therapy.* Boston: Shambhala.

Wilber, K. (2006). *Integral spirituality: A startling new role for religion in the modern and postmodern world.* Boston: Integral Books.

PART III

PLURALISM, PARTICIPATION, AND UNITY IN QUALITATIVE RESEARCH

CHAPTER 10

Comparisons through Five Lenses

I n this chapter, the five researchers compare their own approaches and analyses of Teresa's experience with each of the others'. Through five lenses, the similarities and differences between these approaches and analyses are clarified. In preparing for this exploration, each researcher read the chapters written by the other four researchers and made note of general similarities and differences between their own and other approaches, among choices and procedures used in analyzing the Teresa texts, and among their findings. The researchers sometimes also made note of the sensibilities, analytic style, and written expressions of the individual researchers. In presenting these sets of comparisons in order, the research worldview of each approach and each individual researcher comes through in what he or she looks for, finds significant, and in how qualitative research work is characterized. The researchers agreed to adopt a descriptive and expository attitude, rather than a critical one, in order to clarify their differences and thereby to inform readers' evaluative conclusions. Although the researchers had read, studied, and taught qualitative research methods other than their own, including those employed in this project, considerable revision was required in order to ensure that each approach is described accurately from the standpoint of an "insider." This chapter offers a rare opportunity to delve into the way qualitative researchers in various traditions read and view each others' work in the context of data with which they are intimately familiar and with which they themselves have worked.

The Lens of Phenomenological Psychology:
Frederick Wertz

As I read the work of my colleagues and look for similarities to and differences from my own, I find both. The other four analyses arose from traditions that are intertwined with my own and address a common subject matter. Each analysis contains many procedures that are identical to mine as well as different procedures that can be readily related to mine. The same could be said with regard to the findings: the knowledge generated by the different methods is similar to mine in significant ways, and even the most striking differences can be meaningfully related to mine. Although some of the discrepancies in these analyses and findings are related to our contrasting approaches, many stem from the individual researchers as persons—our relevant past experiences, our sensibilities, our analytic styles, and our background stocks of knowledge. If I were to conduct research using my colleagues' analytic procedures, I would probably arrive at findings somewhat different from theirs due to my own values, ways of thinking, and writing style. Each researcher's distinctive talents as a knower and unique presence as a person appear to be inevitable in and beneficial to human science. Qualitative research invites, encourages, and calls forth the full personal involvement and creativity of each researcher, and our analyses reflect each of us as persons doing research as they also illuminate the subject matter.

I found many similar procedures among our approaches. For instance, all five researchers began with the data and read them openly with a sensitivity to their context and limits. All researchers were reflexive, honest, and critical in describing their own presence and procedures. All of us focused, in large part, on the participant's intentions and meanings, even if we understood them in different ways. All of us allowed patterns and insights to emerge from the data themselves in a process of discovery. Given these similarities, it should be no surprise that our knowledge claims also have many similarities. Others saw, as I did, Teresa's shock, the collapse of her psychological life, the loss of self and meaningful world, the challenge of restoring her well-being, her rational mode of coping, a heroic and creative process of transformation, and new forms of life as outcomes of her cancer—to name but a few.

Grounded Theory and Phenomenological Psychology

Although both grounded theory and phenomenological research begin with concrete instances of human experience and attend very meticulously to their moment-by-moment unfolding, phenomenological analysis remains descriptive and does not construct a theoretical model that yields hypotheses, as does grounded theory. Phenomenology's reflective, eidetic analysis does not "code" data, employ inductive logic, or emphasize the frequency of themes. Phenomenological analysis is more similar to the interpretive approach in Kathy Charmaz's constructivist grounded theory than to Barney Glaser's variable analysis, which reflects his quantitative training. Phenomenology does not explain experience by means of functional relations of variables outside immediate experience, as Glaser does. Despite similarities, phenomenology and constructivist grounded theory do entail divergent philosophical orientations. Grounded theory assumes that meaning must be constructed, hence the importance of theory. Phenomenology views experience as always already meaningfully organized and therefore intrinsically intelligible without theoretical modeling, only in need of descriptive understanding and faithful conceptualization. Grounded theory moves relatively briefly through descriptive reflection toward higher-level abstractions by means of theoretical categories that contribute to building explanatory models of experience.

From a procedural standpoint, there are many similarities. Both approaches use line-by-line analysis. Both approaches require extant concepts to earn their way into the analysis by virtue of their clearly evident relevance to participants' concrete experiences. Grounded theory's "sensitizing concepts" are akin to phenomenology's "fore-understanding," though the latter sometimes suggests more a preconceptual familiarity than received knowledge. Both approaches call for the researcher's critical reflexivity as well as a willingness to modify existing concepts on the basis of fresh encounters with data. All data—every expression of participants—are subject to analysis in both approaches, and each finding is recorded and accounted for in the scientific record. Some phenomenologists "name" (the theme of) each meaning unit, as grounded theorists "code" or categorize the participant's verbal material. However, whereas phenomenologists' key procedure is *reflection* on the meaningful structure of the concrete intentional life of participants, *theoretical model building* is the procedural aim in grounded theory.

Grounded theorists may engage in reflections and record them along with many other kinds of thinking in their "memos" as they move toward abstract theoretical statements. I find many phenomenological procedures, such as insights into the essence of Teresa's experience, employed by Kathy Charmaz in her grounded theory analysis. For instance, by varying the age of the person suffering the loss of self in traumatic experience, she realizes that the regaining of self is dependent on cultural conditions offering opportunities for self-transformation. Kathy's version of grounded theory has been influenced by phenomenology. These similarities are one basis of the considerable convergence between our analyses of Teresa's experience. The meticulousness of our attention to each data point led both Kathy and me to the significance of telling and revealing traumatic experience to others. Kathy's central theme, "losing a valued self," as well as her recognition of how prior skills enabled Teresa to courageously grow in the face of impending death, converge with what I found. I too saw Teresa's loss of her voice as a loss of her "identity" and found a creative process of self-transformation in her resilient recovery. Both Kathy and I recognized the importance of Teresa's acceptance of loss as a condition of the successful formation of a new self. Both analyses claimed that Teresa's tempering of her emotions and her use of dispassionate logic were effective in coping with her life-threatening illness. Both Kathy and I used comparative procedures in order to acquire general knowledge. By contrasting Teresa's and Gail's experiences, we identified general differences between those traumatic experiences in which a person loses self and creates a new identity versus those that involve temporary self-loss and a recovery of one's previous identity.

Grounded theory's constructive theorizing contrasts with pure phenomenological reflection and description. Kathy focused on "losing and regaining a valued self" in part because of its theoretical importance in psychological literature on the illness experience. Whereas this construct became the central category with which Kathy's analysis worked, I focused in a broader way on the variegated concrete phenomena of "trauma and resilience" and reflected on all their constituents and substructures, of which the self is one moment or theme among many others whose overall structure I tried to grasp. Kathy began her analysis after Teresa's diagnosis, upon the dawning of self-loss, whereas I began with Teresa's childhood, in which I saw a sedimentation of meanings that was retained in her later experience of trauma and resilience. In featuring the theoretical category of "losing and regaining a valued self," Kathy builds a model that includes hypotheses of functional, if–then relationships that explain the self-loss and the "continuum of self reconstruction." In contrast to the phenomenological bracketing of realities that are independent of Teresa's experience with trauma and resilience, Kathy's theorizing makes reference to real-world conditions in order to explain the loss and consequent regaining of self. For instance, she focuses on such positions and conditions as chronological age, cultural opportunities, and objective bodily functionality. In explaining the loss and regaining of a valued self, Kathy postulates the influence of such conditions as the loss of function, age, and the availability of societal opportunities for self-change. Phenomenological psychology makes no claims about independent conditions outside experience and does not use them in the construction of a model. Instead, the phenomenologist reflects on the way the world (including a person's "age," "body," and "culture") is *experienced*, that is, on the meanings these have within the person's psychological life. Such meanings are then brought to light as essential constituents of the intentional structure of the phenomenon under investigation. Phenomenological psychological analysis remains purely descriptive of holistic *psychological* structures instead of building a theoretical model based on abstract functional relations.

Discourse Analysis and Phenomenological Psychology

Discourse analysis, also rooted in the antipositivist traditions of continental philosophy, has many similarities with phenomenology. Both acknowledge the social situatedness and potential for agency on the part of the human being, who constructs the world through, and is in turn constructed by, language. Both traditions provide the human scientist with a host of descriptive-analytic concepts and strategies that inform data analyses. Both methods begin with an open reading of the data and gradually bring to bear a sharper focus on material that is relevant to the research problem. Both approaches describe human action by means of recurrent meaningful patterns that transcend their content and the experience of the individual whose particular psychological life (viewed by both as relational practices) is analyzed. However, discourse analysis focuses on circumscribed patterns of verbal performance, whereas phenomenology attempts to more comprehensively understand and describe the intentionalities of subjective experience. Discourse analysis attends to the socially interactive aspects of written and spoken language as the locus of and primary context for analyzing meaning. Unless a phenomenological psychologist is researching "the interview" or "the writing of lived experience," he or she tends not to analyze the text or the interviewer–interviewee interactions except inasmuch as they provide access to prior lived experiences. Whereas the discourse analyst illuminates the interview itself as context that shapes the production of writing and talk, the phenomenologist *sees through* the interview as it expresses examples of the research topic. However, these approaches may converge and interrelate inasmuch as there is a unity and connection between discourse performances and the larger psychological life of interlocutors.

Linda McMullen's incisive findings regarding the pattern of "enhancing oneself, diminishing others" in discourse about trauma deliberately follow from the nature of her approach. Linda was not attempting, as I did, to generate knowledge of Teresa's moment-to-moment lived experience; she did not focus on Teresa's past childhood experience at all. Instead, she viewed the written text and the interview as *accounts* of misfortune, and focused on the practice of accounting. In contrast, for me, the written description and interview provided access to and shed light on a prior experience of misfortune. Seeking only to analyze the latter, I assembled material from the written description and interview, regardless of its verbal context, in a temporally ordered description of the original phenomenal experience. My individual phenomenal description did not include interaction of the interviewer and Teresa, for it was meant only to provide access to the participant's *prior experience*.

Linda focused on the written text and the overall interview in order to analyze psychologically revelatory patterns of writing and talk that constitute culturally valued and prevalent practices. On the basis of an open reading informed by descriptive concepts such as "positioning" and an exploration of the theoretical literature, Linda selected a theoretically relevant category and analyzed a recurrent pattern of discourse found in Teresa's verbal performances in her written text and interview interaction: *enhancing oneself, diminishing others*. Linda's analysis of this discourse pattern remained descriptive and structural rather than building an explanatory model of self-enhancement. Although I too employed a descriptive, structural analysis, I did not focus on the written text or interview, as such, nor did I restrict my reflections to a particular theoretical construct, but aimed to understand the meanings and overall structure of the entire original experience of trauma and resilience. The only discourse that I analyzed was Teresa's interactions with the others whom she encountered in the course of her bout with cancer. For instance, I reflected on Teresa's discursive strategy for limiting her mother's distress by verbalizing only part of her medical condition.

Linda's discourse analysis brought to light something that my phenomenological analysis did not. I had not focused at all on Teresa's speech pattern of "enhancing oneself, diminishing others" and did not relate this to the context of her present interaction with the interviewer or her social situation in school. My analysis moved instead to "what Teresa's discourse describes" and found patterns of meaning quite different from that which Linda brought to light in the written text and interview. For instance, in Teresa's interactions with her surgeon, I found patterns of meaning very different from self-enhancement. In that situation, when Teresa's cancer was first diagnosed, Teresa was initially paralyzed and later reduced to tears as her physician "came up big," providing knowledge, masterful competence, emotional support, and hope for the future. In surgery itself, Teresa was also diminished, to anesthetized unconsciousness on the operating table, while the physician— the center of agency at this moment—performed life-saving surgery. I found a postsurgery substructure of bedridden life in which Teresa's mother rose up and loomed large as an executive managing her situation. These structures of Teresa's intentional life contrast sharply with that of the particular pattern of discourse that Linda analyzed here.

My analysis also found meanings in Teresa's original expereince that are akin to what Linda discovered in her later discourse. For instance, my analysis identified Teresa's coping style of actively handling challenges herself while leaving others in the background. Later, this same style was embodied in her extraordinary expansiveness as she attempted to live the fullest possible life in the face of death. In these moments of Teresa's experience, we see an "expanding self and minimal other" that bears significant connection to what Linda found. However, in the phenomenological analysis these moments are placed in the larger process and historical trajectory of Teresa's personal life. My analysis of Teresa's experience suggested the future possibility of integrating her active, expansive agency with her, at times, helpless dependency on emotionally available and supportive others. For example, in her marriage, Teresa seemed to be moving toward an increasing ability to share her weak neediness and to allow her husband to actively provide her with care. I recognized at least a potential movement toward allowing others to be strong enhancers of her life. Further study would be needed to understand the relationships between "enhancing oneself, diminishing others" and these more integrative intentionalities of Teresa's historically changing life. Phenomenologically, whereas one meaning horizon of the discourse pattern of "enhancing oneself, diminishing others" includes (as Linda asserts) the interview, the class, and the larger audience of her expression, another horizon (constitutive of the past) is the experiential meanings retained, recollected, and verbalized. Linda's insightful explication of the way Teresa distinguished herself as "special, unusual, and extraordinary" eluded me in my original analysis, but reflecting now, I recognize these as important self-meanings not only in Teresa's socially interactive discourse in the interview, but also in Teresa's nonverbal ways of living through trauma that began in her childhood, reached new heights in the music conservatory, and were further developed in her struggle with cancer.

These two approaches share in common a meticulous scrutiny of the participant's expressions, a comparison of different lifeworld examples of the topic under investigation, and a focus on general dynamic patterns of human relational activities that transcend the researched context in which they are found. Discourse analysis and phenomenological psychology converge in similar knowledge because psychological life admits of an overall unitary structure of experience that includes discourse. These contrasting approaches, although divergent, are also therefore complementary. The phenomenological psychological analysis shows how a person attempts, in an effort to overcome the diminishment of trauma at the hands of a destructive "other," to rise up and transcend smallness and vulnerability in an appropriation of power. The speech pattern of "enhancing oneself, diminishing others" both reflects this process and is also its own way of enhancing the person diminished by trauma, as mandated by our individualistic culture that demands that we grow from misfortune. Phenomenological psychology reveals intentional meaning structures in the individual's temporal life, and discourse analysis reveals cultural patterns and imperatives in verbal practices. Both methods may bring to light such general patterns as the individualistic coping with and thriving on tragedy.

Narrative Research and Phenomenological Psychology

Phenomenology and narrative research hold in common the conviction that human science research can articulate valuable knowledge through words and through ordinary language. These approaches utilize close attention to the expressions of research participants. Both acknowledge the potential of the research participants' language to express the meaningful temporal unfolding of life in situations with other people. Both approaches are holistic, insisting that each moment of mental life is dependent on the whole. The modern hermeneutic and narrative movements were led by the philosophers Heidegger and Ricoeur, who were students of Husserl and identified themselves as phenomenologists.

Nevertheless, many narrative researchers take a different direction from phenomenological psychologists, who offer generally applicable procedures for gaining knowledge of the full range of human subject matters, both nonverbal and verbal. Phenomenologists reflect directly on first-person conscious experience, utilize nonverbal expression, and collect diverse kinds of verbal description, including but not limited to narratives. In contrast, narrative researchers resist formalizing a common "method" and, embracing methodological and conceptual relativism, freely draw on various philosophical, theoretical, literary, and social traditions in addition to phenomenology, placing the emphasis on the interpretive power of stories. Whereas phenomenology finds meanings inherent in the intentional structure of both verbal and nonverbal lived experience, narrative researchers tend to view meaning as originating in words. For instance, Ruthellen Josselson states that Teresa "structures her story as one of shock," whereas I take the shock to be an experience existing prior to expression, which may or may not be expressed in narrative form. Phenomenologists attempt to suspend their preconceptions and seek access to the phenomena themselves, whereas narrative researchers self-consciously employ a variety of interpretive frameworks, such as feminism and psychoanalysis. Phenomenology approaches experience eidetically rather than interpretively when it takes the individual experience as "an example of" a phenomenon and describes the essential structure evident in the individual experience. Narrative researchers sometimes undertake the study of persons' lives as such without seeking knowledge beyond cases, and they may assume a greater license of interpretation than do phenomenological psychologists.

Ruthellen's narrative is similar to mine in that we have both paid close attention to Teresa's expression as a whole and in its parts, employing the "hermeneutic circle" as a means of articulating the meaningful interrelations of parts and the whole. I viewed the narrative aspects of Teresa's data as valuable in offering access to the temporal structures of Teresa's experience, as Ruthellen did. I suspended my previous assumptions regarding the word *resilience* (including those concerning physical matter) in order to let the meanings of this phenomena emerge from Teresa's lifeworld example. Ruthellen interpreted the term according to its historical root meaning (as merely "a return to a previous state"), which she criticized in light of Teresa's experience. Beyond semantics, both of us found that Teresa's psychological life involved significant transformation in the course of the late adolescent task of identity development. Many other similarities in our findings include, for instance, the significance of singing in Teresa's identity; her tragic loss of identity in the loss of her voice; habitual coping by means of turning away from emotions toward rationality; and the transformative adventure in which Teresa forged a new identity.

Whereas I attempted to reflect, without a guiding framework, on each meaning unit in Teresa's description, Ruthellen drew on various interpretive traditions as she read Teresa's texts. These traditions included Bakhtin's writing about the dialogical and multivocal character of the self; the psychoanalytic theory of defense; and literary notions of tragedy and romance. Ruthellen's analysis was also informed by her interest in human identity and her clinical sensitivities to human affect and coping mechanisms. Although I too have been informed by psychoanalysis as a clinical psychologist, my phenomenological training led me to suspend this perspective as I reflected on meaning units. With her interpretive lenses, Ruthellen identified in Teresa's expression different *voices of the self* and examined how these voices related to one another. Teresa's self-definitions, with their many aspects (e.g., physical, emotional, logical, student, opera singer, psychologist) were brought to light in Teresa's narrative of transformation and integration. Although my phenomenological reflection identified the overall process of identity transformation and integration, this was viewed as embedded in Teresa's experiential process. Had I adopted "identity" as a theme, as I did "social support" and "spirituality," my findings in this area would have been more detailed and might have looked more like Ruthellen's. However, our different emphases on identity, as lived through the intentionalities of lived experience versus identity as articulated in life stories, would have remained.

Ruthellen focused explicitly on the way in which Teresa's expression depended on its social context, and she analyzed the interview situation as part of a graduate class. She noted Teresa's resistant relationship with the interviewer, who appeared to rigidly emphasize social support. My own interest in the interview was only to analytically discern descriptive expressions of Teresa's previous experience of trauma. I viewed the interviewer's emphases on social support and the topic of God as a legitimate topical interest and viewed Teresa's responses as revealing aspects of her original experience of trauma rather than as artifacts of the research situation. Although I viewed the interview as providing a limited perspective on the original event, I judged its access to be genuine even when I was frustrated by its limits (especially its failure to evoke descriptions of Teresa's closest friendships and marriage). Without specific topical interests in Teresa's habitual modes of social interaction, her identity, her personality, her present psychological health, or her story telling in the interview, I considered her repeated relational patterns with the interviewer irrelevant and did not analyze them as did Ruthellen.

Other differences between Ruthellen's and my analyses stem from our respective relations to psychoanalysis, clinical concerns, and personal theoretical interests. Ruthellen interpreted Teresa's way of coping with her disease by using psychoanalytic defense mechanisms of suppression, denial, dissociation and, without naming them, rationalization and projection. Her interpretations were closely text-bound, supported by Teresa's characterization of herself (after being diagnosed with cancer and losing her voice) as proceeding as though "nothing happened." Also following psychoanalytic theory, Ruthellen traced Teresa's coping strategy to her childhood, in which she handled her family's intense, unpredictable emotionality by separating herself from uncomfortable emotions and adopting a reasoning stance. I identified emotional collapse followed by rational problem solving as moment of the present experience, and I also viewed Teresa's habitual, logical problem-solving strategy as rooted in her childhood relations with mother and father. However, I stopped short of calling these "defense mechanisms," given my phenomenological tendency to describe mental life as situationally related rather then intrapsychic. I viewed Teresa's "rational overdrive" as a context-bound, effective way of transcending uncanny emotions (with their implication of her death) in order to solve her real medical problems. I found an openly lived, even if sometimes tempered, emotionality in other situations. I did not view Teresa as inducing her difficult emotions, such as despair, in others as a way of coping ("projection"). I viewed her perception of emotion in others as having the meaning of "the others'." Though theories are not its starting point, phenomenology can use them heuristically in the process of clarifying essential structures with descriptive evidence. Without further descriptive evidence, I would hesitate to postulate "displacement." I characterized Teresa's intentionality as variously owning, tempering, and at times deliberately turning away from emotion and therefore viewed her emotionality as full, variegated, and relatively functional and progressive rather than projective (in the psychoanalytic sense) and regressive. Therefore I was not "worried" about Teresa's "dissociative" tendencies. Perhaps Ruthellen experienced a sharper sense of Teresa's isolation, disappointment, resentment, and rage about vulnerability in her intimate relationships than did I. This may in part be due to my bracketing of practical, clinical aims and attempting to remain descriptive and atheoretical. Nevertheless, my analysis converged with Ruthellen's in the identification of Teresa's struggle to integrate her intense emotions, vulnerabilities, and dependencies with others.

Both Ruthellen and I conducted thematic analyses, and both of us analyzed the themes with close attention to Teresa's experience as a whole. Ruthellen drew themes of the "tragic" and "romantic" from the tradition of literary study, which illuminated distinctive features of Teresa's lived experience. Ruthellen also viewed Teresa's narrative in accordance with her own theoretical interests in the internal reworkings of self. She highlighted Teresa's interpersonal disappointments, in which others were unreliable and abandoning, except in caring for her physical needs. In reading the narrative, Ruthellen paid attention to Teresa's ways of coping with loss (tragic narrative) and constructing a new life (romantic narrative), statements about self experience, and statements describing relations of self and others. In contrast, I took up themes that were assigned in the research project by the class—trauma, resilience, social support, and spirituality. From Teresa's description, I understood her lived experiences as intentionally related to situations, as ways of relating to the world, rather than as internal work on self. In analyzing Teresa's interactions with her teacher, her physician, and her husband, I found her experiences of others to include their responses not only to her physical needs but also to her personal vulnerabilities, dependencies, and existential strivings. I found Teresa attempting to move toward integrating her independence and dependence, her emotionality and practicality, in her future—for instance, in her marriage.

Intuitive Inquiry and Phenomenological Psychology

The relationship between phenomenological psychology and intuitive inquiry can be quite close in that intuition (used here as defined by Rosemarie Anderson, not Husserl) can be employed in phenomenological research, and phenomenological methods can be incorporated in an intuitive inquiry. However, this overlap is not necessary. Phenomenological psychological research can be conducted without intuitive ways of knowing and without key components of intuitive inquiry, just as the latter can be conducted without utilizing phenomenological methods.

Intuitive inquiry is hospitable to and compatible with the phenomenological method, which may be employed informally throughout all five cycles and quite formally in Cycle 3 (data collection and descriptive analysis) and Cycle 4 (interpretation). Intuitive inquiry has been informed by phenomenology, and many intuitive inquiries have featured phenomenological methods. However, the emphases on the personal significance of the research topic, the free-ranging use of intuitive ways of knowing, and the goals of personal and societal transformation are not necessarily involved in phenomenological research. Phenomenological methodology can be employed with any topic, regardless of its personal significance to the researcher. Phenomenological psychologists do not necessarily practice such intuitive ways of knowing as those found in dreams, art, reverie, spirituality, and meditation. Phenomenology is a reflective method that does not intrinsically entail practical, transformative aims and outcomes.

Rosemarie did not simply accept "trauma and resiliency" as the topic of her analysis, as I did. She engaged a broader, highly personal process of dwelling with Teresa's texts, meditating on them, tracking them in her dreams, and reaching for a personally gripping topic that stretched into the unknown *before* she entered her cycle of analysis. Personal and cultural breakthroughs were the goal of Rosemarie's research from the start. Rosemarie's initial intuitive approach eventually led her to focus on the fascinating topic of "reverse mirroring," which I did not clearly identify as a theme. Rosemarie delved into the mysterious inner reaches of this hidden dimension of Teresa's experience. I worked more prosaically, devoting full attention to each detail of Teresa's description in an effort to comprehensively grasp the structure of her traumatic experience, maintaining even attention to all its constituents regardless of their personal significance to me. My phenomenology followed a more traditional, relatively disinterested, scientific process.

Rosemarie's and my approaches to the data have similarities. We both read Teresa's expressions openly, became immersed in the data, and allowed her experience to resonate deeply with our own. We both differentiated the protocol into meaning units of roughly the same size. However, whereas I maintained and reflected on Teresa's experience in its original temporal order, Rosemarie sorted the data using thematic content analysis, named categories, and rearranged the themes in various ways with an eye to striking patterns. The themes of Teresa's pragmatic coping strategy, emotional shutdown, personal transformation, and the rare aggressive cancer were identified in both our analyses. However, whereas I reflected on the relevance and meaning of these themes along with other constituents of the overall psychological structure of trauma, Rosemarie used interpretive intuition to discover the mysterious topic of reverse mirroring between emotional numbness and aggression (discourses of denial and anger) as a topic in its own right. Nevertheless Rosemarie, in a close textual reading similar to mine, traced Teresa's control of her emotions to her childhood family situation and recognized in Teresa's later adult life an increasing openness to and integration of strong emotions in her academic work, marriage, and recreation. Rosemarie articulated Teresa's impressive ways of integrating bodily emotional resonance with practical challenges in fencing, mountain climbing, and motor cycling, insightfully tracing this integrative learning to her modulation of strong emotions in her vocal training. Although I did not tune in to these subtle body–world processes in Teresa's postcancer transformation, Rosemarie's insights are directly in line with my structural insight into Teresa's aim to integrate her intense feelings with practical action.

Phenomenological research can include key components of intuitive inquiry, such as the study of personally significant topics with visionary potential and the capability for transforming the researcher and society, though these were not explicitly included in my analysis of Teresa's experience. I recognize many intuitive ways of knowing in my psychological analysis. I experience psychological reflection as a nonpossessive form of love, and I am drawn to latent, unnamed, secret meanings. I too allow myself to empathically identify with the participant in an emotionally vital and imaginative way that gravitates to fault lines—the sites of suffering, hospitality to the sacred, and far-reaching possibilities within experience. I empathically paired and joined with Teresa's experience and interrogated not only its obvious characteristics but also explored its further-reaching implications and potentials. One of these involved Teresa's nontheistic spirituality, including her humility, generosity, gratitude, and hope. Through intuition I understood that these primarily emotional moments of faith, which were not based on a belief in God, bear on existence as a whole and on matters beyond the actually given world. Intuition was also involved in my analysis of Teresa's practical–rational coping style, which I approached on the basis of personally assuming Teresa's meanings. I too have experienced complete emotional collapse and have engaged in practical–rational overdrive in an effort to solve potentially overwhelming problems. I retain my lonely desire for greater emotional integration, and I have been fortunate to also experience love in my most broken-down moments. I have learned the importance of surrendering, letting myself collapse, and depending on others' generosity and care, as Teresa sought to do in her marriage. My knowledge of these processes in Teresa's life, especially in her marriage, was limited by the paucity of relevant descriptive data. Even if Teresa and I are not able to fully integrate our polarities in our own relationships, we both live the existential paradoxes of being emotional and practical, weak and strong, vulnerable and agentic, and dependent and self-reliant, which I view as quite general—even *essential*—in human existence. The possibility of integrating these polarities is far-reaching, as a horizon of our personal lives and cultural history. These intuitive–eidetic insights are based on my allowing myself to couple and resonate with Teresa's experience in a manner similar to Rosemarie, who, as a former gymnast, was able to reflect on the way Teresa's bodily discipline as an opera singer and later as a rock climber exquisitely enabled her to rise beyond the horrors of her disease. These intuitive ways of knowing the transpersonal dimensions of human life can flourish at the heart of phenomenological psychological analysis.

The Lens of Constructivist Grounded Theory:
Kathy Charmaz

Reading my coauthors' analyses underscored my belief in the multiplicity of possible interpretations. Standpoints and starting points matter. *Our* purposes, as well as those of our research participants, shape what we do. What we take as evidence is personal and political as well as methodological. Yet the collective lies embedded in the personal. While reading each colleague's paper, I was reminded how rhythms of collective life echo in our individual renderings of these data. We each draw on a fund of knowledge, and we each recreate it and perhaps transcend it in our own way. Graduate school socialization and theoretical allegiances can seep into the deepest levels of consciousness and shape our perspective and method.

In my case, a graduate course in epistemology captivated me and challenged my worldview. Reading about the theory of relativity in the philosophy of science was revelatory for me. At that time, Thomas Kuhn's (1962) *The Structure of Scientific Revolutions* left lasting impressions on theoretically oriented graduate students who began to trace the implications of Kuhn's arguments for theory and method in the social sciences. Symbolic interactionism (Blumer, 1969; Mead, 1932, 1934; Strauss, 1969) and phenomenological sociology (Berger, 1963; Berger & Luckmann, 1967; Schutz, 1970) shaped my nascent social psychological and methodological assumptions. Symbolic interactionist Herbert Blumer (1969) exhorted sociologists to "respect your subjects," and classical theorist Max Weber (1949) contended that to understand human action, we must learn what people intend and how they define their situations and then begin analysis from their beliefs and definitions. All these influences foster an openness to participants' lives, encourage a relativist view of the empirical world, and emphasize multiple realities and varied definitions of situations. Participants' and researchers' meanings and actions arise in specific contexts and situations, thereby shaping inquiry. I strive to learn the logic of research participants' experience from their view and begin analysis from that point. This methodological stance involves empathetic understanding to discover how people construct their lives and why they act as they do. Granted, we cannot wholly separate our understandings of data from ourselves, but we can try to understand what things mean to the people we study.

Interview and personal narrative methods form a silent frame on the material that we study. From my perspective, we cannot separate either findings or analyses of these findings from their frame. My comparisons with colleagues' methodological approaches derive from *constructivist* grounded theory, rather than from Glaser and Strauss's (1967) classic version. Constructivist grounded theory shares more commonalities with phenomenology and intuitive inquiry than the classic version. I have long followed Bergson's (1903/2007, p. 1) distinction between two ways of knowing a thing: one may either go all around it or enter into it. Bergson observed that most philosophers go *around* their studied phenomena, not *inside* it, as typifies what most social scientists do now. Classic grounded theory goes around the phenomena; constructivist grounded theory attempts to go inside it. Researchers bring their subjectivities to the studied experience, and those affect it. Nonetheless, starting from this studied experience, as best we can, profoundly reshapes what grounded theorists can see, sense, and know.

Phenomenological Psychology and Constructivist Grounded Theory

Phenomenology and constructivist grounded theory converge on a number of points. Proponents of both methods have questioned the traditional view of a unitary scientific method and aim to begin analysis afresh, without preconceiving it with prior theories or knowledge. Both phenomenology and constructivist grounded theory emphasize subjectivity and temporality and have strong alliances with the social constructionist tradition.

Both methods have complementary yet distinctive ways of engaging data. Phenomenology delves deeply into experience and views it from the inside. Fred Wertz's phenomenological approach fosters precise analysis of and reflection about the studied experience. Constructivist grounded theory emphasizes slowing down to see and understand experience, as occurs with phenomenological study. Both methods offer ways of focusing our gaze on what we see and how we see it, yet grounded theory also invokes specific methodological strategies for speeding up the analytic process.

Like phenomenologists, constructivist grounded theorists aim to understand experience and its meanings as their research participants do. We both look for tacit meanings and actions. Phenomenologists analyze only those contextual dimensions of experience that the researcher can see and show. Constructivist grounded theorists believe that researchers may miss the hidden implications of social locations and thus aim to preserve differences and variation among individuals and within the processes we study. We assume that we cannot treat either experience or our analyses as separate from the social contexts and conditions of their production.

Both approaches emphasize engaging the studied experience as directly as possible to begin inquiry. The phenomenological method defines and works with meaning units in an exacting scrutiny of the data. Grounded theorists engage in a close initial coding to identify fruitful leads in the data. Similar to phenomenology, grounded theorists employ this close coding to find out what is happening from research participants' views. In contrast to phenomenologists, grounded theorists later identify and use focused codes to move across a large number of cases and thus do not give all cases a close coding. Constructivist grounded theory assumes that realities are not given but are constructed through actions, which we mirror in our coding and analytic practices, whereas phenomenologists are vigilant about making realities explicit through their description of phenomena. From a constructivist grounded theory perspective, researchers' and research participants' views may become entrenched and actions may be limited, but enacting them makes them real. These different emphases impose somewhat different concerns for how we use our respective methods.

Phenomenologists bracket their experiences to study the research participant's experience. Bracketing is fundamental to the phenomenological method because it focuses inquiry squarely on the research participant's experience. Constructivist grounded theorists assume that language and meaning shape and constitute description and, therefore, description itself interprets the studied experience, albeit such description may not theorize this experience. Phenomenologists remain focused on the given experience; constructivist grounded theorists interrogate how *our* language and social locations, such as gender, age, race, situation, etc., may influence our analyses of the experience.

When comparing methodological strategies, several differences stand out. Phenomenology is not a hypothesis-testing method, nor is it a method of theory construction, as grounded theory is. Fred does not offer hypotheses, and he explicitly states that he does not aim to build theory. Grounded theory does use hypotheses in service of theory construction after developing analytic categories. We construct hypotheses only to check and sort plausible interpretations or to develop and assess tentative emergent theoretical categories. Throughout the analytic process, grounded theorists explicitly invoke comparative methods, such as my comparisons of Teresa's and Gail's situations and experiences, which led to constructing the category of a "disrupted self" and highlighted the problems and prospects in "making a comeback." Phenomenologists seek to describe the essence of a given experience and its significance as it is lived. Constructivist grounded theorists aim to look at how experience is constituted, its implicit meanings, and to understand the contexts and conditions that give rise to it. Phenomenologists take a similar view, although they restrict contexts and conditions to those within the studied experience itself and have the responsibility of showing that they constitute the experience. Phenomenologists might see what grounded theorists define as contexts and conditions as being independent of an experience, whereas grounded theorists may view them as linked to, or at times, eliciting the experience. Constructivist grounded theorists delve into the experience but also widen the frame of inquiry to include the relative positions and realities in which this experience is situated, including those that a researcher identifies but research participants may not recognize. "Contexts" and "conditions" differ between these two approaches because constructivist grounded theorists take into account larger social, cultural, historical, and generational realities in which the studied experience is located, whereas phenomenologists recognize and study such contexts only inasmuch as they are found within experience itself.

The grounded theory research quest for the properties of its emergent categories resonates with the phenomenological search for the invariant structure of an experience. Both Fred and I look for tacit meanings and actions that make an experience what it is. However, we differ at this point. Phenomenologists look for essences and thus search for invariants in human experience. Constructivist grounded theorists look for basic patterns and processes but aim to theorize them. We view our theoretical understandings as partial, conditional, and situated in temporal, spatial, and social locations. For phenomenologists, essences of human phenomena are also temporal, spatial, and socially localized and constitutive of the experience itself.

A main difference between grounded theory and phenomenology resides in the respective stances toward theory and theorizing. Phenomenology is a descriptive method; constructivist grounded theory is an interpretive and comparative method for theory construction that begins with an inductive logic. For constructivist grounded theorists, theory means creating an interpretive understanding of the studied phenomenon and establishing relationships between abstract concepts constructed from this phenomenon. Theorizing is a practice based on social actions (Charmaz, 2006). Constructivist grounded theorists acknowledge subjectivity in theorizing and view theory as rhetorical, situational, and embedded in the historical, cultural, and social conditions of its production.

Grounded theorists and phenomenologists likely differ in how they view the context of experience. Fred began with an interest in resilience and considered Teresa's experience of trauma and transformation as a whole and described what constituted it. He then showed how relationships and meanings of the past influence are implicitly retained in Teresa's experience in the present. I also looked inside her experience and considered her past, although not in as much detail. In addition, I considered personal attributes and social characteristics that she brought to this experience. Thus, I saw Teresa's youth and relatively privileged background as a college student who had access to health care as forming the backdrop of her experience.

Phenomenologists describe meaning units in the data. Grounded theorists start analysis with meanings and actions that the participants indicate are most significant—and problematic—to *them*, as revealed through their statements or their actions. The processes involved in how participants grapple with and perhaps attempt to resolve this significant problem become the focus for a grounded theory analysis. Grounded theorists look for the fundamental social or social psychological processes in dealing or coping with this problem, which may be tacit or entirely taken for granted. In these data, I viewed losing and regaining a valued self as the most problematic and fundamental processes affecting Teresa and Gail, and therefore I analyzed these processes. In my view, both women were remarkably aware of what was most significant to them and articulate about the troubles they faced. Readers may examine the data and evaluate whether focusing on losing and regaining a valued self meets the criteria for conducting grounded theory analysis.

In keeping with constructivist grounded theory, I stuck to what came across to me as most significant in Teresa's and Gail's lives, losing and regaining a valued self, and attempted to conceptualize what these processes entailed. Fred stuck to the described experience of trauma and resilience and provided a detailed description of how Teresa lives this experience through her accounts of it. Similar to Fred's phenomenological approach, grounded theorists build their analyses first and afterward consider earlier ideas and knowledge, which I do here. At this point, we treat the literature and, if relevant, our own ideas as data and sources of comparison. I have woven fewer studies and offered less discussion of substantive literatures in my chapter than I would do for a full study but do offer several comparisons in the preceding pages.

Fred's analysis reveals his remarkable openness to Teresa's experience. Both Fred and Rosemarie Anderson express appreciation of this experience but, moreover, enter sacred ground. Rosemarie's experience as a priest who ministered to suffering people sensitizes her to the sacred. Fred and Rosemarie observe with wonder the dignity and fragility of the human spirit. Each speaks of doing research with love. I have felt being in a sacred space during interviews but had not sensed it before in the writing when the analyst of experience did not conduct the interview. Perhaps Fred's and Rosemarie's very methods take them on this journey and allow them to share the experience. Their writings of it contain a resonance that studies often lack when the analyst does not participate in data gathering. My rendering of Teresa's story reflects my starting points of attempting to look at experience from the inside and learning how Teresa defines her situation. This rendering includes compassionate understanding but has not been guided by an explicit frame of doing research with love.

Although grounded theory begins as an inductive method, it also invokes abductive reasoning, which includes forming and testing hypotheses. As grounded theory moves away from concrete experience and into abductive reasoning, it diverges from phenomenology. Abductive reasoning leads the grounded theorist to attempt to imagine all possible theoretical interpretations for a surprising—or interesting—finding. These interpretations are framed as hypotheses to be tested. Subsequently, the grounded theorist gathers more data to ascertain which theoretical interpretation is strongest. From a grounded theory perspective, Fred's description of the surgeon's actions and Teresa's response each pose several possible interpretations. Fred explores implicit meanings through the intuition of essences, a way of understanding invariant characteristics of experience. Like Fred, I sensed that Teresa saw the surgeon as the expert and accepted his urging to join him as an active agent in attacking her cancer. He subsequently became a fellow rational problem solver in saving her voice. It is difficult for me to ascertain from the data we have whether or not the surgeon took on a greater personal meaning to Teresa beyond the primacy of his immediate role in those few moments.

Fred offers an intriguing description of Teresa's response to the surgeon's assurance that they would do everything possible to limit the effects of the surgery. Teresa wrote, "I tried to say something meaningful, expressive . . . all that I could manage was, 'Man . . . I was actually pretty good.' " Fred notes the ambiguity in her statement about whether it meant a retrospective evaluation or present description but also describes it as "a deeply expressive characterization of herself this moment" in facing the truth. I interpreted the same statement as Teresa looking back at the singer she had been in the past and feeling profound loss in the present.

Fred's deeply spiritual analysis of Teresa's relationship with God is sensitive, compelling, and plausible. But does it describe what Teresa felt and thought? I cannot tell. From a grounded theory perspective, Fred's analyses of the surgeon's actions, Teresa's response, and her spirituality provide fascinating "leads." Both Fred and I would seek more descriptive data to clarify such leads, if we were conducting a fully developed research project. However, Fred uses the data we have and describes meanings of these points, whereas I would want further evidence before defining them. The data about Teresa's spirituality are problematic because her interviewer's questions preconceived its significance and forced accounts from her, rather than opening up whatever her experience was. Grounded theorists attempt to limit interview questions and instead listen and look, rather than direct responses from the participant (particularly in a first interview).

Grounded theorists often discover leads in one study that they might wish to pursue in a subsequent study. Among the leads that I saw are the forms of telling "bad news"; emotionality and patient–professional encounters; and forming patient–professional partnerships and the meanings of crucial moments. I did not theorize about such topics per se but instead only touched on them to the extent that they informed my analysis of losing and regaining a valued self. This point brings us to another major difference between grounded theory and phenomenology. My grounded theory processual analysis concentrates on a fundamental part of the experience here; from studying it, we gain insight into the whole of Teresa's experience. Fred's phenomenological analysis concentrates on the whole of Teresa's experience; from examining the whole, we better understand the parts.

Discourse Analysis and Constructivist Grounded Theory

Linda McMullen employs a variant of discourse analysis in social psychology that emphasizes how specific discursive positions are constituted and interrogates the functions and consequences of such positions. Performance is central. Like grounded theorists, discourse analysts view meaning as constructed, situated, and negotiated. Both methods emphasize action, but researchers can use grounded theory methods from varied starting points for varied purposes. Constructivist grounded theorists attempt to explicate research participants' meanings and to scrutinize our own. We look for how our meanings enter the analysis and assess whether their inclusion is justified, which discourse analysts also do.

We can discern numerous significant points of convergence between discourse analysis and grounded theory. Both approaches take talk as a focus of inquiry and view it as a form of meaningful social action. Unlike some ethnographers and conversational analysts, both grounded theorists and discourse analysts see talk as meaningful whether or not it occurs in a natural setting, and thus we both find interviews and documents to be useful sources of data. Constructivist grounded theory attends to the frame of discourse as well as the content and assumes that the frame influences content. As I note in my chapter, class assignments shape Teresa's written account of an unfortunate event and her classmate's intensive interview with her.

Both discourse analysts and grounded theorists view research as a continuing process. A criterion of classic grounded theory is that a developed theory be modifiable as new data shed light on the studied phenomenon. Both discourse analysts and grounded theorists engage in early analysis. Grounded theorists look at key words, statements, and actions in the data. Discourse analysts focus on how the research participant(s) uses a large set of discursive resources. Grounded theory contains several strategies and aims to study processes. Linda's analysis is less guided by specific strategies than grounded theory, but her approach is more guided by analytic concepts. Constructivist grounded theory minimizes steps (but does use specific strategies) and avoids importing extant concepts into the analysis. Linda took into account concepts of "resilience," "coping," and "recovery" as possible conceptual frameworks for her analysis, although she later states that she would interrogate them as taken-for-granted concepts, as I would.

In different ways, neither discourse analysts nor grounded theorists are committed to an analysis of the individual. Linda's analytic engagement resides with the text and the discourses in it, not with the person. Grounded theorists learn from the people whose stories we hear, read, and piece together. We build our analyses, however, on the studied experience; the major process, if we define one; and the collective story. The discourse analyst remains outside the research participant's experience and looks at it from multiple vantage points as to how the performance is given and what it accomplishes. At this point we diverge. I appreciate the elegance of Linda's writing and the precision of her thinking; nonetheless, my analysis contrasts most from hers.

Linda's attention to discourse, word use, and performance makes her analysis the most sociological of the four psychological approaches. Why then would my analysis differ so greatly? Linda's starting point outside the experience contrasts with my intent to go inside this experience and to begin analysis from that point. Going inside the experience makes constructivist grounded theory a profoundly interactional method that relies on developing an empathetic relationship *with* the person but seldom engages in an analysis *of* the person. Discourse analysts also do not engage in an analysis of the person; instead they focus on identifying which discursive resources research participants use, how and for what purposes they use them, and which consequences result. Both discourse analysis and constructivist grounded theory see discourses as positional and situational and may locate them in culture, history, and immediate situations as well as examine the positions taken within the discourse (Charmaz, 2009; Clarke, 2005, 2006, 2009).

Beyond these comparisons, Linda and I define different discourses in these accounts on which to focus. Subsequently, different meanings reverberate through our analyses. Linda sees a discourse of enhancing oneself, diminishing others as one of several discursive patterns that she could have analyzed but was struck most by this pattern and chose to focus on it. Constructivist grounded theorists aim to discover what is most significant to research participants and begin analysis there. I defined losing and regaining a valued self as most significant from Teresa's perspective when reading her discourse of coming to terms with devastating illness through experiencing loss and transformation. I found a similar discourse in Gail's data, although the nature of her injury did not cast the specter of permanent loss and thus altered the context and conditions of her experience. Loss spreads and spirals from the physical to the psychological and social. The discourse of loss in Teresa's narrative resonates with the experiences of other people who have unexpected life-threatening illnesses. When we take this standpoint, Teresa's accounts portray a courageous young woman who dealt with adversity with tenacity, pluck, and an uncommon lack of bitterness. Teresa used the resources she had in ways that she knew. As I mention in my chapter, intensive interviews and autobiographical accounts place the research participant in the center of her story. Being in the center is intensified by experiencing a health crisis because it pulls people into themselves and having a virulent cancer intensifies this process (Charmaz, 1991).

My reading of some of the same statements that Linda saw as diminishing others takes a different turn. Teresa had said about the voice students, "I knew that they couldn't bear the discomfort of being around me under the circumstances." Linda viewed Teresa's statement about the voice students as "constructing them as sensitive and unable to cope" (p. 213) and "not up to the task that was required of them" (p. 212). I agree with Linda's interpretation of how Teresa constructed the voice students as unable to cope. From my reading, the data support this interpretation. Linda states that this construction implies that the voice students were "not up to the task that was required of them," which she presents as one possible reading from the analyst's perspective.

Constructivist grounded theorists, in contrast, would want to test all conceivable readings by gathering more data on research participants' constructions and acts of friendship, as is consistent with the iterative approach and logic of grounded theory. We can treat friendship as a contingent concept and problematic object for further empirical investigation, rather than assuming a shared definition that imposes implicit criteria on other social actors. If the voice program were as competitive and rife with jealousy and envy as Teresa describes, then friendships could well be tenuous, fleeting, and based on temporary alliances and superficial sociability. Tasks and trust would then be limited.

I saw Teresa's statement as reflecting an ability to see the world from other students' view despite having been shunned. Being shunned—and stigmatized—frequently occurs when people bear the markers of visible illness and disability, and it intensifies if others see them as symbols of death. Teresa's tales of being shunned echoed what I have heard repeatedly in interviews with people who have serious chronic illnesses and have read in autobiographical accounts. Arthur Frank's (1991) evocative narrative of having cancer implies that being "cast out" is part of the experience; Robert F. Murphy (1987) and Albert B. Robillard (1999) document how their academic colleagues avoided and ignored them during their illnesses. Frank writes, "The damaged body only fails to perform properly; the stigmatized body contaminates its surroundings" (1991, p. 92).

What Linda sees as enhancing oneself, I see as validating self. This distinction points to a major difference between a focus on discourse as such and a focus on experience. Linda provides an elegant analysis of discursive form independent of Teresa's subjective, experiential meanings. In contrast, I attend less to the form of discourse and more to the experiencing person's subjective meanings of its content. From this perspective, Teresa validates that she took control to the extent possible, that she survived, that she is active in the world. Plunging into new activities, packing her schedule, proving that she can succeed in new ventures all validate that she is alive and can shape her life. People who have had life-threatening crises often engage in such actions, for they realize that they may never have another chance.

Linda views Teresa's narratives as "making others peripheral to the account" and diminished by absence of detail in the discourse. As a discourse analyst Linda does not take a position on Teresa's experience. We both considered how the contextual frames of the interview and personal narrative may affect the research participant's responses, but we emphasize different implications of its influence. Linda notes the production of the protocols and sees her analysis as anchored in her reading of this context. She raises the question of whether the student research participants might wish to present themselves as agents, and thus "doing agency" might be built into the discourse. I raised the point that lack of anonymity forms the contextual backdrop in which these accounts arose. Might not a seeming unwillingness to disclose intimate details be related to this context? In Gail's account, other potentially key actors recede in the background. Her team members remained nameless.

She was reluctant to tell her family and her athletic trainer about her injury. Gail said, "I guess I didn't really need so much emotional support and psychological support from my family because I guess in some way I would say that my mind was very strong." Does that mean that Gail had diminished them as she assumed a heroic role in her own story? Again I find intriguing possibilities for further research that could lead a researcher in new directions. Certainly people perform different discourses for varied audiences and situations. And discourses can be layered, contradictory, and simultaneous. Yet the marked contrast between Linda's and my analyses suggests that our analytic methods and interpretation merge in each approach, whether we approach inquiry from outside or inside the experience.

Narrative Research and Constructivist Grounded Theory

Ruthellen Josselson explains narrative analysis as an interpretive approach that involves the subjectivities of both the researcher and participants and uses a conceptual framework to analyze texts. Narrative analysis draws on varied analytic methods. Constructivist grounded theory considers intersubjectivity but aims to create the conceptual framework from the studied data themselves; it is an analytic method consisting of specific strategies and flexible guidelines. Researchers can use constructivist grounded methods with varied kinds of collected data. Constructivist grounded theory begins with broad concepts but follows leads that the researcher defines in the data. This strategy can lead the researcher to new theoretical terrain.

Both constructivist grounded theory and narrative analysis are explicitly interpretive methods. Like constructivist grounded theorists, Ruthellen acknowledges perspectives that inform her analysis, but the points at which these perspectives are invoked may differ. Grounded theorists attempt to develop their analyses first and then integrate them with other ideas and research. As a constructivist grounded theorist, I engage in reflexivity throughout the research about the perspectives I bring to the analysis, not only from theory and research but also from such sources as social class, gender, race, and embodiment.

How constructivist grounded theorists and narrative analysts render the data has differed in the past but may converge in the future. Grounded theorists typically have fractured research participants' narratives and then reintegrated them into a collective analytic story, whereas narrative analysts have protected the integrity of the individual narrative. Ruthellen states that narrative analysis is distinct because it addresses whole accounts, offering comparisons of Teresa's written and interview narratives. Narrative analysts have adopted grounded theory strategies to analyze narrative content more than narrative structure (see, e.g., Hansen, Walter, & Baker, 2007; Mathieson & Stam, 1995; Salander, 2002). However, I have argued that researchers can use grounded theory for analyzing whole accounts, too, and address their structure and implications.

Both narrative analysis and constructivist grounded theory focus on meaning and context, albeit in somewhat different ways. Ruthellen aims to reveal disguised meanings, and I try to define tacit meanings. Both approaches attend to silences, to what is left out. Ruthellen takes the personal narrative and data into account, as I do, although she adopts resilience as a central theme, which I do not. We both see Teresa's story as one of loss and transformation and draw on many of the same statements in the data.

Our approaches differ in how we engage the data. Ruthellen began with an overall reading and then identification of narrative form, which she saw as tragic and romance narratives. By attending to statements about self experience, she developed broad categories. Ruthellen first worked from general to specific and then worked between specifics and broad categories of "emotion and logic," "identity," and "self with others." I began with broad concepts of self and identity but went directly to a close coding of what I saw happening in these data.

Our respective analyses reveal some differences in the role of extant theory and the place of the individual. Ruthellen looks at Teresa's accounts through a psychoanalytic lens and thus invokes its concepts to analyze Teresa's meanings. Grounded theorists avoid starting with an extant theory. Typically grounded theorists concentrate on processes and phenomena that we define in the data, not on individual psychology. Ruthellen and I converge in our efforts to look for research participants' presuppositions and aim to be aware of our own. Yet it's hard for me to separate presupposition from narrative interpretation when Ruthellen states, "Perhaps I am experiencing what she [Teresa] does with others—avoiding her own feelings by perceiving or injecting them in those close to her" (p. 233). Ruthellen's phrasing "what she does with others . . ." sounds like an established fact rather than an interpretation. Teresa's accounts do not convince me that she avoids her feelings or perceives or injects them into other people. From a constructivist grounded theory perspective, these are possible interpretations but not conclusive statements. Yet, Ruthellen's narrative approach supports making interpretations that reach beyond what is directly ascertainable and may or may not be shared by her readers and research participants. In contrast to Ruthellen's interpretation, I see Teresa as compartmentalizing feelings and attempting to keep them contained, so that she can act. Ruthellen's questions about Teresa's incongruent experiences of "total loss and nothing happened" (p. 18) suggest to me the kind of multiple selves that arise during profound uncertainty (Charmaz, 1991).

Both Ruthellen and I view context as significant and note the situated positions of Teresa's accounts. Sociology and social psychology inform my notion of context, and hence I extend it to consider the larger social contexts of Teresa's life. I find Teresa's views and actions concerning her parents, voice teacher, and peers understandable given such contexts. Teresa is a young American woman who sought an independent path consistent with her generation. Her stance, however, conflicted with her father's wishes and her mother's deference to him. Cultural and generational chasms may have exacerbated the tensions between Teresa and her parents. Further research could trace the extent to which cultural and generational expectations raise tensions and are played out in individual views and actions.

Intuitive Inquiry and Constructivist Grounded Theory

Intuitive inquiry broadens conceptions of knowledge apprehended by the senses. Rosemarie Anderson's recognition—and celebration—of the researcher as an embodied, intuitive being holds the potential of bridging humanistic and transformative psychology with conventional scientific traditions. The researcher's subjectivity enters inquiry at every stage and has the power to reveal hidden truths and multiple worlds. Constructivist grounded theory assumes subjectivity and builds on the researcher's interpretations. It leans toward what Rosemarie calls "a big-picture perspective." Grounded theorists likely build on their intuitive thoughts about the research topic by engaging in the iterative process of gathering and analyzing data in which each informs and refines the other.

Bringing intuitive awareness into a scientific narrative suggests a new direction: the *reënchantment of science*, to borrow David Ray Griffin's (1988) marvelous term for integrating the tacit, elusive, and mysterious into scientific thinking itself. Intuitive inquiry encourages ambiguity, liminality, and mystery to *enter* inquiry. Inner and outer can merge. Hence, intuitive inquiry includes elusive understandings and mystical experiences. Grounded theory fosters explicating, clarifying, and solving mysteries *through* inquiry.

Both intuitive inquiry and grounded theory are inductive methods that provide tools for theory construction. Intuitive inquiry focuses on psychological experience, and its cycles support exploring it. Grounded theory is a general method that researchers adopt for multiple forms and levels of inquiry. To my knowledge, its strategies have not yet been mined for their usefulness in exploring inner and outer worlds in ways analogous to intuitive inquiry. Grounded theory is a systematic method that arose out of positivism as well as an interpretive tradition. Earlier versions of the method are imbued with the kind of objectivism that intuitive inquiry belies. Constructivist grounded theory is substantially more compatible with intuitive inquiry than earlier versions of grounded theory because it assumes that the viewer is part of what is viewed.

Intuitive inquiry not only begins with the topic but also invokes concepts to examine it. Rosemarie uses psychological concepts of denial and coping in her intuitive analysis of Teresa's texts; however, Rosemarie aimed to develop an independent focus rather than to accept concepts such as resilience and coping strategies from the start. Grounded theorists avoid applying specific extant concepts because we stress emergent analysis. Similarly, we do not conduct a literature review to inform our analyses; rather we delay it until after we have formed these analyses.

Grounded theorists only invoke broad concepts early in the research process as a means of opening inquiry. Constructivist grounded theory emphasizes using flexible guidelines in its iterative process. Perhaps ironically, its flexibility makes it a less sequential method than intuitive inquiry, although its emphasis on grounding concepts makes it a more conventional method. Not only do constructivist grounded theorists move back and forth between data gathering and analysis, but we also move back and forth between coding and constructing conceptual categories. These moves arise from the researcher's analytic engagement and thus make constructivist grounded theory less sequential and rule-bound than earlier versions.

Rosemarie speaks of the creative encounter with data in which the researcher's ideas build from the data but differ from them. These intuitive breakthroughs resemble the imaginative interpretations in grounded theory. Feelings of confusion and bewilderment pervade the process, which seems to be a process of discovery, of reaching and learning, and then interpreting. Confusion and ambiguity are part of inductive qualitative research and characterize the process of conducting constructivist grounded theory, particularly as the researcher enters the liminal realm where experience lies beyond words. Yet something magical can happen as we begin to understand.

Intuitive inquiry engenders intimate knowledge of the research topic and intimacy with the research participants. Rosemarie's approach is deeply humanistic in its compassion for research participants. She is unafraid to speak of love and the compelling beckoning of the research topic. Last, Rosemarie reveals her awareness that going inside the experience is transformative for the researcher as well as the researched. The privilege of sharing—and interpreting—changes us. In turn, these shared experiences may contribute to our research participants' transformations as well.

The Lens of Discourse Analysis: Linda McMullen

Discourse analysis, as it is understood in discursive psychology, intersects with and diverges from a phenomenological psychological approach, constructivist grounded theory, narrative research, and intuitive inquiry in various ways and to varying degrees. As qualitative researchers working with written texts for the present project, my colleagues and I share a commitment to focusing on the participants' words, to careful and multiple readings of the texts, to meticulous analysis, and to engaging in interpretation. Beyond these broad strokes, however, the ways and extent to which we intersect and diverge on key aspects such as focus and aim of inquiry, assumptions about what we are getting at and its ontological status, epistemological position, ways of organizing the data, and analytic procedures result in my analytic product bearing little resemblance to those of my colleagues. However, points of intersection do exist, and they can inform us about both the convergences and divergences in our methodologies.

Phenomenological Psychology and Discourse Analysis

Much can be said about the ways in which these two methodologies differ. In the first paragraph of Fred Wertz's chapter (Chapter 5), he refers to his "analysis of Teresa's experience of trauma and resilience" (p. 124). As noted in my chapter, although I acknowledge that the student project from which our data were generated was framed with words such as *trauma* and *resilience*, I considered these words as historically and culturally located, taken-for-granted concepts that are to be critically queried (Burr, 1995). For a discourse analyst in the tradition of discursive psychology, this stance toward such concepts transforms the focus of the research from a study about trauma and resiliency to a study about what people do when they are asked to write or talk about "when something *very* unfortunate happened to you," particularly when this topic has been discussed in relation to themes such as social support, agency, hope, spirituality, and the self, as it was in the present case. That is, as a discourse analyst, I do not assume the topic of the research, but only that participants have been oriented to write or talk about a set of historically and culturally nuanced terms.

Although both a phenomenological psychological approach and discourse analysis eschew positivism (the positing of something or the taking of something as given; Crotty, 1998), this action has radically different outcomes. While Fred discards the tendency to focus on reality independent of the experience, he still assumes the existence of the experience itself. This stance distinguishes phenomenological psychology from transcendental phenomenology, which abstains from all existential positing. In fact, the aim of Fred's research is to describe *the psychology* of the experience faithfully in light of concrete evidence. Discourse analysts would take quite a different position on the notion of experience. Some would deny its existence, and say that all we have is text; what is real is language. Others would not deny that human beings perceive and have reactions to occurrences in the world, but rather would emphasize the ways in which these occurrences are discursively constructed and would consider the invocation of *experience* as a discursive strategy to be analyzed. Similarly, rather than taking psychological concepts such as feeling and thinking as foundational, discursive psychologists would query these terms and analyze how they are used by speakers. So, "*the psychology* of the experience" becomes a doubly critiqued phrase for a discursive psychologist.

With its basis in a constructionist epistemology, a discursive analyst would assume that his or her analysis is only one account or version, that different analysts would interpret the text differently, and even that the same analyst might do so on different occasions. This stance appears to contrast with the notion of faithful description that is at the heart of the phenomenological psychological approach. However, a psychological phenomenological analysis also recognizes and allows for multiple meanings and analyses, and insists that all of these different analyses may still be faithful to what is lived. The difference comes back to the psychological phenomenological analyst's aim of achieving fidelity to experience: In phenomenology, validity requires multiple perspectives. In discourse analysis, multiple accounts or interpretations of discourse are expected, and the validity of these versions is assessed by the extent to which they are warrantable (Wood & Kroger, 2000).

How phenomenological psychological researchers and discourse analysts organize and think about their data also differs considerably. Because Fred is interested, in part, in producing an individual phenomenological description, he focused on all (or nearly all) of the data that were available to us, combined the written account and the interview, and structured the combined data into a narrative, temporal sequence. I looked for discursive patterns in the data, understood the written account and the interview as separate, local contexts, and considered context in my analysis. Because discourse is situated or occasioned, the contributions of the interviewer are considered to be as important as those of the interviewee, so, unlike Fred, I did not eliminate the interviewer's utterances. All of the data available to us informed my construction of the discursive pattern on which I focused, but again, unlike Fred, I left the majority of the data unanalyzed.

The ways in which we worked with the data differ as well. Fred produced temporally organized structural moments or substructures of experience and identified themes in the data. I focused not only on what was said, but on how it was said, on what actions the speech accomplished, and with what possible consequences. Fred's unit of analysis was understood as a meaning unit, while mine was understood as a set of excerpts from which I constructed a discursive pattern. Fred worked at grasping the sense of each meaning unit and conceptualizing what it revealed about and contributed to the psychological experience of trauma, recovery, and resilience, and I worked at showing how a discursive pattern in talk oriented to trauma, recovery, and resilience was structured and what it accomplished. Fred took Teresa's words and wrote poetically, expansively, and psychologically of and from them; it is as if he tried to get inside the experience, to articulate what might be called the implicit and the explicit as fully as possible, and then reflected on his detailed written description. I worked largely with what was explicit, although the implicit (e.g., how a portion of talk might be interpreted by a participant) can be shown by how participants orient to it. In our own ways, however, each of us focused on *showing*: Fred tried to get at how Teresa's experience showed itself, whereas I focused on demonstrating how my interpretations of the excerpts and my overall claims about the variations in the discursive pattern were grounded in the text (Wood & Kroger, 2000, p. 170).

Context is important for both phenomenological psychological analysis and discourse analysis, but how it is understood—that is, what is focused on and how it is focused on—differs. Fred's focus was on context as the familial and the cultural, on what he understood as background information or content that could inform his description and interpretation, and on how meaning units related to each other and to the experience as a whole. I understood context in relation to how the data were shaped by, for example, time and culture, institutions (e.g., a university setting), local arrangements (e.g., instructions for the tasks that were used to generate the data), and what came before or after a particular segment of text. Not surprisingly, our practices with regard to generalizing also differ. Fred's work went beyond detailing the individual psychological structure of Teresa's experience to a set of imaginative variations of the essential and universal constituents of the trauma experience that can be empirically verified. Beyond the necessity of specifying the generality of my claims that form the analysis of this project, I make no assumptions about the generalizability of the particular discursive pattern that I constructed. It is important to emphasize, however, that neither Fred nor I made claims about how widespread the yields of our analyses are; rather, any statements about the extent and limits of generalizability would await further empirical demonstration. Finally, although both Fred and I view our analyses as subject to change, he understands such change as correction in the service of getting a more accurate description of the phenomenon, whereas I understand it as yet another version of a nearly inexhaustible number of ways in which the analysis can be rendered.

Although there is much in Fred's analysis about which I do not speak—for instance, the meaning of trauma, Teresa's cancer, life, death, and suffering, transcendence, the body, rationality and emotionality—there are moments of intersection in our analyses. I provide one such example from his taking up of the assigned theme of spirituality. In reference to what he calls "a kind of faith lived as an attitude of respectful acceptance—love," Fred wrote:

> This attitude is ego transcendent, in sharp contrast to her rational–instrumental modes of relating to others by means of what they have done or can do for her, which, through much of her traumatic experience, is *nothing*. This spirituality is an important part of how she gets along with others harmoniously and also how she transcends their impotence, indifference,

and lack of support. Teresa's acceptance of others' failings is a crucial foundation for cultivating her own agency in the face of trauma while remaining
engaged and connected with others. (p. 149)

Although both Fred and I invoke concepts of agency in relation to Teresa and
of *nothing*, impotence, indifference, and lack of support (in Fred's case) or
of passivity, absence, inability to cope, and disappointment (in my case) in
relation to others in Teresa's life, Fred's analysis is psychologically interpretive, whereas mine shows how these positionings of oneself and others are
achieved and how they can be understood in terms of local, institutional,
cultural, and historical contexts.

Constructivist Grounded Theory and Discourse Analysis

Kathy Charmaz's version of grounded theory and the particular version of
discourse analysis that I employ in this project share certain assumptions.
Both are based in an epistemology that Kathy labels "constructivism" and that
I label "constructionism" (see Burr, 1995, p. 2, for one statement on the difference between the two labels). These terms refer to a set of assumptions—
about what constitutes knowledge, how knowledge is constituted, and the relation between the knower and the known—that challenge objectivist notions
that meaningful reality resides in the objects of study. Rather, meaningful
reality is understood as constructed between persons in interaction, as situated, and as multiply versioned. This shared epistemology leads both of us to
view the data as occasioned and mutually constructed by the participants, to
understand our analytic product as a set of interpretations, and to resist predetermined framings of our project as about resiliency.

However, although both Kathy and I take language as crucial for knowledge construction, I believe we depart significantly with regard to what we
assume we are getting at in our analyses. For Kathy, language is fundamental
for meaning and action, that is, it is a reality in its own right, but it also reveals
something beyond itself—a route to something else, constructed or otherwise. Specifically, the texts from which we worked were used by Kathy to construct a theory about the process of losing and regaining a valued self. Kathy
very clearly distinguishes her use of the term *self* from self-concept when she
refers to it as "an unfolding social and subjective process, the experienced
self" (p. 170), but invoking the notion of the experienced self indicates to me
that language is understood as saying something about something else, and it
is this something else that is constructed or otherwise gotten at. In contrast,
discourse analysis (as I have performed it) takes language as the object of
study. The analyst's task is to show what speakers *do* with utterances and what
effects these utterances have. Language is not a resource or route to something else, that is, to something psychological; rather it is the focus or topic of

study in its own right (Wood & Kroger, 2000). Kathy's focus on constructing a social psychological process and my focus on constructing a social action suggest to me that the relative emphases we place on the expressive and representational versus performative capacities of language differ.

The ways in which Kathy and I approached and analyzed the data are also quite different. Both of us began our work not knowing what our focus would be and by asking ourselves what was most striking in the data. Beyond this opening stance, our paths diverged considerably. Kathy engaged in line-by-line coding of the whole text, compared fragments of data with each other, data with codes, codes with categories, and categories with categories, moving in ever-increasing levels of abstraction in the service of theorizing about the social psychological process that struck her upon reading the data and which, perhaps, was informed by her previous research on illness. Once I had begun to construct the discursive pattern that I found most salient and on which I eventually focused, I intensely analyzed a small number of extracts of text, and, with the exception of my labeling of the discursive pattern, showed concretely how my claims were evidenced in the data. Kathy's inclusion of segments of text from which we worked was for the purpose of showing that her theory was grounded in the data, whereas mine was to show explicitly not only what evidence I was using, but how I was using it. Kathy focused on writing about the "what" of which the participants spoke and on interpreting the "how" and the "why"; I focused on what was said and how it was said in the service of making claims about what was being performed. I made no claims about what the participants were thinking or feeling or about their motivations.

Like Fred's analysis, Kathy's work is much more holistic than mine. Many more of the data are explicitly relied upon and used by both Fred and Kathy. As a consequence, I find few points of intersection between my and Kathy's work. One possible intersection appears in parts of her last two paragraphs:

> . . . Teresa plunged into a new world where she found acceptance and opportunities. Not surprisingly, she found this world preferable to her former life. Teresa emphasized the positive gains she found in this world and viewed the voice students negatively in contrast to the people in her new life. . . . Perhaps Teresa's negative views of the voice students let her relinquish what she had so greatly cherished. Teresa's hierarchy of values had shifted to fit her new life and, by contrast, the voice students failed to measure up. Forming a revised, critical view of the voice students might be one way Teresa could neutralize loss and, simultaneously, realign herself with new sources of identification. If so, then criticizing the voice students likely helped solidify Teresa's belief that her life had taken a better direction and perhaps quelled lingering regrets she might have had. By this time, Teresa's intellectual companions and other cancer patients provided her with new frames of reference and

new measures of self. Both negative judgments and positive measures give an individual the comparative material to articulate a new narrative of self with fresh purposes. (p. 198)

Kathy's references to "a revised, critical view" and to "negative judgments" might be equated with my label of *diminishing others*, while "positive gains" and "positive measures" might be understood as mapping on to my label of *enhancing oneself*. However, Kathy's interpretation is primarily functional and psychological in form; she writes with immediacy and theorizes about these negative judgments and positive measures and about how they are part of the process of losing and regaining a valued self. My interpretation is about the discursive patterns, per se, that is, about how the variations of *enhancing oneself, diminishing others* are accomplished and what the consequences of such patterns are. Because the focus and goals of our methodologies are quite different, how we treat and understand the same data, particularly in relation to the status we accord the data (i.e., as saying something about a social psychological process or as performing a social action) result in very different analytic products.

Narrative Research and Discourse Analysis

One of Ruthellen Josselson's summary statements about her analysis of Teresa's protocol perhaps comes closest to the *what* of my analysis. She states:

Her narrative is one of personal agency and a determination to overcome adversity. Her stories illustrate internal rather than interpersonal realities. Other people in her life are painted, in relation to her loss, as disappointing, emotionally unreliable, betraying, or abandoning—though adequately available to care for her physically when she is in need. (pp. 229–230)

Yet even in this intersection there are subtle differences in how Ruthellen and I write that are important to articulate. First, Ruthellen uses the nominalization *personal agency*, whereas I use *agent* in the sense of reflexive positioning, that is, a discursively produced way of being that Teresa employs at certain points in her written and interview protocols. For me, agency is one of several positions that Teresa enacts through what she speaks of and how she speaks of it. In Ruthellen's analysis, agency is a psychological construct that is used to summarize (at least part of) the content (or "what") Teresa says. I would not understand this content as illustrating "internal realities"; that is, I view agency as something people *do* rather than something they *have* or something that is understood as being inside their experience. The way in which Ruthellen and I "paint" or construct Teresa's portrayal of the people in her life is similar in its epistemology and content, but Ruthellen's version draws on material that I did not analyze (e.g., Teresa's talk of how people physically cared for her when she was ill). Her version is framed within a larger narrative of transformation centered in a process of identity formation, and is, therefore, more comprehensive and far-reaching than mine.

Ruthellen and I very clearly share a commitment to a constructionist epistemology. We understand our respective analyses as constructed, interpretive accounts of the constructed accounts of Teresa and the interviewer. We understand the data as occasioned, as being jointly formed through the interaction of the speakers or of the speaker and an imagined audience. Context informs our analyses, although I explicitly interpret how differences in the control afforded by a written task versus a face-to-face interview might shape the data. Narrative research and discourse analysis also borrow analytic concepts and procedures from each other. For example, Ruthellen states that she "paid particular attention to statements about self experience ('I statements')" (p. 232). Discourse analysis is, then, a strategy that narrative researchers use as part of their analysis. Similarly, discursive analysts sometimes draw on the concept of narrative and on the principles of narrative as part of their work. However, in the case of discursive analysis, narrative is usually understood as a discursive resource that participants use for particular purposes. That is, the data are not understood in terms of narrative content or structure, and the goal is not to identify narrative genres or to produce a narrative from the data.

Like Fred's and Kathy's work, Ruthellen's analysis relies on all (or almost all) of the data, whereas mine focuses on a small number of extracts. I do not claim that any discursive pattern that I work up is the only pattern used by the speaker(s) or that it cannot occur alongside another pattern that might be understood as contradictory. For example, I might have worked up a discursive pattern of *doing gratitude* or focused on what I might have termed discourses of vulnerability and on how they were structured and used by the speaker(s). For me, comprehensiveness and identifying what is most significant are not goals. However, as Ruthellen states, narrative research endeavors "to explore the whole account" and to show "how the parts are integrated to create a whole" (p. 226). I do not work to integrate parts into a whole; however, I do understand the parts that I analyze in relation to the texts as a whole.

For some narrative researchers, particularly those whose disciplinary allegiance is to psychology, the goal is, as Ruthellen articulates, to "capture the lived experience of people in terms of their own meaning making" (p. 225). As a discourse analyst, I do not assume that I get at experience; rather, as noted previously, language or talk is taken as the object of study, and no assumptions are made about what a speaker has experienced or is experiencing. In addition, I do not make use of so-called psychological constructs, such as internal world, psychic realities, identity formation, coping, self, or unconscious defenses, and would only do so if they were invoked by the speakers.

Another point of intersection in our analyses illustrates how we use some of the same parts of the texts in different ways. Under the theme *relations with others*, Ruthellen writes:

> As she [Teresa] speaks of the role of others' actions in relation to her ordeal, we see that other people are variously resented for being solicitous of and upset by her illness (her mother, her voice teacher, her father) and resented for not being solicitous or concerned enough (her fellow voice students, her father). This pattern may suggest that she locates expressions of her rage about her vulnerability in her intimate relationships. (p. 237)

This part of Ruthellen's analysis might be seen as mapping on to what I have called *diminishing others*, but our work differs in significant ways. Ruthellen's analysis re-presents the data not as a chronology but more as a psychological analysis and interpretation that are organized according to a theme named *relations with others*, which she identifies as central to Teresa's narrative. In contrast, I do not make psychological interpretations about the speaker. Rather, I make interpretations about the functions of various discursive resources or discourses and about the social actions that are being performed by their use. In many ways, my analytic product might appear decidedly unpsychological to many readers. Despite these differences, both Ruthellen and I suggest that our respective analyses challenge existing theory on resilience.

Intuitive Inquiry and Discourse Analysis

On the basis of my and Rosemarie Anderson's analytic products, I might conclude that discourse analysis and intuitive analysis have very little in common. I say nothing about Rosemarie's Theme 1 (Pragmatic and Dispassionate Use of Reason and Logic as a Coping Strategy), Theme 2 (Emotional "Shutdown" of Feelings and Physical Sensations of Numbness), and Theme 5 (Anaplastic Cancer Portrayed as an Angry Cancer), or about the overarching theme of reverse mirroring that Rosemarie creates when she considers these three themes together. Even when it is clear that we are using some of the same parts of the text, our analyses differ. For example, to illustrate Theme 3 (Personal Transformation from "Fat Girl with No Friends" to a Transformed Self with Accompanying Emotions of Anger, Relief, and Gratitude), Rosemarie uses part of the text that forms my extract 1, specifically lines 7–16. In relation to this meaning unit, she says:

> For me, an interesting aspect of Teresa's postsurgery life is her participation in fencing, motorcycling, and rock climbing. All of these sports require extreme attention to outer and inner bodily sensations. One cannot be a

novice fencer, motorcyclist, or rock climber without paying attention to what
is happening inside and around one's physical body. That a "fat girl with no
friends" who used to "numb out" in the face of emotions and bodily sensations would even try these sports is surprising. Teresa's exploration of these
sports is extreme, but then Teresa is strong-minded. Teresa's courage is a raw
form of spirituality, grounded in the nitty-gritty of taking life on just as it is.
(p. 261)

Although Rosemarie uses some of the same lines as I do, she combines
these lines with other parts of the texts (which she refers to as *meaning units*)
and augments her scholarly understanding with intuitive and experiential
knowledge about emotions, physical sensations, and the use of one's body in
sport to describe and interpret them. In my analysis, I included the part of
the written text that immediately preceded lines 7–16, and it was the conjunction of this preceding text (lines 1–6 of extract 1) and lines 7–16 that formed
my analysis of extract 1 and, in part, my construction of the first pattern of
enhancing oneself, diminishing others. That is, my argument about Teresa's use
of a discourse of agency and independence was formed, in part, via the jux-
taposition of this discourse with Teresa's talk about others. As mentioned
previously, one of the core features of discourse analysis is situation, or how
discourse is organized sequentially; attending to how written accounts or conversations are sequenced is, then, an important task of discourse analysts. So,
differences in our analyses result, in part, from how and to what extent we
slice and combine portions of the text and from how we use them in relation
to, or in combination with, other portions of the text.

Although the first six lines of my extract 1 are not included as an illustrative example in Rosemarie's Theme 3, they do appear in almost their entirety
in Rosemarie's Theme 4—Intense Emotions Expressed by Others. However,
while I read and interpreted these lines as Teresa constructing her voice
teacher as "deeply affected by her circumstances," but as whose actions were
"invariable and passive" (p. 212), Rosemarie read them as evidence of Teresa
being at the center of much emotional tension and interpreted them as giving
Teresa "an emotional workout that she could not easily ignore and hopefully
could integrate intrapsychically" (p. 262). Because Rosemarie and I rely on
analytic concepts that derive from very different traditions—hers from phenomenological and heuristic research, psychoanalysis, feminist and womanist
scholarship, and mine from symbolic interactionism, ethnomethodology, and
speech act theory—we use different vocabularies and we speak differently. It
should not be surprising, then, that we do very different things with the same
piece of text.

What might be surprising is that I do see a connection between intuitive
inquiry and discourse analysis, at least in terms of how I understand what

I do. When I analyze a text, I engage with it in different ways. I use many of the strategies outlined by Wood and Kroger (2000): For example, I ask myself how am I reading the text and why am I reading it in a particular way; I take note of my impressions and reactions; I play with the text; I take nothing for granted; I read for what is not said; I deliberately do not deliberate. Being trained as a psychotherapist, I often ask myself "What is going on here?" Answering this question comes, in part, from deliberate and focused analytic work. But I believe it also comes from another sort of knowing. It comes from imagining, from less consciously sustained thought, from attending to bodily sensations, from identifying empathically with the text. In other words, it comes from what Rosemarie calls *intuition*.

That Rosemarie and I focus on two quite different discourses speaks not only to our ontological and epistemological commitments and to the nature and scope of our analytic and interpretive activities. It speaks to our intuitive sensibilities. The ways in which we attend to, interact with, and live in the data are shaped by a dynamic interplay of method and researcher, of person and technique, all of which are located in particularities of time, place, and history. It should not be surprising, then, that our analytic products touch, yet are distinct.

The Lens of Narrative Research: Ruthellen Josselson

Teresa's story is fairly straightforward in its details. A young, promising singer gets thyroid cancer and loses her singing voice. Her entire sense of identity had been rooted in her singing and in her hopes for an operatic career. When this becomes impossible after throat surgery, she recreates her primary sense of identity as a psychology graduate student. Then her voice starts to come back, but not with its former capacity, and she has to decide which avenue to pursue. By anyone's account, it is a painful story and a story of courage and perseverance. The differences among us, as researchers, center on what we do with the narrative.

It is interesting that four of us extract and quote Teresa's central and moving line, "My voice was gone, so I was gone, and I'd never been anything but my voice." This sentence poignantly epitomizes the history and nature of Teresa's sense of loss. Teresa's story could be the plot of a novel or a movie. The challenge to this group is to analyze Teresa's story in such a way as to conceptualize or at least locate her story in a scholarly theoretical context.

Narrative analysis draws on aspects of each of the other approaches. It tries to detail the *phenomenology* of experience as represented in the narration; that is, to see the world from the point of view of the narrator. It is attentive to the structure of the *discourse* as it creates and shades meaning and considers what social and identity locations the narrator may be performing by structuring the narration in a particular way. It organizes material into themes that resemble a *grounded theory* mode, reading line by line to note and categorize primary and secondary themes. And it is intuitive in that, through empathy and free association, it invites an examination of the subjectivities of the researcher. The process of iterative readings is not very different from what Rosemarie details as the procedures of intuitive inquiry. Beyond these shared perspectives, the narrative analyst tries to stay focused on the intersection of layers of meanings, much as one might analyze a literary text. The narrative researcher also remains mindful of going beyond description and keeps in mind the question of how a close reading of a text can advance knowledge and understanding at a more conceptual level. Thus, a narrative research reading is guided by some conceptually framed research question; the individual (or individuals) under consideration provides an instance for study of this theory-based investigation.

My analysis begins with a consideration of how this may or may not be a story of resilience (the initial research question), and I suggest that Teresa's narrative is more about processes of transformation in response to trauma and loss. I argue that Teresa does not return to a previous level of functioning, although she briefly tried to do so. Instead, her response to her loss is a sense of rebirth. Thus, I frame my analysis in terms of the conceptualization of resilience. This conceptual starting point is different from where my colleagues began.

In comparing my findings to those of my colleagues, my attention is particularly focused on what we each discovered as important "truths" about Teresa. I therefore briefly summarize the main points of my analysis in order to be able to compare them to what others emphasized in their readings. My analysis focuses on three main themes that I constructed as central tensions in regard to Teresa's coping with what was framed by the opening question as a "very unfortunate" event. These themes involve the intersection of her late adolescent developmental task of forming an identity with the loss of what had defined her identity throughout her life. This first theme, then, concerns Teresa's transformation of identity in response to the loss of her previous self-definition as a "voice."

A second major tension involves Teresa's experience of thinking and feeling and how she has balanced or interwoven the two. While she focuses on her cognitive efforts to manage the tragedy that befell her, there is also an undernarrated but nevertheless clearly marked self that is periodically out-of-control emotionally. The nexus between thinking and feeling is a central aspect of Teresa's experience as feelings threaten to overwhelm her, and she manages to cope with threat and loss through a determined application of logic and dispassion.

The third tension I discussed relates to her experience of self with others. Although Teresa regards herself as fundamentally alone in coping with the repeated threats of death and loss of function, she nevertheless must live in a world of others. Although the interviewer set out to investigate how social support from others assisted her in coping, Teresa resisted this idea in favor of stressing her own internal efforts to find the resolve to recreate herself and cope with her loss. In my analysis, I commented on how the other people in her life played complex roles in reflecting her shifting identity definitions and, at a deeper psychological level, seemed to express emotions that she could not bear in herself.

In order to try to create a holistic psychological portrait of Teresa's account of her coping following her tragic loss, I then explored how these themes were interconnected. I suggested that Teresa's privileging of thinking and her distancing of feeling were related to her use of others in the process of coping. I tried to show that she locates the more disruptive ("freaking out") feelings in others while she remains coolheaded. This process is itself connected to her narrative of rebirth and transformation. Identity, for Teresa, is entwined with her spiting of others: She had opposed her father by being a singer, and she spited the rejecting musical community by becoming a psychologist. Her emotional life, especially her anger, is thus enacted interpersonally with important consequences for her identity.

Thus, my analysis endeavors to go beyond naming primary themes in trying to detail how they are interwoven. I also stay alert to how these processes could be of interest in the context of the conceptual literature. Every person, as Kluckhorn and Murray (1953) famously said, is like all other people, like some other people, and like no other people. Every person, like Teresa, has a powerful and meaningful life story. How can these stories be heuristic in social sciences and help us learn something about what is true about others as well? How can the individual interview be read to lead to new and interesting questions about human experience?

Teresa's is an "unfinalizable" story, one whose ending is not yet known, especially as Teresa continues to be threatened by other cancers and continues to be in the process of balancing her intellectual/academic and musical selves. As Bakhtin (1981) said, every story points toward the future and carries the potential for revision. Therefore, I offer my analysis as a way of understanding Teresa's current assessment of the effect of this "very unfortunate" event on her life and her view of how she has coped with this. I leave open, however, the possibility that this could well be reframed and revised at a later time.

As I compare my own reading of the texts to those of my colleagues, I am most interested in what we each think we learned about Teresa and what implications this learning might have for an understanding of, or further research on, resilience and trauma. Do their approaches yield conclusions or interpretations similar to mine or very different ones? Are our goals and intentions different in terms of what we are hoping to elucidate? Are our "methods" different routes to the same place?

My narrative reading of Teresa differs in emphasis and form from the other readings. In contrast to my colleagues, I seem to be more interested in problematizing the text, looking for internal dialogue as a way of discovering what may be of conceptual interest in order to extend or critique theory. In general, narrative researchers are primarily interested not just in themes but in the interrelationship of themes. In my view, Kathy, Fred, and Linda retell Teresa's story in a more linear form than I do, since I am more interested in the tensions and internal contradictions in the story, the hidden subtexts, the possibilities of what may lie beneath the surface, and the interconnection of the elements. I think the narrative approach, with its concern with layered meanings in texts and its differentiation between the telling and the told, nicely dovetails with psychodynamic models (my personal theoretical grounding) of psychological experience, but there are other models that could well be employed.

Phenomenological Psychology and Narrative Research

Narrative research makes extensive use of phenomenological reading of the text to try to discover the meanings of the lived experience to the narrator. Like phenomenologists, narrative researchers begin with a highly empathic approach to both the interview and the text, attempting to see the person and his or her experienced world from his or her perspective, moving what was Other into relation with us. We aim to reach the internal array of an Other's experience, bounded always by our shared participation in a matrix of signification. Although we recognize that we can never fully know another person, empathy is premised on continuity, recognizing that kinship between self and other offers an opportunity for a deeper and more articulated understanding. Empathy becomes an attitude of attention to the real world based in an effort to connect ourselves to it rather than to distance ourselves from it (Buber, 1965; Josselson, 1995). Phenomenology and narrative research share a philosophical heritage and an assumptive world about subjectivity and experience.

Narratives, however, are not records of facts, of how things actually were, but of a meaning-making system that makes sense out of the chaotic mass of perceptions and experiences of a life. Narrative researchers read closely for both apparent and camouflaged meanings (Josselson, 2004), but perhaps not quite so elaborately as in Fred's demonstration. Fred's empathic, evocative, and lyrical rendition of Teresa's existential crises brings us very close to the "essences" that form the core of her experience of trauma and resilience, as he attempts to distill, amplify, and re-present the array of her perceptions and experiences.

Narrative researchers are mindful that any narrative is just one narrative, a storied form of experience that could be told a number of ways. (Indeed, we witness Teresa telling her story somewhat differently in written and oral forms.) The meanings of the past are constructed by (and in) the present (see Josselson, 2009), and the telling is created for the listener. Teresa would likely tell her story differently to her therapist, to her best friend, or to a classmate interviewing her for this assignment. She tells it differently now than she would have 3 years ago or 3 years hence. Narrative researchers take the narrational context into account as we consider the meanings of the narration. In the search for "essences," these considerations are absent in Fred's phenomenological account.

Fred's method strips the interviewing conversation from the text and considers only Teresa's words. Doing this, for example, misses the fact that the importance of God to Teresa was introduced by the interviewer. Teresa fairly clearly says that this is not a context in which she spontaneously thinks about her experience. Indeed, she describes herself as agnostic, but Fred stresses her spirituality and the intricacies of her relationship to God. I think that Teresa might not have even mentioned God had this not been framed by the interviewer. She does, however, mention her reading in many religions, suggesting a spiritual quest that she has not yet resolved. I think that Fred's writing here amplifies spiritual experience in what he terms an "imaginative" reading that may well be consonant with Teresa's felt way of being in the world. To his credit, he details the bases for his reading and acknowledges his "imaginative variations."

Fred offers many images that aim to express the essence of Teresa's existential dilemmas, and he writes Teresa's story as an encomium of life-affirming triumph. I, too, admire Teresa. I am perhaps more attentive than Fred to her internal struggles and the conflicted aspects of her, which may reflect my positioning as a psychodynamically oriented clinical psychologist or as a narrativist interested in the polyvocality of experience and life stories. This is always the challenge of an interpretive enterprise such as qualitative research; the best we can do is to try to name our horizons of understanding.

Constructivist Grounded Theory and Narrative Research

Kathy Charmaz, like Fred Wertz, offers a poetic account of the text, drawing on her own language to dramatize Teresa's suffering. I stay closer to Teresa's words and add my own voice only to conceptualize or comment on my relationship to the text or my reading of it at a different level of analysis.

Kathy's reading focuses on losing and regaining self as two ends of a continuum of reconstructing self. She emphasizes the conditions under which loss of self develops, as well as those necessary to effect *intentional* reconstruction of self. My focus is more on loss of identity, reflecting the ways these terms are used in psychology. Psychology has a long history of trying to distinguish between "self" and "identity" (Lapsley & Power, 1988), a distinction that is perhaps less problematic in sociology. I think that Kathy uses the term *self* in much the way I use *identity*. In detailing the loss and regaining of self in Teresa, Kathy breaks down these processes into component parts, from receiving and telling bad news to drawing lessons from the past and learning to live with uncertainty. I have no disagreement with Kathy's analysis, but I find it to be a highly detailed description, and I miss an interpretation of what new knowledge might be produced from this analysis. I am also, I think, more interested than Kathy in where the "lost" self still resides in the "regained" self and would not depict them conceptually as a line. Although not all narrative researchers think from a psychodynamic or self psychological framework, I do. The difference illustrated here perhaps reflects the difference between the relatively atheoretical starting point of grounded theory and the more theoretical embeddedness permitted in narrative research.

Kathy frames a set of research questions that she sets out to explore: "What is loss of self? How might it be related to a disrupted self and a changed self? Which experiences contribute to suffering loss of self? How do people who suffer loss of self regain a valued self?" She offers a lyrical and evocative meditation, using both her own and Teresa's words related to these questions, detailing Teresa's pain and angst. She then uses Gail's experience (an interview I did not take up) to show a contrast between a self that is lost and one that is disrupted. Indeed, differentiating, especially with reference to trauma, between "lost" and "disrupted" selves may be theoretically highly valuable. I particularly appreciated Kathy's focus on Teresa's efforts to live with uncertainty, which, I think, speaks to the same issue of fluctuation of self-states that I tried to discuss.

Discourse Analysis and Narrative Research

As a narrative psychologist, I aim to understand the individual, whereas Linda McMullen stresses understanding the processes of social construction through discourse. Her focus is on how Teresa positions herself in regard to others, which relates to a theme that I also explored but arrived at through a different route. We both notice how, in the narrative, Teresa devalues the input of others in stressing her own agency and coping resources, but we make somewhat different interpretations of this—differences that ensue from starting with different assumptions and goals.

I was intrigued by Linda's comments on the relationship between Teresa's "instrument" (her voice) and "instrumentality," and I found this a creative and productive line of analysis. This thinking leads her to ask about what social actions Teresa might be performing and concludes that her narrative performance serves, in part, to "enhance oneself and diminish others." Importantly, Linda states, "I understand my analysis not as evidence that Teresa is a 'self-enhancer,' and that this trait serves as a pathway to resilience. . . . Rather, I see the variations in how this action is performed as serving specific ends, and as having a variety of social consequences in the particular contexts in which the data for this project were generated." I understand this to mean that Linda's aim is to explore how agency and its self-enhancing variations might be socially constructed and have social consequences in this particular context. So Linda and I are seeing similar phenomena but interpreting them in relation to different conceptual contexts. I would agree that Teresa stresses her instrumentality and agency, that she sees herself as being in charge of her own life and tends not to rely on others, who, in any case, don't feel very reliable to her. As a psychologist who is interested in relational interaction, I focus on how Teresa makes internal use of what she experiences as others' reactions to her loss, and I suggest that this may serve her internal psychological balance by projecting into others that which she cannot bear. This perhaps represents the differences between a psychological reading and one that is focused on the function and consequence of particular social actions.

Intuitive Inquiry and Narrative Research

Like intuitive inquiry, narrative research honors the hermeneutic circle and modifies the conceptual context in light of the data, modifies the interview focus in light of changes in the conceptual context, and refashions the interpretive stance in light of these changes, and so forth. Rosemarie Anderson stresses the researcher's "personal engagement with the data," taking what I consider reflexivity to its extreme limits—but she keeps it in bounds and it works. Rosemarie's analysis primarily focuses on my second theme, Teresa's experience of affect and reason and the way she recruits both her body and other people into managing this balance. Rosemarie also details a theme that I found among the most interesting—the possibility that Teresa enlists others to carry emotions that she finds intolerable—but she seems to arrive at this theme by a different route.

Unique to the group, Rosemarie intuitively creates a conceptual hypothesis about disease as a "mirroring discourse," which I find quite intriguing and a promising avenue to pursue in other interviews. My own analysis focused very little on the body, partly because I wasn't especially attentive to the embodied aspects of Teresa's experience, although they are certainly very important. I thought that Rosemarie's insight that Teresa may locate her anger in her cancer was brilliant. I appreciated Rosemarie for pointing this out to me; it is not at all obvious and leads me to new thoughts—a hallmark of good research, in my view.

This lesson is perhaps one of the most important ones from this comparisons project: Our analyses of interviews are strongly affected by who we are as interpreters and to what we can be attuned. What we emphasize and conceptualize has much to do with what we bring to the enterprise, regardless of our method. As a result, narrative researchers habitually read interviews in collaboration groups in order to take advantage of different sensibilities and to hold in check the potential to "read in" to the text. Method, I think, is just a way of ordering our capacity for insight—but does not produce it. In the end, I think, research is just a form of conversation in which we try to detail and justify our interpretations of whatever data we have in view. None of us is, in any sense, "right" about Teresa, but we have each, in our own way, offered ways of seeing this interview that may lead to greater understanding of human experience.

The Lens of Intuitive Inquiry: Rosemarie Anderson

To prepare this comparative analysis of the five qualitative analyses presented in the chapters of this volume, I first read all the analyses as though I were reading them for the first time. Earlier, I had prepared preliminary drafts and heard my colleagues Fred Wertz, Kathy Charmaz, Linda McMullen, and Ruthellen Josselson present their analyses at various conferences. Nevertheless, as I reread the analyses, I observed what attracted my interest or challenged me in some way. Following this, I read each analysis one more time, noting in the margins unique properties of our analytic procedures as well as the commonalities and differences between my colleagues' analyses and my intuitive inquiry analysis. In other words, I began this comparative analysis much like I might prepare to analyze a set of interview transcripts.

What struck me first is that the five analyses read like a mystery, as though each of us discovers a unique piece of a puzzle. Each analysis highlights, interprets, and "unpacks" various aspects of the Teresa texts. While the analyses overlap considerably in procedures, identified themes, and interpretations, there are also many differences in procedures, themes, and interpretive emphases. Each analysis is also written, at least in part, in a manner that engages the reader personally and immediately, thereby communicating to readers the relevance and importance of the findings.

In the comparative analysis below, I first describe the unique features of phenomenological, grounded theory, discourse analysis, and narrative research analyses of the Teresa texts presented in this volume and then compare each analysis to my intuitive inquiry analysis. Following this, I conclude with a discussion of four distinctive features of my analysis (Anderson, 1998, 2000, 2004, 2009) that are not already covered in the comparisons.

Phenomenological Psychology and Intuitive Inquiry

Phenomenological psychological research is well known for in-depth analyses, and Fred Wertz's chapter provides a comprehensive phenomenological analysis of the Teresa texts. Like many phenomenologists, Fred has a love for words and the nuance that language conveys to human understanding. Words seem to "fly" off his fingers as he types. Throughout the chapter, Fred examines every nuance and imaginative variation on the Teresa texts in detail and reminds the reader that he can only provide examples of the steps he took in the analysis because of the length of his analytical texts. At the end of the chapter, Fred states the intent of the phenomenological research to explore "the inexhaustible diversity, depth, complexity, and fundamental mysteriousness of lived experience [that] always exceed our knowledge." Indeed, like intuitive inquiry, the character of Fred's phenomenological analysis points inescapably to the fundamental mystery of lived experience.

To invoke an analogy from the natural world, Fred's phenomenological analysis reminds me of the difference between the visual perception of an eagle and that of a hawk in a Native American tradition passed down by Patricia Underwood Spencer (1990). According to her Oneida ancestors, the eagle looks for prey by scanning the entire field, searching for patterns that vary within the whole field, whereas the hawk sees minor details, such as a single moving object, perhaps a mouse scurrying across a meadow. When I read Fred's analysis, I experience the kinesthetic sense of him going back and forth between the scanning modes of the eagle and the hawk in order not to miss a single thing. For example, Fred's individual phenomenal description, comprised of 55 meaning units presented in temporal order, seems to be an example of scanning across the entire field so that patterns may become apparent. Subsequently, Fred reflects on each one of these meaning units in detail. After these reflections, Fred generates the individual psychological structure in which he scans these reflections, looking for pattern variations, and identifies 11 temporal moments of substructures in Teresa's experience. Step by step, Fred's phenomenological analysis could be viewed as procedural shifts that alternate between these two perceptual modes.

Given Fred's obvious thoroughness, I was surprised to note that I had identified and worked with more meaning units (77) than he had, suggesting to me that I am more exact and analytic in my use of intuitive inquiry than I had imagined. True enough, intuitive people do not ordinarily think of themselves as detailed and methodical. However, I have long believed that the analytic procedures of intuitive inquiry should not be skipped (as beginning researchers are sometimes wont to do) because these procedures are essential to intuitive or creative interpretation, setting a context or spacious "container" for intuitive insights to "drop in" as interpretation proceeds. As I describe in the chapter on intuitive inquiry, intuitions do not ordinarily "free float" outside of an individual's intention, focus, and context—and if they do, they are difficult to interpret. That said, the way in which Fred uses imaginative variation is related to, but also different from, the imaginal processes embedded in the procedures of intuitive inquiry. Fred's imaginative variations and interpretations are closely aligned with variations in the data. In contrast, intuitive inquiry invites a wide spectrum of symbolic and unconscious processes (see section on modes of intuition in Chapter 9 on intuitive inquiry), including night-dream and day-dream insights, whether or not the insight is based directly on the empirical data being analyzed. Intuitive inquirers tend to trust right-brain processes to evoke imagery and embodied senses that lead them to creative insights about the topic of study and, over time, to breakthrough insights.

Fred's phenomenological analysis also contains two features not found in the other four analyses in this volume, including intuitive inquiry. First, Fred presents a discussion of the role of religion and even spirituality within Teresa's response to trauma and ongoing recovery. Within phenomenological psychology, there is a long tradition of interpretation, and Fred's discussion of the role of religion and spirituality in the Teresa texts falls within this tradition. Second, based on imaginative variations of all the features of Teresa's experiences, Fred presents a long list (but not the entire list!) of the "general" constituents of Teresa's experiences of trauma and recovery. He then compares these constituents with the interview about Gail's experience and builds toward possible conceptual generalizations about trauma and recovery. Fred carries the trajectory of descriptive conceptualization further than any of the other analyses. In comparison to intuitive inquiry, I did not intend to provide a comprehensive set of conceptualizations about trauma and recovery but to explore in depth the ways in which new insights might be brought to this topic by following the patterns in the data that intrigued me the most as the analysis continued.

Constructivist Grounded Theory and Intuitive Inquiry

Grounded theory has a reputation for analyses and interpretations of qualitative data that inductively build toward middle-range theories. Kathy Charmaz's constructivist grounded theory analysis in this volume follows in this tradition. The analytic coding procedures that Kathy describes are meticulous and varied, furthering the generation of emergent categories that coalesce into theoretical constructs over time. In reading Kathy's chapter, I sense much deliberation and thought occurring behind the scenes during her various coding procedures, probably reflective of her extensive study of individuals who have survived chronic illnesses of various types. After line-by-line coding, she chose to focus her analysis on the theme of losing and regaining a valued self. She explores this particular theme comprehensively, based on commonalities and differences between the Teresa and the Gail interview texts.

Kathy's analysis seems to me to provide a kind of "surround sound" on Teresa's experience, articulating the interviewee's experience from many angles, especially Teresa's self-understanding. If I were Teresa reading each of the qualitative analyses presented in this volume, I would probably recognize parts of myself portrayed within each of them. However, I might feel that Kathy's analysis aligns closely to my self-understanding. Kathy does not interpret Teresa's words and actions beyond what Teresa says or implies. What is interesting about this is that Kathy is a social psychologist trained within the field of sociology. The rest of us were originally trained in the field of psychology as researchers or clinical psychologists. As I considered this, I began to wonder if psychologists are trained or selected for their penchants to infer nonobvious or unconscious processes. Kathy's analysis was so "clean" of such discussions that at the end of her chapter I found myself laughing at myself. That is, I could not help but ask if Kathy would ever get around to a discussion of those deep, inner processes that psychologists tend to find so intriguing.

By comparison, in my use of intuitive inquiry analysis of the Teresa texts, I scanned for what is not explicit, as though intuitive insights express themselves via a subtle perceptual process slightly out of sight, or outside the obvious, because intuitive inquiry functions well in the generation of new and even breakthrough insights. To borrow a metaphor used in digital technology, I seem to have a double focus in data analysis and interpretation as though the "linear processor" in my left brain is looking at details and organizing them and the "parallel processor" in my right brain is looking for patterns, both implicit and explicit, that shimmer against each other in my visual and kinesthetic perceptual fields. Both analytic and intuitive processes are embedded in this ongoing ebb and flow. I am not so much looking for unconscious processes, per se, but for aspects of the data that speak toward possibilities in human nature not heretofore explored in depth. I seek the trajectories toward which the data point. Rather like watching a ball thrown into the air, I am looking to where the ball is likely to pass and land, knowing well that a strong breeze may come along and divert its path. Intuitions present possibilities, not certainties. In my mind, all qualitative analyses, and especially analyses derived via intuitive inquiry, present possibilities for theoretical consideration and follow-up empirical analyses and not certainties per se. Within a postmodern or ultramodern perspective, intuitive inquiry is designed to explore possibilities embedded in the data that allow for new understandings of present and future events.

In addition, while both constructivist grounded theory and intuitive inquiry are inductive methods that build toward theory, Kathy and I created theoretical constructs quite differently. Kathy built her theoretical constructs by carefully linking data with emergent codes. In contrast, based on an intuitively derived content analysis of the Teresa texts, I cultivated my own personal resources to gain intuitive insights, weighing them carefully against the data at hand. Therefore, in analysis and eventual theory building, my findings go beyond what is obvious, at the surface of the texts, to other elements that are more covert but also discernible. Expressed phenomenologically, the analysis seems to arise intersubjectively *between* me and the data. Although many qualitative researchers, including grounded theorists, actively employ intersubjective processes in analysis and interpretation, in intuitive inquiry analysis and theory building are confidently placed within a self-reflective, hermeneutical circle, which cycles back and forth between personal insight and data.

Discourse Analysis and Intuitive Inquiry

Linda McMullen's discourse analysis of the Teresa texts reads more like a detective story or investigative journalism than any of the other qualitative analyses. Linda focuses on the instrumentality of Teresa's words in relationship to herself and others and follows this focus to conclusion, step by step. Rather than exploring Teresa's use of language as an indicator of personal traits or characteristics, Linda examines the way in which Teresa's discourse functions relative to trauma and recovery. Specifically, Linda's analysis proposes that Teresa's words function to enhance herself and diminish others as Teresa endeavors to cope with cancer and the loss of her singing voice and subsequently revitalize her life. What is examined is how actions in the written text and interview are performed and function to meet particular ends. In reading Linda's analysis of Teresa's use of language, I could not help but reflect personally about how I have used language, especially in stressful situations, to shape others' understanding of me, if not my own self-understanding. Since the unit of analysis is Teresa's discourse and not the person of Teresa, readers of Linda's analysis are able to examine the inherent fluidity and performative aspects of language in the social construction of meaning.

Although Linda's discourse analysis and my inquiry analysis come to different conclusions about the Teresa texts, two aspects of our analytic procedures are surprisingly alike. First, both of us followed that which intrigued and interested us in the data rather than analyzing a full spectrum of interpretive possibilities explicit and implicit in the texts. In following our intrigue, both Linda's and my analyses point beyond what Teresa might have said about herself. Second, while I did not set out to focus on the instrumentality of Teresa's discourse, my findings do. In essence, my findings suggest that Teresa's discourse mirrors the nature of the illness itself, whether or not the "mirroring" discourse is intentional or conscious. My analysis also suggests that the language about the body may voice aspects of felt embodiment, ordinarily subliminal to cognitive awareness. Inherent in my analyses of both the Teresa and the Reno texts is the possibility that the language we use to talk about our bodies and disease may function in some inchoate way in relationship to disease symptoms.

Narrative Research and Intuitive Inquiry

Ruthellen Josselson provides a narrative research analysis of the Teresa texts that weaves the elements of Teresa's story into an integral "big picture." Aligned with the intent of narrative research to make the invisible apparent and return meaning to the text, Ruthellen's analysis synthesizes various elements, especially linguistic elements, of Teresa's experience into a narrative that feels meaningful, sympathetic, and whole. I sense that Ruthellen weaves and reweaves selected elements of Teresa's narrative until she feels assured that the "tapestry" renders a satisfying portrayal of the texts, both emotionally and conceptually, including narrative elements that may seem inconsistent or discontinuous from the whole at first glance. In Ruthellen's language, narrative analysis is "not a record of what 'really' happened," per se, but rather it attempts to bring "forth something new—something not apparent in the surface of the text." Her use of the hermeneutical circle involves an ebb and flow between selective narrative elements and the whole until a rich and multilayered interpretation has been rendered. In my own language, her narrative analysis of Teresa's experience is an integrated whole that is greater than sum of its constituent elements or even the whole itself.

Generally speaking, narrative research and intuitive inquiry seem to share more in common with each other than intuitive inquiry shares with any of the other qualitative approaches in this volume. Epistemologically, both of our analytic procedures are grounded in the tradition of European hermeneutics. Procedurally, we both make use of the hermeneutic circle, a process that flows between specific aspects of the texts and the whole, and back to specifics. The differences in our analyses are probably not methodological so much as they reflect the differences in our intuitive styles and what we bring to the analysis by way of personal and professional experience. These differences are subtle. Ruthellen seems to attend more than I do to the "layering of voices (subject positions), their interaction, the continuities, ambiguities, and disjunctions expressed." I would describe this as a sophisticated and particular form of pattern recognition that emphasizes meaning making. In contrast, in my analysis, I tended to look for structural, misaligned, and missing themes and patterns in the Teresa texts and how these themes and patterns are interrelated. My analytical penchant for looking for missing and interrelated elements is based on life experience. As a quantitative researcher I have been analyzing the structural components of statistical patterns for more than 30 years, so looking for the structural, patterned components in qualitative data and their interaction seems natural to me. In addition, Zen Buddhist meditation has taught me to observe the interstitial spaces between objects and events, sometimes known in the West as "negative space," in order to free the mind from preconceptualizations. In Japanese aesthetics, this practice is known as *ma* (Matsumoto, 1988; Mellick, 1996). Over time, I have come to apply the practice of *ma* to data interpretation as well.

Ruthellen's and my analyses of the Teresa texts are also aligned in our tendency to emphasize the potentially vulnerable aspects of Teresa's story. Throughout Ruthellen's analysis, her experience as a psychodynamically oriented psychologist, accustomed to hearing accounts of personal tragedy, seems close at hand in the selection of narrative elements that inform her analysis. For example, she notes the contrast between Teresa's lack of affect about the recurrence of cancer and her placement of grief and worry in the words and actions of others close to her, exemplified in Teresa's remarkable statement that she might "hold her breath until it ended." My own sensitivity to human vulnerability and suffering comes from attending to my own personal suffering and the suffering of the world as a contemplative. Like Ruthellen, I also note that Teresa uses the actions and emotions of others around her in ways that seem to reflect back to her feelings that she does not express overtly as her own. In addition, my analysis describes the implicit vulnerability potential in reverse mirroring between Teresa's discourse of dispassionate logic, numbing of feelings and bodily sensations, and the projected anger of her descriptions of her cancer symptoms as described in the next section. Both as an Episcopal priest and a transpersonal psychologist, I have also heard many stories of recovery and transformation. Often in these stories, the challenges and "lost parts" of the stories—these in-between, *ma*-like moments—convey the greatest potential for recovery and transformation. Therefore, I gravitated toward looking for the discontinuous or missing aspects of the Teresa texts that may point toward resolution and healing.

Unique Characteristics of Intuitive Inquiry

Of course, I am enthusiastic about intuitive inquiry—I developed the method! That said, what distinguishes my intuitive inquiry analysis of the Teresa texts is primarily the originality of some of its findings. I was pleased that my analysis demonstrated the power of intuition to invite new insights on a topic. As I have indicated in my chapter on intuitive inquiry, one of the primary purposes of the method is to invite breakthrough insights on any topic of study— and that is precisely what happened.

The intuitive inquiry analysis of the Teresa texts identified several themes also identified in one or more of the other qualitative analyses in this volume. Specifically, the themes of Pragmatic and Dispassionate Use of Reason and Logic as Coping Strategies (Theme 1); Emotional "Shutdown" of Feelings (first part of Theme 2); Personal Transformation from "Fat Girl with No Friends" to a Transformed Self with Accompanying Emotions of Anger, Relief, and Gratitude (Theme 3); and Intense Emotions Expressed by Others (Theme 4) were identified in one or more of the other analyses. However, my analysis is also unique in two important ways. First, I focus on somatic numbness as well as emotional distancing from feelings in Theme 2. Repeatedly Teresa describes feeling numb to physical sensations or parts of her body, including the tumor. Second, in Theme 5, Anaplastic Cancer Portrayed as an Angry Cancer, I notice that Teresa describes her cancer as an angry cancer, perhaps adopting what she had heard from others regarding its fast-growing nature. Linking Themes 1, 2, and 5 together, I then suggest an overarching theme of Reverse Mirroring between Teresa's Use of Dispassionate Logic; Numbing of Feelings and Bodily Sensations; and a Somatic Discourse of Anaplastic Cancer, an Angry Cancer.

Aside from the analytical findings, there are two characteristics of my intuitive inquiry analysis of the Teresa texts that distinguish it from the others that I have not discussed in my other comparisons. First, whereas many qualitative approaches require specific forms of data analyses, a wide variety of analytic procedures can be used as the basis for data analysis in Cycle 3 of intuitive inquiry. In Cycle 3, data are presented in descriptive form prior to the researcher's interpretation. To date, intuitive inquirers have relied primarily on thematic content analysis, participant portraits, or highly edited interview transcripts for Cycle 3 analysis and presentation. Hypothetically, however, all the qualitative analytic procedures presented in this volume—as well as those of action inquiry, case study, focus group, ethnographic, heuristic, and participatory research—could be employed in Cycle 3 data analysis. I am aware of two researchers who are currently combining the analytic coding procedures of constructivist grounded theory in Cycle 3 within the overall framework of intuitive inquiry's five cycles.

Second and of foremost importance, I would characterize intuitive inquiry as a hermeneutics of potential, reflective of the method's historical origins in the fields of transpersonal and humanistic psychology. As a hermeneutics of potential, intuitive inquiry points to the unknown capacities that come into form through human lived experience and participation in the world. The title of Abraham Maslow's *The Farther Reaches of Human Nature* is a case in point. Epistemologically and methodologically, a hermeneutics of potential complements a hermeneutics of faith, originating in the writings of Paul Ricoeur, and a hermeneutics of suspicion, originating in the writings of Karl Marx and Sigmund Freud. All three hermeneutical modes are essential to research praxis. Of course, historically, a hermeneutics of potential is inherent to the writings of many of the world's greatest thinkers in philosophy, theology, spirituality, and psychology. To name a few, phenomenological and existential philosophers Edmund Husserl, Soren Kierkegaard, and Merleau-Ponty; existential psychologists Ludwig Binswanger and Medard Boss; philosopher Alfred North Whitehead and process theologians Charles Hartshorne and David Ray Griffin; philosopher and poet Owen Barfield; existential theologians Martin Buber and Carl Tillich; Islamic scholars Al Gazalli and Henri Corbin; psychologist William James; and transpersonal psychologists Abraham Maslow and Anthony Sutich all point to the unknown potential in human nature—something yet to be discovered or revealed about who we as humans are and could be. In contrast, in looking for common characteristics and repeatable findings, much of psychological research clings to a repetition of the past and takes scant notice of the nascent potentials arising in human experience. In averring a hermeneutics of potential, intuitive inquiry invites a direct exploration and attention to what is becoming possible in the present. What is nascent now may in time become commonplace. What is anomalous now may meet challenges approaching from the future. While distinctly applicable to intuitive inquiry, a hermeneutics of potential urges the development of a renewed scientific discourse that explores the present *and* potentiates the future for all approaches to human science research and scholarship.

Similarity and Difference among Analytic Approaches

Comparisons of the analytic practices characteristic of five qualitative research traditions challenge us to sort out their similarities, differences, and relations with each other. These five approaches share common intellectual roots and overlap with each other in practice. They may be likened to members of a family with common parents and considerable resemblance. And yet each is unique, has its characteristic style, moves in its own way, and takes a different direction. To make matters more complex, none of these research traditions is monolithic. We learned in the general descriptions of each approach that there are variants among the ways it is applied, and each of the researchers in this volume uses one of the various approaches to phenomenological psychology, grounded theory, discursive analysis, and narrative research. Finally, even within these subtraditions, each researcher has his or her own individual personal style and has appropriated the subtradition in his or her own unique way. We have attempted to acknowledge and explicate the personal values and the intellectual and expressive styles of each researcher. One of the most important conclusions of these comparisons is that the approaches share much with each other. We now draw attention to some of these commonalities that arise through the comparisons, despite the many kinds of differences we see among the five ways of qualitative analysis.

Significant Commonalities

Each researcher, in comparing his or her approach to others, noticed significant commonalities. To a great and perhaps surprising extent, the five researchers, in keeping with their respective traditions, share significant views about the human being. Human beings are linguistic meaning makers engaged in complex situations occurring in multiple contexts. Human performances are multifaceted, make meaning, and shape the world; they are at once embodied, cognitive, practical, emotional, interpersonal, social, cultural, and temporal. The human being is never a "finished factual thing" but rather has potential beyond the actual and is able to creatively refashion him- or herself. The person, inextricably embedded with others in culture, is also an agent who shapes his or her ways of being in the world. This basic conceptualization of the person is shared not only by these five researchers but has been systematically elaborated by the founders and systematizers of these five traditions. Moreover, it could be strongly argued that, even if this understanding is not always reflected in the theories of the great virtuoso qualitative researchers of the past, such as Freud, James, Maslow, and Kohlberg, this very image of the person is implicit and operative in the concrete analyses they performed. This view of the person is not limited to psychology; it is also deeply shared by qualitative researchers across the spectrum of human science disciplines in their common recognition of "what a person is."

All five qualitative researchers place great value on speech, both written and conversational, in their study of the human being, as the virtuoso pioneers of qualitative research also did in practice and as the human science methodologists have explicitly recommended in their writings. All five researchers began their analysis with an open reading of the verbal expression of the research participant. As noted, Freud called this attitude "evenly hovering attention" and Kohlberg reported that he read over the interview transcripts prior to carrying out any specific analytic procedures. This common approach to speech and more generally to human expression has been delineated by philosophers in the continental traditions following from Dilthey, who emphasized *Verstehen*, the fundamental practice of understanding in human science research.

Qualitative researchers' attempts to understand their participants' linguistic expressions lead them to read the verbal data as a whole and to sensitively distinguish their various facets. With understanding, the researchers all attend to the data's internal organization, content, modes of meaning construction, and relation to such multiple contexts as the immediate situation in which the data were generated and the larger life historical and cultural backdrops. These contexts form important reference points for the researcher's critical understanding of the texts that are used in analysis and may themselves be taken up in the analyses. A process of understanding that moves back and forth between wholes and parts, which has been called the "hermeneutic circle," appears to be fundamental across multiple individual practices, systems, and traditions of qualitative research.

All five qualitative researchers became personally involved with the text. Each drew on his or her own human experience and meanings, which resonated with the participant's expressions. The researchers understood the subject matter as presented in the written descriptions and interview in a connected, relational way. Although qualitative analysis involves the engagement of the researcher and a relationship with the subject matter, it is not a projective test in which anything goes. In their readings, understandings, and analyses, the researchers not only identified empathically with the participant and responded to her in a personal way but also viewed her as an *other* in her own right. The researchers, as they inhabited the participant's discourse and meanings, stepped back, assumed a certain distance, became interested in the ways in which the participant constituted, organized, and lived her life. In this way these qualitative approaches are radically empirical, data based, and their results are emergent rather than projected or imposed. All the products of analysis—descriptions, interpretations, and theories—have their reference to the textual expressions of another person to which they continually refer. This qualitative principle of emergent knowledge is a basic and unifying one that assures that the findings of qualitative research have an evidentiary base. We pursue these unifying fundaments of qualitative research practice further, along with the differences of these approaches, in the final chapter.

Next: The Participant's Experience of the Analyses

In this chapter we have delved intimately into the anatomy of five approaches to qualitative research as well as the sensibilities and styles of five experienced qualitative researchers. Light was shed on the alternative philosophies, aims, choices, procedures, findings, sensibilities, and reporting styles that take place in qualitative research. This exploration was grounded in and made continual reference to the data and life situations of another person, whom we called Teresa, who is, after all, not a fictional but a real, living person, a *participant* in this project, and whose life is, and is understood to be, implicated in these analyses. Readers might well wonder, as did our audiences in professional conferences where this work was presented, how the person herself, Emily McSpadden, would respond to these analyses that have based themselves on what she wrote and said about her life. How would she see and what would she think of these researchers' work? That is the topic of the next chapter.

References

Anderson, R. (1998). Intuitive inquiry: A transpersonal approach. In W. Braud & R. Anderson, *Transpersonal research methods for the social sciences: Honoring human experience* (pp. 69–94). Thousand Oaks, CA: Sage.

Anderson, R. (2000). Intuitive inquiry: Interpreting objective and subjective data. *ReVision: Journal of Consciousness and Transformation, 22*(4), 31–39.

Anderson, R. (2004). Intuitive inquiry: An epistemology of the heart for scientific inquiry. *The Humanistic Psychologist, 32*(4), 307–341.

Anderson, R. (in press). Intuitive inquiry: The ways of the heart in human science research. In R. Anderson & W. Braud, *Transforming self and others through research: Transpersonal research methods and skills for the human sciences and humanities.* Albany, NY: State University of New York Press.

Bakhtin, M. M. (1981). *The dialogic imagination.* Austin, TX: Univeristy of Texas Press.

Berger, P. L. (1963). *Invitation to sociology: A humanistic perspective.* Garden City, NY: Doubleday.

Berger, P. L., & Luckmann, T. (1966). *The social construction of reality: A treatise in the sociology of knowledge.* Garden City, NY: Anchor Books.

Bergson, H. (2007). *An introduction to metaphysics.* New York: Palgrave Macmillan. (Original work published 1903)

Blumer, H. (1969). *Symbolic interactionism: Perspective and method.* Englewood Cliffs, NJ: Prentice-Hall.

Buber, M. (1965). *The knowledge of man.* New York: HarperCollins.

Burr, V. (1995). *An introduction to social constructionism.* London: Routledge.

Charmaz. K. (1991). *Good days, bad days: The self in chronic illness and time.* New Brunswick, NJ: Rutgers University Press.

Charmaz, K. (2006). *Constructing grounded theory: A practical guide through qualitative analysis.* London: Sage.

Charmaz, K. (2009). Shifting the grounds: Constructivist grounded theory methods. In J. M. Morse et al. *Developing grounded theory: The second generation* (pp. 127–193). Walnut Creek, CA: Left Coast Press.

Clarke, A. E. (2005). *Situational analysis: Grounded theory after the postmodern turn.* Thousand Oaks, CA: Sage.

Clarke, A. E. (2006). Feminisms, grounded theory, and situational analysis. In S. Hess-Biber & D. Leckenby (Eds.), *Handbook of feminist research methods* (pp. 345–370). Thousand Oaks, CA: Sage.

Clarke, A. E. (2009). From grounded theory to situational analysis: What's new? Why? How? In J. M. Morse et al. *Developing grounded theory: The second generation* (pp. 194–235). Walnut Creek, CA: Left Coast Press.

Crotty, M. (1998). *The foundations of social research: Meaning and perspective in the research process.* London: Sage.

Frank, A. W. (1991). *At the will of the body.* Boston: Houghton Mifflin.

Glaser, B. G., & Strauss, A. L. (1967). *The discovery of grounded theory: Strategies for qualitative research.* Chicago: Aldine.

Griffith, D. R. (1988). *The reenchantment of science: Postmodern proposals.* Albany, NY: State University of New York Press.

Hansen, E. C., Walters, J., & Baker, R. W. (2007). Explaining chronic obstructive pulmonary disease (COPD): Perceptions of the role played by smoking. *Sociology of Health and Illness, 29*(5), 730–749.

Josselson, R. (1995). "Imagining the real": Empathy, narrative and the dialogic self. In R. Josselson & A. Lieblich (Eds.), *Interpreting experience: The narrative study of lives* (Vol. 3, pp. 27–44). Thousand Oaks, CA: Sage.

Josselson, R. (2004). The hermeneutics of faith and the hermeneutics of suspicion. *Narrative Inquiry, 14*(1), 1–29.

Josselson, R. (2009). The present of the past: Dialogues with memory over time. *Journal of Personality, 77*(3), 647–668.

Kluckhohn, C., & Murray, H. A. (1953). *Personality in nature, society, and culture.* New York: Knopf.

Kuhn, T. S. (1962). *The structure of scientific revolutions.* Chicago: University of Chicago Press.

Lapsley, D., & Power, C. (Eds.). (1988). *Self, ego and identity.* New York: Springer-Verlag.

Mathieson, C., & Stam, H. (1995). Renegotiating identity: Cancer narratives. *Sociology of Health and Illness, 17*(3), 283–306.

Matsumoto, M. (1988). *The unspoken way.* Tokyo & New York: Kodansha.

Mead, G. H. (1932). *The philosophy of the present.* La Salle, IL: Open Court.

Mead, G. H. (1934). *Mind, self and society.* Chicago: University of Chicago Press.

Mellick, J. (1996). *The natural artistry of dreams.* Berkeley, CA: Conari Press.

Murphy, R. F. (1987). *The body silent.* New York: Henry Holt.

Robillard, A. B. (1999). *Meaning of a disability: The lived experience of paralysis.* Philadelphia: Temple University Press.

Salander, P. (2002). Bad news from the patient's perspective: An analysis of the written narratives of newly diagnosed cancer patients. *Social Science and Medicine, 55,* 721–732.

Schutz, A. (1970). *On phenomenology and social relations: Selected writings.* Chicago: University of Chicago Press.

Spencer, P. U. (1990, Summer). A Native American worldview. *Noetic Sciences Review,* 14–20.

Strauss, A. L. (1969). *Mirrors and masks.* Mill Valley, CA: Sociology Press. (Original work published 1959)

Weber, M. (1949). *Max Weber on the methodology of the social sciences.* Glencoe, IL: Free Press.

Wood, L. A., & Kroger, R. O. (2000). *Doing discourse analysis: Methods for studying action in talk and text.* Thousand Oaks, CA: Sage.

CHAPTER 11

The Participant's Response

I n many psychological research projects, participants have been given the opportunity to receive and read the final report. Traditionally, research- ers have rarely followed up by contacting participants and inquiring about their responses, let alone presenting them in publications. The findings of qualitative research may be highly personal and often include interpretations supported by quotations in which participants can readily recognize them- selves. Some forms of qualitative research have begun to deliberately engage participants in the research process, even in the evaluation and formulation of findings. In action and clinical research, the participant's ownership of, active contribution to, and benefit from the findings may be primary research goals. The present demonstration of analytic practices was not undertaken with the intent of sharing the findings with participants nor of benefiting them per- sonally. However, we believe that it is important for qualitative researchers, as well as psychologists in general, to understand how research participants are affected by and respond to research findings that concern them.

In light of the unusual focus of this project on a single individual, we asked Emily McSpadden to share her responses to our findings here. When she agreed, we gave her no specific instructions and encouraged her to freely express her responses, as fully as possible, in any way she chose. We have not altered the content of Emily's original written response. Readers will note that Emily's narrative addresses the five analyses in the order in which she read them rather than in the order we have used in previous chapters. We all agreed that fidelity to Emily's experience is more important than a consistent order of presentation across chapters.

Our purpose in inviting Emily to respond to our analyses was not to seek validation of the findings. None of us five researchers believes that a participant has interpretive authority regarding knowledge claims based on research. Rather, we have been interested in participants' responses to research as a topic in its own right. In the final chapter, we explore the general meanings of participants' responses to research reports, and we address the question of interpretive authority. As a basis for exploration and discussion, Emily McSpadden offers the following narrative of her experience of the research process and of reading the five analyses.

Of My Voice, in My Voice: Emily McSpadden

From my standpoint, it all began innocently enough. . . .

While taking a graduate course on qualitative research, our class was given an assignment. We had all agreed that we would study the phenomenon of resiliency in the midst of adversity and/or trauma, and that everyone in the class would pair up and interview one another. We were to conduct our interviews using open-ended questions, allowing the resulting data to be as rich and free flowing as possible; we were also to consider themes of possible strengths drawn from social supports or spiritual beliefs and practices, in the event that either or both of those were relevant to the interviewee's described experience. With those basic instructions, we went to it. My partner and I spent an afternoon conducting our interviews, recording them, and later transcribing them, verbatim, to submit to the class. We would then, as a class, choose one interview in particular on which to perform our analyses.

Like I said, innocent enough.

It didn't take any time at all for me to decide on a traumatic event to describe for the interview. I'm not sure if everyone else found it so easy, and I almost hope they didn't. I'd like to think instead that traumatic experiences are harder to come by. During the interview, I found myself disclosing much of the information aloud for the first time, finding words as best I could for things I had never outwardly expressed before then. The experience of being interviewed, then, proved to be far more powerful than I had expected, though not at all disturbing, damaging, or unbearably uncomfortable. When our class decided that my interview would be the one analyzed by the entire class, the choice was made while I was still anonymous to everyone but my interview partner; it wasn't until the choice was finalized that the question arose as to whether or not I would, or even could, remain anonymous for the remainder of the course. It might prove helpful, for instance, for our professor and members of the class to ask further questions of me in order to gain additional context for the original data. This was therefore the first time I found myself grappling with the question of anonymity, although it wasn't at all a difficult grapple. Rather, I was eager to help, and I never found it uncomfortable, even if it meant potentially delving further into what could prove to be painful personal memories, and before an audience of peers. Nevertheless, I considered it a rare and exciting opportunity.

For one, I'd be helping fellow students understand and perform qualitative research methods, something I considered invaluable. Second, I was able to share this quirky story of mine, in the hopes that, if I were in fact an example of someone who had successfully shown resiliency through trauma, others might see how I'd managed and find strength to weather the storms in their own lives. Finally, I found myself having to confront the numerous issues surrounding the event of my traumatic experience in a very personal yet public way, a challenge that I slowly came to experience as deeply satisfying and profound. A series of e-mails was exchanged, first between our professor, my interview partner, and myself, ensuring that my comfort level was established regarding discussing my experience openly. Afterward, an e-mail was sent to the members of the class (with my blessing) to inform everyone that the protocol that had been chosen was mine, and that I had agreed to answer questions about the protocol during class. From then onward, we had two or three class discussions during which I not only answered questions regarding the protocol itself, but also responded to preliminary analyses from classmates, and even spoke to the issue of my experience in the course as the participant at the center of the discussion.

Throughout the process of the class project, I remained at ease with answering personal questions from my classmates, discussing issues that arose in the data regarding my personal relationships, and never once did I feel that things became too difficult or personal to continue my participation. Upon completion of the course, I found myself pleased with the overall experience, glad for the opportunity to test myself in this novel manner. When I was approached to take part in the current project, it was as though I had a sense of what was to come. And yet, given the distinct nature of the project and the implications of a publication, a presentation of the findings, or both, the stakes naturally were a bit higher and certainly worth more careful consideration on my part. This, after all, would be no mere class project.

From the beginning of our conversations regarding this project, there was always concern that I never feel pressured to participate due to my status as a student, perhaps doing a favor for my professor in order to remain in his good graces. Honestly, I never felt any such sense of coercion or pressure. There were thoughts that crossed my mind, at the initial decision-making period, when I considered a hypothetical refusal, more as an exercise than anything I was drawn to as a preference. As I did so, I found myself instantly regretting even an imaginary "no" to the question of participating. How could I pass up such a rare opportunity to take part in a project I found so fascinating, not only as a student, but as a participant? I was personally curious to see how it would evolve, how much the analyses might differ or converge, and whether or not I might see my story do some good. It wasn't long before I found myself agreeing wholeheartedly to participate. Since my previous experience with the class project and our professor, Fred Wertz, was such a rewarding one, I was eager to participate in this new opportunity that he described to me, and my reasons remained the same: to further research, to possibly help others who were seeking to understand their own horizons of resiliency, and to challenge myself yet again to grow through a careful exploration of my own traumatic experience. I was made well aware, via the consenting process, that the project would involve my previously transcribed interview being analyzed by several experienced qualitative researchers, each utilizing a different methodology. I was also given to understand that, upon completion of the analyses, I would have the opportunity to read them and, should I choose, to respond to them. The analyses and my possible contribution would then be compiled for publication and presentation. Most importantly, I was told that I could stop the entire process at any time if I chose to, that my data were still my own, and that my comfort level was always of paramount importance.

As time passed, I naturally became more and more curious as to what the analyses would be like. The previous class project had been an open forum, and we all spoke freely to one another regarding the data in real time. The first thing that struck me as different about this new scenario was the fact that I would not personally be present for the analyses as they took place, and that there would be people analyzing the data who wouldn't know who I was; they would have never met me or necessarily feel any obligation to extend any kindness in their view of my words or their meaning. In the class setting, my fellow students had a shared context with me beyond my interview protocol. Although this had added to my level of comfort, the new project provided no such cushion, and I suddenly felt a bit vulnerable. It was still a tolerable circumstance, however, as I felt myself fully committed to being genuine and aiding the cause. It was not because I had anything to gain for myself by staying onboard, nor did I feel pressured to remain in a situation that caused me discomfort; I was genuinely intrigued to know what would come of the analyses, and felt some comfort in knowing that, should I find anything wholly objectionable, I could literally pull the plug at any time. I knew it would have been a grave disappointment to the researchers, and I would have felt a bit uneasy about that particular side effect, but my own reputation and comfort were (and are) valuable enough to me that I could walk away from the project with a perfectly clear conscience if I ever felt the need. Additionally, there was constant contact with Dr. Wertz, repeated renewals of assurances that my comfort was most important throughout the process, and that everything could, in fact, come to a screeching halt if I ever felt it should. Apart from concern for me as a research participant, he was always also checking in with me as a grad student in the throws of course work, and, knowing my story as well as he did, he acted out of concern for my health and its maintenance in light of my increasingly stressful graduate student schedule and workload.

His consistent and genuine outreach certainly went a long way in creating for me a feeling of assurance in my involvement with the project, particularly my ever-present sense of control as participant. I never felt that, should I decide to stop the mighty research wheel turning, that any of his concern for me, not only as his student but as a person in my own right, would be in any way lessened or retracted from me.

Further concerns emerged with time, both in my own reflection and through conversations with Dr. Wertz; these were concerns I hadn't previously considered but began to give me pause as the project continued to take shape. For instance, I wasn't the only person depicted in my telling of my story; there were others mentioned who didn't necessarily have a say, at the time of my initial interview, as to whether or not they wanted any part of this. I chose to reveal my identity during the class project, but this situation was significantly different, and the implications of my revealing my identity for this project were certainly more complicated. When I learned that the researchers doing the analyses for the project (with the exception of Dr. Wertz) knew me only as "Teresa," my reaction was a bit confused. I found the concept of a pseudonym, while perfectly legitimate as a means of concealing my identity for my protection, altogether strange nonetheless; it seemed, in an odd way, as though my experiences were being taken from me and attributed to another person, one I didn't even know (as I know no one by the name of Teresa). It wasn't so much the prospect of not receiving credit for my own experiences that bothered me, but rather the assumption that I needed protection, and that this required a kind of distance between my identity, my "self," and the events of my life.

I chose to participate in the project, in great part, to become closer to the experience, to explore it further and perhaps own it in different ways by reading what the researchers might say in their analyses. Further, if I were to respond to the analyses, would I do so behind the mask of "Teresa," or from the standpoint of my own identity? To speak from the position of a pseudonym, while I understand its purpose to be protective and perhaps liberating, I feel instead would be a bit disingenuous. I do think that I could speak as Teresa in my responses, but I also feel, given the type of data and my feelings about it, that I would feel more comfortable (and no less likely to be candid) speaking as myself. (If I felt the data to be either too personal or somehow damaging to my reputation, perhaps I would be more comfortable with a pseudonym, but I didn't find this to be the case.)

On the other hand, there was still the issue of the people in my life who were mentioned in my data, and whether they had any interest at all in my airing my feelings about them in this very public forum. The issue first became apparent to me while casually sharing the premise of the project and my involvement in it with my husband; he asked me, at one point, if he was mentioned and joked about hoping I spoke well of him. At around the same time frame, Dr. Wertz mentioned exposure of my parents and husband within my data as a possible risk for me to consider, especially in terms of whether or not I should disclose my identity. If I were to remain anonymous throughout the process, this would be less of an issue, as my parents' and husband's identities would be blurred by the fact that my own identity would remain unknown in the final published work. If, however, I wished to disclose my identity fully, this would also require that those closest to me, those I discussed fairly intimately in my interview data, would have to be considered. This decision, then, was no longer just my own, but a shared one; I took it upon myself to explain the situation to my husband first, then my parents. This also led to my personal choice of offering to share my interview protocol with them, which actually proved to be more daunting and awkward than I ever imagined, and not only for myself, but for them. In all honesty, I never imagined my parents would read the data. Nevertheless, nothing that I said in the interview was novel to them. I had voiced those opinions many times before in their presence; the only possible issue would have been disclosing those opinions to a wide world of strangers. Thankfully, my parents and my husband have been supportive of me ever since they first heard of my involvement in this project, and all graciously agreed to support me if I decided to disclose my identity. With their blessing, and with my continuing feelings of awkwardness surrounding being distanced from my data, I have remained ever inclined to use my own name, thanking Teresa for her time. That is, of course, as far as I understand my choice to go; I know the researchers can likely choose to keep me anonymous, and I respect their expertise on the matter, just as they have been respectful of me.

When I received the analyses, it took me some time before I could bring myself to read them. I had eagerly awaited their completion, yet I was oddly nervous about reading them once I finally had them in hand. Mostly, my apprehension seemed to arise not from fear that I would be angered or hurt by what I read (although I won't deny it was present, just not nearly enough to dampen my curiosity), but from the real possibility that I would read something that trespassed my sense of safety and would force me to back out of the project. By that point, I had become even more enthusiastic about the collaboration of these esteemed researchers being brought together in this way. It was the very sort of project I would be eager to read even if I had nothing at all to do with it. The fact that my protocol was being used was an honor; I was, however, prepared to honor my own right and privilege as a research participant to walk away from the project if I felt the need. Such was my commitment to the process rather than the project; I knew, as a student of research, the importance of upholding the most rigorous of ethical principles in work of such a sensitive nature, regardless of how thick-skinned I might have considered myself to be.

Another element of the project brought me some comfort and was a major incentive for my continued participation. Oftentimes, in my limited exposure to research given my status as a graduate student, I have noticed a dynamic that does not hold analyses directly accountable to those whose data have been analyzed, whether the results are quantitative or qualitative in nature. While qualitative methods seem to be more conscious of the participant on the whole, they nevertheless exhibit a lack of dialogue with the person or persons who provided the initial data, or at least no such dialogue is ever disseminated to the reader as a fundamental part of reporting the results. In terms of research ethics, I have always found this a problematic element in every methodology I've encountered to date: namely, that the "debriefing" process was not somehow a more explicit element of the research and find- ings themselves, but rather a mere procedural component of what constitutes the proper conduct of a scientist working with human subjects. Even in the case of analyses where face-to-face interviews were the sources of data, the voice of the participant remains ever behind the veil of the analysis, filtered in some way or another from representing itself as such. While I firmly believe that qualitative methods honor the voice of the participant in a much more rich and intimate way than quantitative methods are able, the voice of promi- nence remains that of an expert/narrator, despite the most genuine and authentic attempts to allow the data to speak for themselves. When I realized, then, that this project would provide me an opportunity as research subject to respond to the analyses, I felt empowered in a way that overshadowed any of my emerging feelings of vulnerability. I can say with great confidence that, were I not offered the chance to respond to the researchers' analyses of my experience, I might not have felt so comfortable with my level of disclosure, or my continued participation at all, especially as the questions of anonymity and inclusion of family members arose.

The researchers can rest assured that they have in me a willing partici- pant who would gladly do it all over again, so long as it provides an opportu- nity for me to do some good with the unpleasantness of personal trauma. In addition, I can't help but think that some may feel I had something to gain, whether professionally or monetarily, from my participation, and therefore was unduly encouraged to remain attached to the project. Granted, royal- ties, coauthorship on a publication, or a note on one's vita are indeed things to be grateful for; anonymity would remove two of those possibilities. Even the thought of these "incentives" as primary motivation for my participation is a little laughable to me; when I think of the amount of courage I found myself having to muster at times during my participation, including sharing my interview with my family and reading the analyses for the first time, I can assure the reader that I seemed to have more at stake than to gain—yet I felt compelled to remain involved, even if anonymity were deemed necessary by the researchers. It seems important that I lend my voice to this project, both through my data and my own voice in response, not only to further the science of qualitative research but to contribute to the research literature on resiliency, hopefully in some meaningful way for researchers and non-researchers alike.

Reading the Analyses

When considering how best to respond to the analyses for this project, my aim was never, under any circumstances, to challenge them. I trust the expertise of the researchers to not only take a respectful approach toward my interview data, but to know a great deal more than I do about how to conduct their respective research. If there was ever any disagreement between the analyses and my own opinions, I don't believe it was such that resulted from feeling any personal affront, but an honest disagreement in conveyance of meaning in a given passage, phrase, or even word. Beyond that, I realize that I have a privileged standpoint on the data, being that they were my own, and that I therefore knew more regarding the originating motivations for my words than any of the researchers could have, making anything that I considered a misunderstanding by the researchers interesting to me rather than personally offensive. That all being said, I didn't feel it was ever my place to analyze my own data in this case, nor to contest the analyses, but rather to provide, to the best of my ability, a glimpse at my reactions to reading what they had to say.

It is often a question that goes unasked in much research on human emotional and behavioral phenomena: What did the participant think about the analysis? How did reading it make him or her feel? Did he or she agree with the findings? And then who, in the end, is the authority? Is it the researcher, the expert on the subject of defining the phenomenon according to the literature and science available, or the research participant, the source of the data and the person who lived it? Some may argue that this sort of information is irrelevant to the findings of this or any research; on the other hand, others may find it to be the very core of its meaning. That issue can easily be left up for later debate; in either case, these questions do arise in the minds of a reader, researcher or not, and in light of the analyses already having been completed, I can see no harm in providing a response that cannot influence their formulation.

In addition to my investment as a research participant who has provided very personal data, I am also concerned with the process as a future researcher myself, having recently learned, through my time as a graduate student in psychology, more and more about what good research entails. I wish to contribute, therefore, a kind of validity to these data that they often don't have an opportunity to access. If an analysis seems entirely off the mark to me, it would only be logical for me to say so. I would likewise be obliged to speak to what I consider an accurate analysis, as best I can. In an odd way, it would be much like peer review, though by not so much a peer as a well-informed party with arguably equal stakes in the project. It is not a model without its flaws, to be sure, and likely would fall prey to arguments of bias. Nevertheless, it stands as an intriguing opportunity to shed light on the accuracy of data analysis in qualitative research in an interesting new way.

The following are my responses to the analyses as they were presented to me. I made these observations upon my initial readings of the analyses, in no particular order, and added comments occasionally upon subsequent readings and reflections. I remained confident, with each rereading of the analyses, that my initial responses were consistent enough with my later observations that I didn't feel the need to change any of my original tone or sentiments. The responses are not addressed directly to the researchers, although I at times found myself pondering what questions I might ask of the researchers in regard to one or another of their findings (I include those musings in my responses). I chose to address the nonresearcher audience, just as the researchers have done. I also chose to include some wording that I felt came naturally to me not as a student of research, but as a person of some education who uses terminology such as *hypothesis* without meaning it in a specific research-oriented light. Therefore, when I chose terms that seems laden with meanings attributable to research, I mean them instead in the layperson's sense. I do not presume to have an equal function in the work by providing my voice in this way, but I do hope to somehow contribute meaningfully to the discourse as a whole.

Intuitive Inquiry

This was the first of the analyses I read; I chose to read them in no particular order. As I read the chapter and the analysis, I first appreciated the researcher's honesty in mentioning the incorporation of personal experiences and beliefs in the analysis process. Getting to know something of the researcher's history aided in calming my fears about reading her analysis. Further, I felt the researcher's disclosure was a sort of offering, conducive to opening a discussion of a kind. I appreciated the care and understanding expressed by the researcher, and I found that same sentiment demonstrated in her treatment of the text. I was also rather surprised by the visceral nature of reactions described, such as the researcher's reports of having dreams and musings about my data. At one point, I was most pleasantly taken aback to find that I was assumed to be one of the readers of the analysis.

As for the analysis, I found myself thinking that, had I been asked simply about the different traumas over the course of my life, my responses would have been very different. I was asked, instead, to choose one example, which I elaborated on. "Reno," the other participant whose data are discussed by this researcher, has a far broader scope for his account, and it took me a bit of reading into the account to remind myself of that when considering the comparisons made by the researcher. Because the scope of Reno's account, as described in the analysis, was so broad, it would stand apart in its simplicity from what I produced in a very different interview setting. Mine might have been very similar in those terms if I had been asked the same questions in the same way, leading in turn to a significantly different analysis on the part of the researcher.

The meaning units chosen resonated with me notably; the researcher's reading of them indicated to me an attunement, empathy, and understanding that I found myself valuing, in addition to keeping what I said tied to its originally intended context. I did note a seeming disconnect between the five primary themes that surfaced (denial, emotional shutdown, transformation of self, intense feelings of others, angry bodily feedback) and the ensuing overarching theme of reverse mirroring. For me, the concept of reverse mirroring was a little confusing, only because it seemed to draw from "disease discourse," as described by the researcher. What was this "disease discourse," and is it specific to disease? For reasons I still don't understand, I found myself at odds with this concept of my data, because while the disease was certainly central to the situation, it wasn't so much the adversary to me, in my own mind, as other factors combined with it. I was also intrigued by the statement that I handled things differently after surgery than I might have done prediagnosis: "Teresa describes herself in ways that seem to me as more emotionally resolved and accepting as she moved forward through treatment and recovery." I wrestled with this conception a little because it surprised me, and I tried to understand it further in terms of the concept of my acceptance as time went on. Personally, I felt the entire ordeal to be a struggle against acceptance of my disease and its possible repercussions, and I now wondered if I had conveyed things differently in my interview. I continued to question whether or not this was the case for me in my experience, though it certainly brought to mind a reasonable reading, one that I could easily understand someone having arrived at and, as such, did not find it disagreeable. I was also struck by the "preliminary lenses" discussed by the researcher, particularly the first two, "life challenges and crises often signal a need for personal change and transformation and, therefore, are sometimes blessings in disguise" and "somatic, psychological, and spiritual states of awareness represent a fluid continuum rather than separate experiential states." Are these meant to be taken as the researcher's hypotheses, or were these evident in what I said? Are these beliefs that the researcher holds, or are they assumed to be held by me as well? Noting that, in the words of the researcher, "these 'flights' into intersubjectivity (e.g., Wilber, 1999, 2006) gave me intuitive insights that I may not have cultivated otherwise," is this an example of such insights, and are they intended to represent mine as well? While I was willing to entertain the possibilities they presented, I admittedly found myself having trouble recognizing my own experience in these lenses. If nothing else, they certainly invited some pondering on my part.

Constructivist Grounded Theory

Again, I found myself appreciative of the researcher's incorporation of personal experience as lending to the analysis, namely her former role as an occupational therapist and her current research on chronic illness. I was also comforted to know that the researcher's aim was "to learn research participants' concerns from their perspectives rather than to impose a preconceived structure on them," thereby gaining optimism that I would be allowed to speak for myself trough my data rather than fall prey to rampant interpretation. I was likewise intrigued by the researcher's impression that the "power" of just one brief statement I made during the interview could guide the entire course of the analysis: "My voice was gone, so I was gone, and I'd never been anything but my voice." When I made that particular statement during the interview, it's the sort of totalizing statement that I suppose artists are sometimes guilty of making, and sometimes seeming overly dramatic as a result. The fact that the researcher was so attuned to this statement brought me not just surprise but also a contented relief that I wasn't being regarded as overstating things by saying this the way I did.

In reading the analysis, my initial gut response was a sense that the "retelling" of my data through the work of the analysis was all very *dramatic.* Initially, it was almost *overly* dramatic for me to read, yet I couldn't deny feeling that, given how "dramatic" the events were, the tone was indeed fitting, and if it were not my own story that I was reading an analysis of, I would have been more at ease with the tone from the onset. The following statement really resonated with me, because I feel it captured so much: "Perhaps time collapses as Teresa returns to the crucial event. Perhaps we catch a glimpse of the 30-year-old woman becoming again the 19-year-old girl who lost the only self she had known and valued." Again, it seemed to me a rather dramatic telling of things, but not to suggest exaggeration or distortion of the data. Rather, I found as I read that this kind of account was warranted, given the circumstances I had described. As a result, however, this analysis proved difficult for me to read; it seemed idealized and aggrandizing, maybe because I was reading about myself in such a positive light, and it's always been awkward for me to receive praise. I found myself almost wincing while reading lines such as, "Teresa's handling of her diagnostic search showed her initiative and ability to take control over her life at an early age. Teresa's willingness to struggle and fight poor odds had long exemplified her stance toward the world." Further reflecting on my discomfort, though, I feel it's perhaps more a result of my overall sense that the researcher struck a significant level of understanding, attuning well to what I was trying to convey. While reading the analysis, I felt that my words and their meaning were being carefully considered, even felt, by the researcher, who felt more like a concerned friend than an inquisitive scientific explorer. Moreover, she was a concerned friend who was really listening. In the end, the main theme of "losing and regaining a valued self" struck me as very much on the mark with how I see things now, in hindsight, when reflecting on what I went through then. I couldn't have seen things that way when I was in the midst of the losing and regaining, though perhaps being able to might have helped to make my process all the more manageable.

Narrative Research

This particular process and analysis seemed to me rather intuitive, and appeared to be true to the data, albeit less structured than the previous two methods. I found it appealing that I was regarded in this analytic perspective as a storyteller, but I was still curious to see if my words would be construed as "story" rather than conveying "fact." It was *my life*, after all, and not just a story, which might as well be fiction. It didn't bother me that the researcher focused on the story itself rather than on the events described, because the events could only have been communicated well if the story made sense, so looking at the story didn't seem such a far-fetched endeavor. I noted that the method would "also take interpretive authority for going beyond, in carefully documented ways, its literal and conscious meanings," and that began to put me slightly ill at ease, only because interpreting what I'd said *beyond* what I'd said made me a little nervous . . . did I not say enough? Or did I hide something that's visible between the lines?

As I read the analysis, I noted that, according to the researcher, I *suppressed* quite a lot when I was ill. This claim didn't strike me as exaggerated, just not entirely reflective of what I'd experienced. On the other hand, perhaps that wasn't the intent of the researcher to address that aspect of the data, since events were not being considered in quite the same way as in the previous analyses I'd read. The idea of different selves seemed to me a good way to depict the way I saw myself during the time I described; to step outside of my experience as a singer was in fact moving into another self. Unlike the grounded theory analysis, this one was never difficult to read, never going too deep under the surface; not that any of it didn't ring true, but none of it seemed to say anything I didn't already say rather explicitly in my interview data. In other words, I didn't really find the analysis going beyond what I said on my own, or at least to the degree I suppose I'd anticipated. In a way, I rather appreciated that, since it didn't challenge me while I read, and it honored what I had to say. On the other hand, was it too kind? I appreciated my story being viewed as "a narrative of existential aloneness"; I felt it to be an appropriate description of what the experience I described in the interview was like for me, along with my sense of resiliency as a relatively lonely experience at times, or at least in my own experience thus far.

Nevertheless, I was left feeling as though I had never been challenged to consider my experience in any particularly different way, as though an "analysis" had almost not quite taken place. Perhaps I was looking for an interpretive lens to show itself and didn't find it, or perhaps it didn't show itself in a way I recognized but others might. Further, the researcher's personal concern for me was interesting, given that sense I had of the analysis. When the researcher said that my "avoiding [my] own feelings by perceiving or injecting them in those close to [me]" was emergent in my interview, and that I spoke "without much affect" about my condition and its possible recurrence, I was left with a sense of being misunderstood in my telling. I feel emotion connected to these things, yes, but as I said in the interview, I have to keep moving forward. To dwell on the emotional elements of these problems day to day, though they are relevant, would serve only to drain me. Must I speak "with affect" to have feeling? Also, it wasn't as though I somehow fabricated social situations in an effort to nest my emotions into other people in my life. My emotions were quite present in myself. Even apart from my illness, others play their roles in my life in ways that carry for me numerous emotions, but I do have, and demonstrate, my own emotions without the need for other people to carry them for me.

Discourse Analysis

The language of "instrument" and "instrumentality" instantly made an impression on me. I found this choice of focus on the part of the researcher not only appropriate, but inspiring me to continue reading more eagerly, so resonant was the concept when I encountered it in my reading. From there, though, the reading of this particular analysis was a strange one. To begin with, I felt almost instantly embarrassed. Had I really been such a self-aggrandizing braggart (or "self-enhancer") in giving my interview? Perhaps so; the excerpts this researcher brought forth certainly seemed to portray the data as such. When I gave the interview, I answered the question of how I got through my trauma, and if it seemed I relied on myself rather than on others, I suppose that would be an accurate representation. "Diminishing the other," however, didn't feel as adequately representative. To be fair, the other was not really there to diminish. The absence of others' actions was evident in my data because those actions were also absent from my experience. The analysis seems to claim, instead, that I exaggerated the smallness of others' roles, and that they were actually greater than I admitted in my interview.

For instance, no one reached out to me from the music school, save one or two people, and quite awkwardly and not so extensively that they had anything to do with my treatments or illness. As another example, my husband was entirely unaware of most of my difficulty resulting from my transition between the worlds of music and psychology as fields of study, likely because I kept it to myself as much as I could during those days. While I didn't mention the involvement of these people in certain elements of my experience of my illness and resulting hardships, I didn't see how it might imply I was really ignoring a presence and support that were actually there. Yes, in terms of undertaking this fundamental change in my life from music to other pursuits, it did feel like a solitary endeavor, and I took it up in that way. Therefore, I can't say the analysis is off the mark in that respect.

What I did find interesting is that my account should be considered potentially exaggerated. Was it so unbelievable that students from the music school or my voice teacher would have difficulty interacting with me in light of my circumstances? If their presence in my life at that time had been notable, I would have gladly reported it; it was, rather, their absence that was more remarkable to me, especially relative to their previous presence. It isn't so much that I minimized people when I gave the interview, but rather that they diminished themselves during my illness. They were less present in my account of events because they were less present in the events themselves. While, at the time it was happening, I did try to relate to their absence as an understandable discomfort, it was still very much the case that they were, for whatever reasons, no longer present in my life, actively or otherwise. In short, it seemed to me, in my reading of the analysis, that the researcher felt I was either misrepresenting the availability of offered support from those around me, or that I simply failed to recognize it. I sincerely hope the first of these is not the case, as I did my best to be completely honest in my account and would hope no deceit was assumed. As for the second possibility, while it's possible, it doesn't change the fact that my perception of events was such that, no matter how much support might have imperceptibly been offered me, it would have been imperceptible to *me*. That is, if I was, in fact, so blind as to miss those offerings, they would not have "existed" for me. Reflecting on that possibility today, I am still unable to recall any such potential event or circumstance that might have been subject to that sort of misinterpretation on my part. Besides, is it not possible that my data, as I gave them, were accurate as they pertained to my experience? It felt, to me, that this researcher did not entirely think so, and it made me question myself, even so far as to reread my own interview.

Something else mentioned in this analysis brought me to a position of confronting myself in a stark light: Do I consider myself "to be unique, unusual, especially talented," as the researcher described my depiction of myself, and if so, is it wrong of me to do so? I suppose I sensed something of a value judgment on the part of the researcher, at least in my considering myself gifted or superior to others musically, and therefore arrogant. Beyond that, does that make what I've said less credible? These questions of self-perception are difficult for any artist to take in. We are told all our lives as artists or performers to be both proud and humble, to balance striving for excellence and recognizing it in ourselves with negotiating the opinions that others have of us. (It also dawned on me at this point that none of the researchers had ever heard me sing; might that piece of data have made a difference in this analysis?)

My entire lived memory prior to the surgery was literally filled not only with music and singing, but also with praise and recognition encouraging me to believe that I was a better singer than other people in my environment. No one ever told me otherwise; in fact, it was likely one of the only things throughout my childhood that was noted as a positive attribute of mine by peers. Losing that could only be matched, in my mind during that period of recovery, by wildly and desperately seeking out everything I could to occupy my time and "talent," if I even had any beyond music (at the time, I truly didn't think I did). So yes, I think I do consider myself unique, because I don't know anyone who has chosen to do what I've done or in the ways I've gone about it all. I feel anyone is perfectly capable of doing the things I do, but I think they are likely either too wise or not as pressured by the ever-present thoughts of mortality to take on so much. Unusual? Yes, I suppose I would say I'm unusual, and for the same reason: I don't know anyone who does as much as I do, who has the history I have. Talented? I was, yes, before the cancer and the surgery. I have retained some of that talent in a different guise, so I do continue to think of myself as talented, just as I did before cancer and surgery. In order to succeed, I would advise anyone in a music program, or any field of study, to believe in the existence of his or her own talent. If I had not eventually found in myself other recognizable "talents," I don't know that I could have later succeeded at much of anything, and not just as a way of coping with hardships or trauma. Then again, whether or not I truly ever succeed does yet remain to be seen, as it is certainly an ongoing process. Meanwhile, I don't necessarily feel that this analysis intends to presuppose a reality that I've potentially distorted, although my reading of the analysis was such. And if using talk that enhances the self and minimizes others is instrumental in being resilient, I wonder if accuracy of events, as they are told or remembered, even matters.

Phenomenological Psychology

As I read this particular analysis, I found the reflections and comments being particularly concerned with my personal transformation through the process that *was* my traumatic experience. The fact that this process was reflected on by the researcher, along with "the world meaningfully presented" to me, made me curious to know what this "world" might look like to an outside observer, at least inasmuch as the observation took place through my telling of things.

In the course of reading through the process of analysis, I found myself a little overcome by the fact that, although elements of my data were obviously considered quite thoroughly, it almost seemed to compartmentalize my experience in such a way as to cut it into sections that captured so much more about me than what I originally thought was in the data. Could what I said really be so revealing about who I was, despite the fact that my description focused on one specific event in my life experience? Could so much of my intentionality be gleaned from what I mentioned? Then, when the thematic findings were presented, I found myself asking aloud, "Really? Do tell! You saw *that*?" I also placed myself in the position of a reader who had no personal connection with the data, wondering at the plausibility of these findings as being extant in the data. Readying myself for bouts of eye-rolling, I continued to read for grounding of these themes. Despite remaining skeptical about one's ability to analyze data like mine to such a depth, and to do so accurately, I found at the end of my reading that I had little argument with the themes. In truth, I never felt that I was being misrepresented. (This continued to seem counterintuitive to me, but reasonable, if in fact no meanings outside of my experience were being imposed after all, as per the researcher's claim.)

In addition to this, I had the very distinct sense that the analysis had been undertaken in so very detailed and elaborate a manner that I was left with feeling all at once that I had said too much and should also have said more. In other words, it seemed to invite me to conversation—not to clarify, but to continue. The discussion of the role of spirituality, for instance, as it was presented in my data, led me to ponder yet again my spiritual conflicts at the time of my diagnosis as subsequent undertakings related to treatment. My personal sense of how I lived my spirituality changed dramatically at this time, and I found myself thinking that I had so much more to say about that than I did in the interview. Such, however, were the circumstances of that particular interview. Also, there was a distinct focus on my interaction with my surgeon, an experience that I've often considered painful but, for both pragmatic and emotional reasons, direly necessary. While reading the reflections and analysis in this section regarding that day in the surgeon's office, I revisited those feelings of discomfort, resignation, and hope all over again.

In the end, however, while I feel quite satisfied that the analysis accurately addressed my experience, I fear I would likely be the only person to think so, and therein I find a strange conundrum. While, in my view, the researcher understood what I was trying to say and accurately depicted the meaning of my experience (from my standpoint), it seems unbelievable that one should be able to do so to such depth and degree. It was, in fact, so unbelievable that *I* could not be convinced until I read the analysis (and reread the specific places in my interview data to which it referred) for myself. How, then, could someone who has not lived through my experience possibly make such a confirmation? The analysis captured so much, but was it too much? Can it, therefore, lead to a greater understanding of an experience in a more general sense if it remains so concerned with the aspects of the individual that it can only speak for that individual, no matter how accurately? On the other hand, perhaps I'm being presumptuous, and any reader could find in such an in-depth analysis enough threads of their own experience when reading through an empathic lens.

I did feel that the depiction of a kind of dying and being reborn was striking, one that seemed for me a better way of saying what I had tried to verbalize at the time of the interview but didn't want to, for fear of being too dramatic. Throughout the whole of my reading of this analysis, I felt as though I was reading a kind of translation of what I wanted to express about my experience but somehow could not. It was not a matter of my words being changed or reinterpreted, but a clarification, using language I was not able to employ at the time of the interview. Here, more than in the occasions of reading any of the other analyses, I felt the most conflicted about the tone I chose in giving my interview. I was keenly aware of the audience of my classmates that it would eventually reach, including the fellow graduate student I spoke to during the interview itself. I now began to wonder why I had attempted to hold back from divulging what, at the time, might have seemed to me more dramatic embellishment than necessary facts. Even when describing my feelings about the experience, I remember trying to be casual rather than effusive, in part because I felt the story was dramatic enough on its own, and also, in truth, to protect my fellow classmates. It was never as a result of embarrassment or trying to keep things to myself because I found them too personal to divulge; I only thought that others might balk at my telling things too dramatically. I felt that, if I were to allow myself ample liberties in telling of the more arduous emotional elements of my experience, it would simply be over the top. In this analysis, much like in the depiction presented by the grounded theory researcher, I found dramatic, emotionally charged language everywhere, and it seemed fitting. If someone else had been conducting the interview, perhaps a professional I felt was more experienced and somehow less vulnerable to pitying me or becoming uncomfortable, I would have perhaps been more forthcoming in providing emotional "embellishment." Oddly, I realize now that I could never have given the interview in that way for the class project, in light of the circumstances, and found myself grateful that these researchers were able to somehow release my data and its meaning from my own strange censure.

Final Thoughts

The importance of words to a researcher performing qualitative analysis, regardless of his or her particular methodological persuasion, cannot be overstated, and is surely not lost on any reader of such research. However, when one's own words are the data being scrutinized and mined for relevant information informing the research at hand, it obviously brings about a very different, far more personalized meaning for the reader. Apart from mere curiosity to know what "experts" think of what you've said, there is the undeniable sense that some kind of judgment is being passed on the words, on the telling of an incident, even on you as a participant. These are not only human words, but words being read by humans, intended to be heard and thought upon by humans. Humans, too, are performing the research, and judgments come naturally, sometimes even unconsciously, to anyone, researcher or not. I am grateful to the researchers here for being frank about their own very human involvement in the project, their reading of my data, and, oftentimes, their personal emotional responses to what I had to say. I also feel that all of the researchers treated my words, and me in turn, with the utmost respect and concern. The fact that they were able to connect with my experience, in spite of my physical absence at the time of its communication, is rewarding to me in its own right, as a communicating being who has accomplished that particular task to some degree of success.

After reading the different analyses of my data, I find myself asking an interesting question: What was being studied? Resiliency? Me as a person who exhibited resiliency? Or both? Perhaps a blurring of this sort is what makes qualitative research important. If, for example, resiliency in the face of trauma is being studied in its function as a human experience, is it right to somehow extract the human being from it in the analysis of the experience? Again, I find myself thinking of words, particularly mine. I think of how each researcher placed such a crucial emphasis on paying careful attention to my words, and whether the focus was on their conveyed meaning, the patterns of their use, the themes they communicated, or the story they told, the words were always the key to understanding that which had been lived, sometimes without words at all. My inability to sing, and at times, to speak, during the course of my illness changed the way in which I had to communicate, even conceive of myself as a person among others in the world. To say in words what I underwent during that time became an interesting task for me, given that so much of my very communication with the world had been altered, and had effectively altered me. I don't know, even now, if the words I spoke and wrote, as they appear for the purposes of this project, can ever adequately convey my experience on the whole. I can at least attest to the fact that they faithfully represent at least some aspect of it, the one I was able to communicate in this way. If this has proven enough to shed some light on the research and its questions, I can ask for no better than that.

Did I walk away from these readings with a fuller understanding of resiliency, whether in a general sense or my own? Yes and no. I knew my own story well enough, and so much of what the researchers found was already embedded there, so the fact that I lived it all gave me some idea as to what I might eventually read in the analyses as pertaining to the experience and nature of resiliency. As for the more general, I see now that so much can be ascertained from one experience, that several different readings of a story, with an aim to understand what has been lived in it, can often bring about crucial insights about the human condition. To be resilient, as I've learned in my reading of these findings, is to undergo a process of change. This change occurs at various levels of experience, and is comprised of both external and internal factors, things within and completely apart from one's control. I have also learned that resiliency is not necessarily the sort of thing that one can judge within oneself, and that it perhaps takes the keen observer's eye to see the makings of it.

While my cancer is in remission at the time of this writing, cancer remains without cure, and I must therefore remain a cancer patient, albeit a survivor thus far. If I exhibited resiliency once, my hope is that I can do so again and again, hopefully improving on my previous efforts with some of the things I've read here. And, in the earnest belief that qualitative research on topics such as this can bring human beings to a place where personal growth can be informed and even inspired, I hope that others can perhaps do the same.

CHAPTER 12

Ethics, Participant Involvement, and Analytic Methodology

I n this final chapter, we address central issues that confront qualitative researchers in a pluralistic world. Our intent is to promote social and scientific responsibility by squarely facing the general challenges that have arisen in this project. We first discuss ethical issues in highly personal qualitative analysis, including the role of guiding principles and flexible conversation in addressing and resolving dilemmas, the mutual obligations between researchers and participants, the ownership of the data, the protection of participants and their social networks, and the values of confidentiality and disclosure. We then discuss the implications of involving participants in research as sources of data, as objects and evaluators of knowledge, and as coresearchers, including the inevitable power and knowledge asymmetries, the question of interpretive authority, and the mutual accountability between scientist and nonscientist. Next we focus on the commensurability of methods among diverse qualitative analytic traditions. We consider the extent to which commonalities of practice among different approaches offer a basic foundation and a unified set of optional, compatible procedures for qualitative analysis as well as the ways in which divergent specializations suit particular research interests and goals. Following from these methodological conclusions, we demonstrate the unity and complementarity of this volume's five approaches to qualitative analysis by examining the coherent and multifaceted character of the knowledge achieved by the various researchers' separate performances. Each of the five researchers describes the lessons learned in the course of this project. Finally, we offer conclusions that open avenues for further reflection and research.

Ethical Perspective: Relational Craft

Ethical perspectives have informed this project from the beginning and throughout. Ethical issues in research are often challenging. Some issues are more complex in qualitative than in quantitative research, and even more so when research adopts unconventional forms. Kvale and Brinkmann (2009) suggested approaching qualitative research, including its ethical engagements, as a *craft*. This means that rather than only applying abstract principles and procedural rules, researchers use ongoing, flexible judgments and creative responses to the complex challenges that arise in research situations. Our ethical perspectives have been informed by the APA's code of ethics as well as by commonly used practices and their variants. Our approach is rooted in such ethical principles as beneficence and nonmaleficence, fidelity and responsibility, integrity, justice, and respect for peoples' rights and dignity as well as the specific standards of conduct (American Psychological Association, 2002). The abstract nature of these principles, the importance of context in the rules of conduct, and the ambiguities of their application in concrete situations require a relational and conversational approach to concrete ethical praxis (Gergen, 1992; Josselson, 2007). Therefore, we, the researchers, have discussed what is good, what is right, not only among ourselves but with the research participant(s), professional colleagues, university institutional review boards, and others willing to lend an ear and a voice to the issues. We made decisions as a group, and sometimes consensus was difficult to achieve. We view consensus as ideal because of the social nature of ethics, rooted as they are in the *common good*, which requires and demands taking multiple perspectives and collective resolutions.

Ethics of Collaboration

Prior to formalizing our ways of protecting human participants in this research, there were ethical dimensions of our collaboration as researchers. In the original invitations to become involved in this project, as well as in virtually every decision during its course, we were sensitive to each others' personal and professional interests, values, and rights. Each researcher's participation was voluntary, and each treated the others in a way that embodied principles of justice, care, and wisdom. Self-interest was subordinated to our individual and collective welfare. In choosing the data to be analyzed, in formulating plans for our tasks, and in shaping our presentations and publication, decisions were made by open, sensitive, and respectful consultation with each other. Sometimes we all agreed to decisions that we would not have made alone. The ethic of mutual understanding, care and collaboration among scholars from different traditions paradigmatically contrasts with research practices that are driven primarily from an interest in promoting one's individual contributions and one's own approach through competition with other approaches and researchers.

Starting Point: Principles and Procedures of Human Protection

The conversational approach to crafting ethical relations in this research began traditionally with an attempt to protect human participants. For instance, our concern for the freedom and well-being of the participants led us to assure that their participation was voluntary, that their privacy would be protected, and that they would retain the right to withdraw their participation at any time during the course of the project. We proposed our plan in an Institutional Review Board (IRB) protocol with consent forms that followed standard operating procedures in research. Both participants who supplied data (as well as their interviewers) were informed in writing of the nature of the project, including its goals and procedures. They were assured that their privacy would be protected by strict confidentiality, that no personally identifying information would be included in the data or in the publication of the research. Among the researchers, only the principal investigator, who safeguarded the consent forms, knew the identity of the participants. Because the data were generated in a graduate class where one participant voluntarily disclosed her identity, the class members, who had agreed in class to adhere to confidentiality, were aware of her identity. The project's IRB protocol received an expedited review and approval, and the consent forms were signed by both participants.

Some ethical complexities of this project arose from its unusual focus on data offered by the single participant we called "Teresa." It is typical of qualitative research to focus on highly personal experience. In communicating and offering evidence of findings, even when numerous participants are included, publications often contain material in which participants can recognize themselves, with which they identify, and which may make them recognizable to others. The possibility of unforeseen consequences of the personal nature of qualitative research requires careful consideration not only among the researchers but in conversations including the participant and others.

Ownership of the Data

One ethical issue we faced in this project is the question of *who owns the data?* Because data are a joint construction of researchers and participants, the answer is "both." Consequently, difficult issues can arise from conflicts about their use, for instance, in publication. According to our consent form, participation could be voluntarily withdrawn at any point during the research. As Emily McSpadden mentions in her chapter, she could have not only withdrawn her active involvement but requested that her data not be used in publication. This possibility raises interesting issues. One set of issues that is rarely addressed in any ethical discourse concerns what our participant experienced as her own ethical obligation to the research. Emily understood that her participation was being counted on by the researchers, who made a large investment of time in a project that depended on her data. She experienced the data as given to the researchers with a commitment on which they could rely. If she, for any reason, objected to our use of the data and wished to withdraw them, she would have had to face an ethical conflict of her own that would require thoughtful resolution. Fortunately this did not happen, but Emily's mention of the issue led us to think about the ethical issues involved.

One ethicist whom we consulted expressed the view that once a participant signs a consent form and voluntarily completes participation in the research, the data are owned exclusively by the researchers, and the participant is not free to withdraw data. The consent form could be considered a contract that irreversibly entitles the researchers to any use the data, including in publication. This traditional view would appear to apply nonproblematically to research in which the data are more or less impersonal and used in aggregate analyses. However, in the case of qualitative research, especially when it involves in-depth personal expression of individual participants, the researchers' claim to exclusive ownership is questionable even if the participant at one time formally agreed to their use. Our team of researchers was troubled by and disagreed with this strict contractual approach. One expressed the strong view that personal data are owned only by the participant, that consent *could* be withdrawn at any time, and that this is part of the risk undertaken by a qualitative researcher. In discussing this issue in an APA convention forum, the consensus among experienced human scientists was that neither researcher nor participant has exclusive priority in the ownership and use of the data. If there is a conflict, a dialogue with ethical obligations on *both* sides is required in order to find the best solution, or at least one that is acceptable for each and all.

Confidentiality and Disclosure

One issue in this project that did involve a conflict concerns the use of the pseudonym, which was originally employed to protect the privacy of the participant. This valuable, standard practice in social research was undertaken routinely by the researchers, one of whom suggested the name "Teresa." Complications arose when this participant, for her own reasons, preferred that her real name be used in publication. A final decision was postponed until the results of the analysis were complete, so that the participant could view the actual reports prepared for publication. At this time in the current project, the issue was complicated by the participant having already accepted the researchers' invitation to respond to the analyses in a chapter and to become a collaborator and coauthor of the publication. When Emily initially read the analyses in preparation for her response, she had a strong negative reaction to the pseudonym and even more resolutely requested that her real name be used. The researchers' immediate reaction to this request was an equally strong concern for Emily's protection and for the minimization of her risks. Some of us worried about the potentially harmful consequences of publically revealing her medical history, for instance, in the context of future applications for employment or health/life insurance. We were also concerned that using her real name in the publication could compromise its scholarly integrity and pedagogical value. The research was initially undertaken and conducted with the assumption of participant anonymity, which is consistent with the project's purpose as a methodological rather than a biographical work. Although the analyses focused primarily on one participant, the researchers did not view their practice as a study *of this particular person* but rather as a demonstration of how to gain *general knowledge of a topic*, in this instance living through misfortune. We were concerned that the use of the participant's real name might erode the social research institution of privacy protection, which is important to convey in a pedagogical text, and might introduce unnecessary dilemmas on the part of students when conducting research without any biographical intent.

One respected ethicist pointed out to us that for the personal identity of the participant to be made known, ethical safeguards would have had to be planned beforehand, approved by an institutional review board, and employed from the outset in order to protect her. Such safeguards could not be established and reviewed retroactively; therefore, the participant's identity should not be revealed in this book. Another researcher-ethicist defended the participant's right to use her own name. This scientist argued that researchers must honor a participant's desire to use his or her real name even after an original premise of confidentiality has been established, as this professional has, in fact, done in publications. This ethicist asserted that persons' life stories are their own and their desire to be identified (as long as no one else is harmed) is a matter of their humanity. We struggled with both sides of this dilemma and discussed it extensively among ourselves, with colleagues, and with the research participant. It became increasingly evident to us that this project was unique, especially in that our research participant was now entering the new role of collaborator and coauthor. One ethicist, also an attorney, suggested that as a coauthor of our publication, the participant has the right to personally identify herself as the originator of her creative product. We attempted, as best we could, to understand the participant's desires and reasoning in making her request. We shared all our reservations with her, including our concern about the well-being of her family members, who could be identified if her real name were published. Some of us were strongly reluctant to grant the participant's request, and others thought the benefits of self-determination outweighed the risks. We all saw the legitimacy of both sides of the issue.

We became increasingly comfortable with what we came to view as our best option. Ruthellen Josselson suggested that the name of the sixth coauthor of this publication be Emily McSpadden, the participant's real name, whereas the pseudonym "Teresa" continue to be used in connection with the data and analysis, which were collected and undertaken with the presumption of confidentiality. This action would honor the participant-collaborator's desire to own her story and creative work in this project. It would also mark the original conditions of the researchers' analyses, reflect their intent to seek general rather than biographical knowledge, and symbolically respect the protective institution of confidentiality in research. Although unconventional, this solution is indicative of the uniqueness of the current project and was agreed on by the researchers and participant-collaborator as the best for each and all, including readers and the research community. The Fordham University IRB, after initially expressing serious questions and doubts, accepted our solution.

We learned that ethical decision making, notoriously difficult in social science research, is even more complex in highly personal, qualitative research and is most difficult when collaborative partnerships and other unconventional roles are undertaken by researchers and participants. Researchers are to be informed by general ethical principles and professional codes of conduct and to be prepared to use standard safeguards, and they should also consider the desires and interests of a wide range of individuals and groups extending from those directly involved in the research to the larger communities related to both participants and researchers. *Craft*, involving ongoing ethical reflection, consultation, discussion, and inventive decision making, is necessarily embedded in an ongoing, relational process.

The Involvement of the Participant in Research: Scientific, Social, and Personal Horizons

Human science research involves both researchers and participants. The research participant's responses to the analyses in this project introduce a host of general questions and considerations about the role of the participant, the significance of the participant's response to the research findings, and the best way that researchers might respond to the participant in turn. Qualitative research typically focuses on more than one participant, seeks general knowledge that goes beyond the individuals involved, and addresses topics that may primarily be relevant to the scientific community rather than to the participants. Nevertheless, increasing attention is focused not only on the ethical but on the scientific, practical, and social significance of participants' responses to research findings. When qualitative research employs participatory and emancipatory approaches, and in some action and evaluation research, participants' understanding, acceptance, and use of the findings may be an essential part of the research process and may be a goal of the research. However, when research aims to offer more general knowledge to the scientific community, the meaning and value of the participant's response raise questions. Some researchers have called on participants in order to confirm the scientific validity of findings, but are participants properly qualified to do so? Even when participants are not viewed by researchers as a legitimate source of validation, participants may read and be affected by research reports, and their responses may inform and concern scientists.

We have invited the participant in this project to respond to the analyses, and she has shared her responses with us and with our readers. Therefore, the present project enabled us to grapple with the meaning of the participant's responses to qualitative analyses, and a number of puzzles and paradoxes came to light. Although the participant sought to respect the expertise of the researchers and did not assume she had the expertise to evaluate the legitimacy of their scientific practices and the validity of their knowledge claims, she inevitably found herself being attracted to and repelled by various practices as well as even judging "the accuracy" of the analyses. Although the researchers, on their part, viewed their analyses as concerning general psychological knowledge that was not intended to match with, and in some cases was intended to go beyond and even contradict, the participant's self-understanding, they could not deny that the participant's life is embodied in her data and implicated in the analyses.

"Researcher" and "Participant" as Positions Assumed by Persons

In addressing these complex issues, it is important to clarify that *researcher* and *participant* are roles or positions and that research is a project of knowledge. Typically, the researcher is the agent of that knowledge, the one who achieves the goal, brings the knowledge into being through a special set of activities. The participant is immersed in the project of living and, by engaging in research, consents to become an object of and a means to the production of this knowledge. There is an inevitable distance and asymmetry between the researcher and participant, between the knower and known. Paradoxically, research involves both a closeness to, and a distance from, life as it is lived by participants.

Relational Asymmetry

As the initiator and agent responsible for the research project, the researcher has a certain privilege. Such activities as determining the topic, methods, findings, and report are distinctly the researcher's. As a helper in service of the research, the participant is in a subordinate position. In consenting to participate in research, the participant depends on, cooperates with, and is there for the researcher. An asymmetry, subservience, and power imbalance are intrinsic to the research relationship. Ethics are the researcher's first priority and trump every other aspect of the research because this power asymmetry requires an existential counterbalance that honors the participant as a free, sovereign, and self-determining being—for instance, one who gives informed consent and has the right to withdraw participation. Nevertheless, the participant's role in the research is to be known—to be observed, interviewed, or recorded—to provide data for analysis. Even though data are given freely, they are subordinated to, subsumed by, the researcher's project of knowledge.

Participant as Person

Because the participant as a person is not reducible to data and to knowledge, human science involves a potentially risky paradox: A sovereign subject is made an object; a person voluntarily submits to become a means to another's end. Research requires that participants are living subjects, original sources of meaning and purpose, as they express themselves in the research. The very intent of psychological research is to achieve closeness and fidelity to the spontaneous living of persons, and yet in the very process it inevitably assumes a distance from and objectifies the person's subjectivity, renders a free meaning-making subject an object first in the constitution of data, then in analysis, and finally in the report of knowledge. The participants' expression in the research situation is the crucial interface between relatively unexamined life-as-lived and life-as-known by the researcher. And yet inevitably, in getting closer to the unknown life, science assumes an analytic distance, goes beyond the relatively unknown life, and offers knowledge in a specialized, expert voice of the scientist that is potentially unanticipated and alienating for participants.

Position Reversal and Sharing

Traditionally one person or group of persons occupies the position of researcher and another occupies the position of participant. However, it is also possible that the same person or group can engage in both sets of activities, and doing so may have both scientific and social benefits. The reversal and sharing of roles may bridge the gap between knower and known, potentially bring knowledge closer to life, equalize the power balance, and even democratize knowledge. The history of psychology is filled with fruitful and well-justified examples of one person engaging in both roles of researcher and participant. Freud's greatest breakthroughs in psychoanalysis resulted from his self analysis and his investigations of his own dreams (Freud, 1900/1965). In psychophysics and memory research, experimenters have collected data from themselves and from other researchers. Kahneman (2003) reported activities with his collaborator Tversky, in which they playfully engaged in decision making, described their experiences with each other, and analyzed their own and each other's psychological processes in the development of theory. Qualitative research has demonstrated the value of one person occupying both positions, engaging in both sets of activities, and has offered innovative arrangements that integrate researcher and participant in the same person— for instance, in enlisting participants as "coresearchers" and in autoethnography. Even when these activities are assumed by the same person, they are distinct and involve the paradox of distance and closeness, a tension between the knower and the known. Partnership research has shown the value of engaging laypersons with a minimum of knowledge and social power, sometimes with special training, in such research activities as determining the topics and aims of knowledge, designing the study, designating data sources, conducting analysis, and reporting findings. Although these different positions and activities require different qualifications and remain distinct in their subjectivity, privileges, and responsibilities, persons can adopt both positions.

The Participant's Response

Even if a person who consents to participate in research has no experience as a researcher, the participant in research is not mere data, is not only an object for the researcher but someone with his or her own interests, purposes, meanings, self-understandings, and self-knowledge. The participant who has provided data for analysis, and has been affected by the research, can try to follow and understand the researcher's practices, can read the researcher's report, and is entitled to evaluate the research from top to bottom in his or her own way.

Some shifting in the usual relations between the participant and researchers took place in this unusual project. Emily McSpadden had been a student of psychology and had conducted research herself. Her written description and interview about her struggle with illness were undertaken in a class where she was gaining expertise as a researcher and exchanging roles of participant and researcher with her interviewer and her other classmates. Emily's reading of the analyses of the Teresa texts is thoughtful. She responded both from the position of a participant, one who lived through the experiences and was personally interested in the analyses, and from the position of a beginning researcher/scholar. At times the boundary between these two positions seemed to collapse. From Emily's standpoint, she is what is known and is presented to the world in the research report. Even though the researchers may have been aiming to communicate a general kind of knowledge with which Emily is not familiar, Emily understandably experiences the knowledge claims as "about her" personally.

We can learn much about the participant's responses to research reports from Emily's responses. Understanding participants' responses to qualitative research enables us to better grasp the implications of the paradox of closeness and distance of this kind of knowledge to the lives of persons. Emily is initially apprehensive and vulnerable, anticipating the way she will be known. She appreciates the honesty of the researchers, the way they allow her to see them as persons with their own sensibilities, preferences, and past experiences. She is grateful for their humanity, their kindness in the way they view her. Her well-being is at issue in being known, and she is aware of the possibility that the researchers, in their analyses, will trespass on the precious ground of life that is uniquely hers. She has given the researchers the gift of her life story, and being known to the researchers and thereby to the world through the research report is a very personal, interpersonal matter. Experiencing the researcher as a concerned friend is gratifying and reassuring for Emily. In reading the analyses, Emily is sensitive to whether the researcher seems to like or dislike her, whether the researcher understands or misunderstands her as she wants to be understood by other people. Her inevitable frame of reference is: How does this feel, what does this research report do for me, and how do the researchers' understandings of me fit with and serve my understanding of myself? In so responding to the research report, Emily is in all likelihood expressing the concerns of many research participants. From the participant's point of view, no one may be in a better position to judge the accuracy of the researchers' report than the participant himself or herself.

The Issue of Interpretive Authority

Should participants find themselves, as they understand themselves, in research reports? One common and understandable response from qualitative researchers is to answer: "In the data—yes, but in the knowledge that results from analysis—no." Participants are viewed as having a certain authority in accessing and reporting their experience. They have the privilege to freely author written accounts of their lives and to elaborate or revise interview data in an effort to express the truths of their lives as lived. However, in the production of knowledge, self-knowledge, even knowledge of the very experiences that only participants can describe, they do not have the same authority. Participants may not have sufficiently examined their experience, may not be in possession of analytic methods or conceptual tools, and may not have facility in producing knowledge, even self-knowledge. Moreover, they may not be familiar with the goals of a researcher or the technical language used by the scientist. After all, the five researchers involved in this project found their knowledge of each others' analyses and traditions, even after careful study, deficient and in need of correction. Authority in interpreting and evaluating each others' knowledge claims—an authority that is developed and cultivated by education, training, and critique—cannot be assumed on the part of a research participant. Therefore participants may not find themselves in the analyses and are not privileged in judging the validity of the researcher's knowledge claims. Participants can only offer additional data, which would give greater access to their lives as lived and thereby possibly motivate the researcher to redirect or revise the analyses and the resulting knowledge.

Both assumptions that the participant has authority in data generation and that the researcher has authority in knowledge production can be questioned. After all, no data are a perfect, unequivocal expression of psychological life, and no knowledge claims are beyond critique. Verbal descriptions are partial, affected by context; they may be contradicted by nonverbal expression and even by further verbal description. Sometimes behavioral observation or extended interviewing reveals psychological processes and social actions that participants did not initially disclose or enact, ones that they would be reluctant to acknowledge and might even unwittingly deny. Because data reveal and conceal, they are problematic, and so even here, there is in principle no absolute authority. The same may be said of science: No researcher is an absolute authority in the analysis and interpretation of data or in the resulting knowledge claims. Scientists are also fallible and subject to authority beyond themselves in the forms of both new data and in the criticisms and alternative analyses of other scientists. Descriptive and interpretive authority are both achieved and established in an ongoing historical process.

There is a strong tradition in human science research of investigating processes of which persons are typically not conscious. Such research may be *consciousness raising.* Freud revealed a "repressed unconscious" and Marx a revealed "false consciousness." An arduous course of psychotherapy and even a political revolution may be required for persons to accept and utilize the insights of scientific knowledge. The very service to humanity performed by human science research may sometimes involve the transgression and painful overturning of individuals' defacto self-understandings. Psychotherapy clients may vehemently resist these interpretations and may take time to acknowledge the applicability of an insight initially grasped only by the scientist. People may benefit in the long run (or perhaps be hurt, as in the case of the suggestion of "false memories") as a consequence of their appropriating social science knowledge of themselves that was initially alienating and disturbing. A person's self-understanding is not immutable nor entirely his or her own possession, and it may change through time and through communication with others.

Emily acknowledges that her understanding of her experience changed between the time of the original event and that of the research. When we invite participants to read and respond to our analyses and reports, it is not simply that they are in a position to know the accuracy of the report. Their responses therefore do not possess interpretive authority or the privilege of invalidating the analyses. They may be limited by their current self-understandings and may not have spent time studying and analyzing their data, as have the researchers. And yet it cannot be denied that social science knowledge is about them and that their appraisal of it is one context for its evaluation.

Scientific knowledge itself changes through time in response to human interests and the self-understandings of laypersons, who have the potential to assume the role of knower and whose utilization of knowledge rightly concerns scientists. Some qualitative research aims at knowledge that directly benefits participants and indirectly benefits others. Grounded theorists have long emphasized usefulness as a criterion of a grounded theory analysis. Here *usefulness* means providing the participants and nonscientists with an analytic tool that they may not have previously had for understanding their experiences and situations. Although participants are not positioned to assume interpretive authority, their responses to analyses are important for psychologists to consider according to the purpose of the knowledge.

Emily's Response to the Analyses

The goal of discourse analysis, as Linda articulates it, is not to understand the person's experience as a whole, to reflect the participant's self-understanding, or even to provide comprehensive knowledge of all the patterns in a participant's talk. Discourse analysis is not about the person, but rather about particular patterns of speech with characteristic social consequences that are culturally common and revelatory. The aim of this kind of analysis is to challenge and expand the ways we interpret our verbal expression. Discourse analysis can easily be misunderstood because its characteristic and exclusive focus on language patterns is different from the way we usually view language in everyday life, that is, as an expression of personal experience and a reference to reality. Linda did not intend her analysis to suggest that Emily was ignoring the presence of others during her recovery or exaggerating her own self-importance. Linda focused on the value, the instrumental consequence, of the diminishment of others and the enhancement of self in Emily's talk. This talk was understood as occasioned by, and as an instance of, a culturally relative discursive pattern. Whereas Emily took these findings in reference to real events in her life, Linda was studying talk as a cultural rather than individual pattern, a virtually anonymous one, without reference to Emily's personal meanings or surrounding realities. It is understandable how Emily could take this analysis personally, because she herself said those things, and in doing so, her intent was to express the reality of her individual situation.

Although the researcher's focus differs deliberately and dramatically from that of the person in everyday life, the two can be related.

Rosemarie's concept of reverse mirroring is also confusing to Emily. The notion deliberately points, in accordance with the goals of intuitive inquiry, to something that is not easily grasped by anyone. The concept is related to literature in health sciences, and Rosemarie develops it through her intuitive understanding of the Teresa texts in order to help move forward general theory and research. In contrast, a research participant such as Emily may not share this background knowledge, the intuitive presence required for the articulation of this kind of concept, or the theoretical goals of such knowledge. Reverse mirroring, which the researcher viewed as an unconscious process, is not expected to correspond with Emily's understanding of herself and may or may not be foregrounded in or relevant to her awareness. Similarly, the spirituality that Fred finds implicit in Teresa's experience may or may not be credible to Emily. A participant might, on the basis of his or her personal experience, identify spirituality with a specific set of beliefs or social rituals (that he or she may reject or avoid), for instance, concerning God and church ceremonies. However, Fred's description of spirituality in Teresa's experience is consistent with a longstanding scholarly tradition that acknowledges an agnostic or even atheistic faith that has little or nothing to do with intellectual dogma and religious organization. Emily was jarred and captivated by the dramatic quality of the knowledge claims made by Kathy and Fred. Although at times the analyses fit with her self-understanding, she acknowledged that her way of viewing herself made it difficult for her to appreciate the way this language articulated meanings implicit in her experience and that, even if disruptive, it is deeply correct. Here Emily was stretching her self-understanding in new ways in her encounter with the special knowledge that remained at a distance from her usual self-interpretation. Another participant might not understand or appreciate this dramatic language and might therefore feel it is "inaccurate." Ruthellen and Rosemarie wrote about ways that Emily kept her troubling emotions at a distance and of how these emotions were carried by Emily's significant others. Might this ever make sense to Emily?

Although participants have a certain privilege in generating data, providing texts, and describing their own lived experience, their self-analysis and knowledge are limited, may also change over time, and are not necessary for research. Participants' "expertise" and "authority" are located in the realm of personal expression, including their response to and use of knowledge. Participants contribute to research by opening their spontaneous living to researchers rather than by engaging in the labor required to create and evaluate scientific knowledge. Nevertheless, individual persons can shift from the participant position to that of a researcher who offers scholarly critique as members of the scientific community, although the roles of researcher and participant are distinct, the boundaries between them are not fixed or absolute.

The Researchers' Relation to Participants' Responses

How did we, the researchers, respond to Emily's response to the analyses? To a person we appreciated what she wrote. We were grateful for her honesty, enjoyed the clarity of her writing, and were deeply moved by the way she experienced our analyses and expressed herself. As persons and not just researchers ourselves, we anticipated Emily's responses with our own vulnerabilities, not unlike those Emily felt in reading our analyses. We wondered: Will she like what I have written? Will she feel I was fair and true? Might what I have written confuse or hurt her? Just as Emily identified with her textual expressions and took our analyses personally, we "took personally" and "took professionally" Emily's response to our work. We felt misunderstood at times. Without an intent to invalidate Emily's experience and yet reluctant to devalue our rigorously developed and refined analyses, we came to the conclusion that Emily did not always understand the findings in the same ways that we did. Some of us did not view our findings as being about Emily as a person but as being about a general subject matter (trauma, embodiment, resiliency, selfhood, discourse, narrative structure). Some did not see Emily as a peer, a methodologist, but as a student who had a limited and evolving grasp of the methods employed; as a person who did not necessarily share the interests and purposes of the analyses; and as a person, like all of us, with limited and changing self-understanding. Some of us felt compelled to clarify ourselves, so that Emily might view the analyses from the more distanced standpoint of the tradition and scientific community whose purposes and norms guided them. We were concerned that readers, especially students, might take Emily's responses as a final authority regarding the value and truthfulness of the findings rather than as a personal response of an individual with her own values, self-understandings, background learning, and preferences. The researchers also noted that Emily had an ongoing relationship with one researcher, who had been her department chair and her teacher, who might one day become her mentor—a thick web of relations in which her responses were situated.

The researchers resisted any inclination to cast doubt on, let alone to "correct" Emily's responses, as if her personal experiences of the analyses were invalid. After all, she was asked to respond to the analyses and did so honestly. However, once Emily became a collaborator, stepped out of the position of providing data, and read the research findings as one becoming a peer, even a budding methodologist and an educator of readers and students, was she not in a sphere where critique and revision are a justified norm? Would it be unfair of us not to clarify our activities as researchers with Emily, as we did with each other, in order to promote rigorously educated understandings of the nature of our knowledge and traditions? We did just this. We wrote our responses as researchers to Emily's responses to the analyses. The result was a document in which we added our own comments to Emily's original text, each researcher's in a different color font, for Emily's consideration (with the exception of Ruthellen, who felt that Emily should be able to say whatever she wanted, and she wrote only general, appreciative comments). We offered Emily the final say in expressing her own experience and responses to the analyses in her chapter. Although she found the conversation with the researchers interesting, she decided to include her initial writing in this book almost without revision. The only revision she made, a significant one, was to add sentences stating that in her reading of the analyses and in her chapter, she was not viewing the material as a psychologist and was not using technical vocabulary with its precise scientific meaning, as was sometimes thought by the researchers. She was writing from the standpoint of a person spontaneously responding to the analyses in whatever language expressed her experience and not as a methodologist or an educator about research methods. We all view this interchange as a conversation, one in which no one has the final word and in which each has spoken for him- or herself. The tension between the participant and the researchers, between living and knowing, between everyday life and science in this ongoing conversation remains.

An Ongoing Conversation between Scientific and Lay Communities

We six authors leave you, as a reader, to draw your own conclusions. The boundary between the scientific and lay community is, after all, not rigidly fixed. Each of the five traditions in this volume has developed special expertise and is capable of criticizing the others from its own point of view. We live in a world where no one point of view, no tradition, and no individual has an exclusive authority concerning the truth. This is a world where discourse and power have been problematized, pluralized, and democratized. The point of view of the scientist is not ultimately privileged over the layperson, for after all, whose interests are to be served by scientific research in the end? Scientific inquiry is rooted in prescientific human interests. It is important for researchers to be reflexive and to care about the impact of analyses on those who might not understand or wish to share their perspectives. That is how relational responsibility works in a pluralistic world.

Foundations, Compatible Options, and Specializations of Qualitative Methodology: Unity among Multiple Commensurate Approaches

The analytic approaches we have explored in this volume share much in common, and yet each has a distinctiveness that is not found in any of the others. In this section, we first delineate the foundation shared by all five approaches. These practices, also clearly evident in the work of pioneering qualitative

researchers such as Freud, James, Maslow, and Kohlberg, appear to be fundamental in qualitative methodology. Then we focus on constituents of qualitative research practice that were not employed by all five researchers and
have not been emphasized in the methodological works of all five traditions
but that are fully compatible with all approaches. These potentially common
practices, many of which are clearly evident in the work of the great, pioneering qualitative researchers in history, can be integrated into each of the five
approaches and utilized by researchers who do not identify with any specific
qualitative tradition. Finally, we focus on what is distinct in each methodological tradition in order to highlight the special contributions that each can
make when employed exclusively and when specially developed in combination with other approaches. These distinctive aspects of each approach may
not be employed, at least to a great extent, in all qualitative analysis. These
special practices are most relevant for researchers working exclusively in or
aiming to develop a high level of sophistication in a particular qualitative
research approach and tradition.

This section aims to clarify practices that are necessary as well as those
that are optional in qualitative research. The practices discussed below are
highly flexible and require adaptation to particular research problems and
researchers. It should also be kept in mind that these procedures of qualitative analysis are differentiated and ordered in this presentation to promote
comprehension, whereas in practice they are by no means enacted separately
or in a rigid sequence. In practice, the procedures and principles below may
be modified, merged, combined, and ordered in various ways.

Foundations of Qualitative Analytic Practice

As we look upon the analytic practices of the five researchers, we find common ones on which more specialized procedures rest. These may be considered fundaments of best qualitative research practice and common norms.
We noted in the conclusion of Chapter 10 that these commonalities are far
from trivial. They may be, in themselves, sufficient to yield significant and
sound scientific knowledge. Following from this, qualitative researchers do
not necessarily choose one specific tradition over the others and may use
these generic practices in order to achieve significant research aims.

Critical Evaluation of Data

The first moment of qualitative analysis on which all others are founded is the
reading of the data with comprehension. As this reading is enacted, one oper-
ation that is carried out, as a prerequisite for further analysis, is the *critical*
evaluation of the data. The researcher examines the constitution of the data
and checks whether they are suitable for analysis. Data are positively evalu-

ated to the extent that they are topically relevant, concretely expressive of the matter under investigation, and complete enough to enable the researcher to answer the research questions and to fulfill the goals of the research. The researcher examines the character and limits of the data, with special attentiveness to the personal and social contexts involved in its constitution. No data are perfect, and all data both reveal and conceal the subject matter. The question is whether they are *good enough* to proceed with a fruitful analysis.

The researchers in this project devoted special attention to the social situation in which Teresa wrote her description and engaged in the interview. The social context of peer relations in the class, the interviewer's presence, the qualities of the verbal interaction (e.g., Teresa's tenacious resistance to the emphasis on social support), and the content of the data themselves were scrutinized by the researchers. Emily also commented on this context in conveying her own experience of the research situation. For some researchers, these limits were viewed as part of the researched phenomenon itself, as in discourse analysis and narrative research, which approached the interview as a linguistic practice to be analyzed in its social context. For others, such as grounded theory, in which theoretical sampling is stressed, and intuitive inquiry, which emphasizes theory building, the data were accepted as a provisional access to the subject matter, which could be supplemented by further data collection (that was actually carried out in a subsequent interview with the participant but was not used in this project). The phenomenological researcher, judging both data sets to offer genuine, albeit limited, access to an example of trauma and resilience in the life of the participant, accepted their limits and viewed the data as an access to past experiences without further regard to the context of its production. All researchers, in their preliminary approach to the data, first critically evaluated them in accordance with their general approach, their research interests, and their goals.

Human Science Attitude

The second foundational aspect of qualitative analysis is the open reading of the data with empathic understanding of the meanings expressed by the participant. All five researchers approached the Teresa texts as human expression, which required the researchers to enter a kinship with the participant in which they coexperience her life situations. Throughout the research process, all researchers focused on the participant's words, read the data openly, resonated with them personally, assumed the participant's meanings as a fellow traveler, and empathically understood the participant's point of view. All researchers entered a *connected form of knowing* with sensitivity to words as personal and collectively sharable expressions. In this procedure the researchers drew on their ability to comprehend ordinary language in all its richness. Rosemarie drew on her experience as a gymnast to enter Teresa's experience of mountain climbing and to understand Teresa's vital bodily attunement during her recovery from cancer. This unique attitude is what Dilthey (1894/1977) called *Verstehen*, understanding the meaning as experienced by human beings.

Focus on the Uniquely Human

In the reading of data, prior to the application of specific analytic procedures, the researchers' understanding involved a focus on the participant's aims and meanings as manifesting the relativities of the psychological world. All view the participant as an active agent and human life as a practice and a performance. All understand psychological life as embodied, emotional (valuing), socially situated, purposive (teleological), meaning oriented, linguistic, interpersonally interactive, evolving through time, and consequential (practical). These common conceptual coordinates, which are viewed together in a holistic way, constituted a substantive, common view about Teresa held by all five researchers. This core qualitative sense and vision of human science subject matter is quite general, shared by the researchers across various philosophical, theoretical, and methodological orientations. Dilthey (1894/1977) articulated this fundamental, qualitative ground of human science, and Husserl (1962/1977) characterized Dilthey's conceptualization as an insight into the essential characteristics of the human being that is prior to and informs specific theories. As such, it may be quite implicit—more assumed than directly stated, as sometimes occurred in the pioneering research of Freud, James, Maslow, and Kohlberg.

Identification of Relevant Expressions

Another key fundament in qualitative analytic practice is identification of the constituents of the data that are potentially relevant to the research: those that enable an answer to the research question. This identification is an extended process inasmuch as the data are complex, and numerous different statements are relevant to the research problem. Fred organized the data into "meaning units" in order to differentiate and systematically consider them, as did Kathy prior to her coding. Rosemarie wrote Teresa's data constituents on index cards. Linda identified various discursive patterns in Teresa's text and began to consider on which she would focus in her analysis. Ruthellen read for themes and grouped them.

Emergent Ideation

As each of the five researchers posed his or her research questions to the relevant data, understandings emerged and conceptualizations formed *from the data.* This emergent ideation occurs in all qualitative research. The most exciting and mysterious moment of qualitative analysis is that in which insight is evident. It is exciting because knowledge is generated; progress is made in answering the research question or solving the research problem. Whether dramatic or ordinary, this involves something of an "aha!" experience on the part of the researcher. This moment of research is mysterious for many reasons, partly because the knowledge is emergent; it arises from the unknown, from the subject matter, and was not previously a possession of the researcher. Although insight involves discovery, a *finding* (and may possess a surprising or "gift-like" quality), it is neither passively received nor independent of the researcher. Emergent knowledge depends on the researcher's intelligence, reflective ability, training, and all the preparation that has taken place in the research process. Emergent ideation takes time. Understanding a text for the purpose of research is the product of extended hard work and sometimes struggle. Emergent ideation, on the one hand, involves a movement beyond the researcher's prior knowledge and, on the other hand, reflects the researcher's questions, approach, sensibilities, background knowledge, and existential familiarity with the subject matter. The process is therefore irreducibly relational. This is a moment in qualitative research may be likened to that in which the quantitative results of a statistical test of significance or a structural equation model appear on the screen of a researcher's computer. However, in qualitative research, newly emergent ideation is not the result of a standard calculation but is an outcome of human reflection and thinking immersed in concrete life.

Emergent ideation of the phenomenological sort begins in the extended process of reflections on each meaning unit of data and continues in their synthesis, in comparisons among individual structures of experience, and in the most general structural conclusions. For instance, when Fred is reading Gail's description of her gymnastic accident and reflects on her *fall*, the idea emerges that trauma involves a vertical dimension, not just a physical fall but a plunge in the context of personal aspiration and goal achievement. Turning to examples from Teresa, Fred recognized how she too *fell* from the upward trajectory of her opera career and suffered a *collapse* of her overall existence, which also involved an emotional *descent* and even a bodily loss of the upright posture on the operating table and in bed during her recovery. Grounded theory develops emergent ideation in activities ranging from its line-by-line coding to its memo writing in which categories of experience are explored (defined, analyzed) and eventually theorized. When Kathy views Teresa's statement about her loss of voice as the fundamental psychological process of self-loss, she is developing an insight into the subject matter that will play a role in her overall work on "losing and regaining a valued self."

After Linda formulates her research questions about the instrumentality of self and others, she finds important issues concerning self-enhancement in the literature on resilience, and selects extracts of Teresa's text that appear to embody one pattern of discourse that is relevant to exploring these questions. She develops her insights into "enhancing oneself, diminishing others" in her detailed examination of these textual excerpts. She finds in these excerpts two different patterns: the first claiming self as in charge, with others unable to cope, and the second claiming self to be unique, unusual, and talented with others having adverse consequences for oneself. Ruthellen finds in the Teresa texts internal reworkings of the experience of self in the story of her having lost everything. Ruthellen finds multiple stories, including one of shock, loss, and reconstruction in the written text and another one of her new identity as a psychologist in the oral interview narrative. Comparing these, she understands both as stories of transformation and integration. As Rosemarie sorted and resorted her 77 meaning units with an eye toward emergent patterns, she named themes and experienced such breakthrough insights as those into Teresa's pragmatic and dispassionate use of denial, logic, and reason as a coping strategy, and eventually the more synthetic and mysterious notion of "reverse mirroring."

The process of emergent ideation does not occur all at once and typically involves extended work. Data may be read and reread, and patterns that are recognized at various points in the analysis may be compared, conceptually distinguished, and synthesized. Modification and self-correction of insights are the norm rather than the exception. Finding the right words to express emergent conceptualization may be difficult and may require a long process of trial and error with many revisions. Researchers may utilize various specific analytic practices that can be developed to high levels of expertise. Such analytic practices were overlapping in the work of the five researchers in the current project. For instance, phenomenological *intuition of essences*—the grasp of "the what" of the subject matter, the recognition of something "essential" to the subject matter—was at least informally employed at one time or another by all the researchers in their respective analyses. All five researchers were also attuned to the *recurrence of structured patterns* in the data and placed considerable conceptual importance on these in their attempts to articulate what was variant and invariant in these recurrences. The *hermeneutic circle*, in which prior familiarity with the subject matter enters a dialectical, iterative process of reformulation in the encounter with the data, including a spiral movement back and forth between parts and wholes, was employed at least implicitly and often quite deliberately and extensively by the five researchers. What is the goal of these modes of analysis? All researchers had an eye out for what could be construed as *fundamental psychological and social significance*, matters important for general psychology. They achieved identification of this significance by *attending to key words, statements and actions* on the part of the participant that possessed especially pregnant, important meanings. The narrative and discourse analytic researchers used *concepts and procedures* that each had borrowed from each other's traditional crafts, demonstrating that in principle these five traditions can mutually inform each other and enrich each other's procedural and conceptual resources.

All the researchers brought to their analyses a wealth of prior understandings of psychological life in general and of the subject matter of this investigation. These "fore-understandings" included the researchers' psychological knowledge and personal life experience. These understandings functioned as sensitizing, conceptual tools that were sometimes reaffirmed and sometimes modified and reshaped in the fresh encounter with the data. Among the very common active operations involved in this process were an attention to tacit, implicit meanings; a meticulous attention to detail; and multiple readings in search of new insights. In this encounter with relevant data, all researchers resisted predetermined and immediate framings in their comprehension and held themselves open through this series of readings, allowing emergent ideation to arise in connection with the data themselves. Articulated well by grounded theorists, extant concepts had to *earn their way* into the analysis by virtue of their *goodness of fit* with the data themselves. Intuitive inquiry requires explicit documentation of the transformation of previous knowledge that takes place in this process.

Check for Evidence and Counterevidence: Adjustment and Refinement of Emergent Ideation

Qualitative analysis shares with all science a skeptical outlook that was also utilized in the analysis of all five researchers. This attitude and related procedures are not an absolute, dismissive skepticism but rather are relative, productive, methodically employed in order to assure that knowledge claims are soundly evidence-based and trustworthy. Not only when findings were in the process of formulation, but also after they had been fully articulated in writing, all five researchers carefully *returned to the textual data* and checked their claims in order to evaluate their goodness of fit, with attention to potentially contrary evidence, and to revise their statements accordingly.

Critical Reflexivity and Transparent Account of Procedure

All five researchers commonly employed *reflexive activity* that monitored the involvement of both personal processes and scientific procedures in the course of the analysis, lending the entire process a *self-critical attitude*. A *transparent account* of personal presence and procedures was offered by all five researchers. This procedure was used in shaping findings themselves throughout the analytic process and was also employed in reporting the research to the scientific community and in *acknowledging the limits* of the respective analyses.

Contribution of General Knowledge

In their knowledge outcomes, all five analyses achieved some level of generalizability. All five sets of analyses yielded knowledge of patterns that transcended the content of the data and of the research participant's life particulars. Although based on the analysis of these particular data, the goal of inquiry in each case was *general psychological knowledge.* Even though the analyses focused primarily on a single case, none of these researchers conducted a "case study," for a case study of this particular person (one genre of qualitative research) would typically require more data collection from the single participant than the current demonstration included. The researchers all aimed, even in this limited context, to *extend existing psychological knowledge*—general psychological theory and practice.

Writing, Engaging the Reader

Our enumeration of common fundaments would not be complete without including writing as a moment of analysis. Much could be said about this. We will only point out that the way each analysis speaks to a specific audience and readership is another relational aspect of qualitative research that shapes the findings. In their writing, all five researchers attempted to *conceptually engage the reader* and to address readers' concerns. In this sense research is thoroughly intersubjective and conversational. Table 12.1 summarizes the foundations of qualitative analytic practices.

Potentially Common Variations of Analytic Praxis

Each researcher employed some specific practices that were not used by all five but that are consistent with and could complement the procedures of all five approaches. These analytic moves have been articulated in the methodology of at least one (but not every) approach, are employed to some extent in various approaches, and are compatible in principle and practice with all five analytic traditions. Many may be identified in the research conducted by the great historical pioneers. These potentially common practices extend and expand the necessary fundaments of qualitative analysis beyond those that are already routinely employed in all traditions. Like the common fundaments of analytic practice, they may be used by researchers who do not identify with any one particular qualitative approach. For instance, the subject matter and purposes of a qualitative analysis can be determined in a variety of ways. Guidelines and procedural steps can be used in carrying out the analysis. Researchers can analyze protocols line by line or in more free-ranging ways. The analytic process and emerging findings can be meticulously recorded. A variety of forms of reasoning may be used in the analysis. Comparisons of data from various sources may be utilized. Additional data

TABLE 12.1. Common Foundational Practices and Norms

♦ Collecting concrete examples of the subject matter: observations, descriptions, expressions
♦ Evaluating the data critically: personal and social context and limits
♦ Employing human science attitude: open empathic understanding of ordinary language
♦ Attending to the uniquely human: teleological, embodied, emotional, practical, social, linguistic, cultural, and temporal
♦ Identifying relevant expressions: text that fulfills research interests
♦ Forming emergent ideation
  • Explicating significance through multiple readings
  • Using fore-understanding and stock of knowledge/procedure
  • Attending to key words, statements, and actions
  • Identifying recurrent patterns through data
  • Explicating implicit meanings
  • Comparing and synthesizing insights
♦ Checking, revising, and refining emergent knowledge by returning to data
♦ Reflecting self-critically on the limits of analytic perspective and achievements
♦ Writing general knowledge that transcends and reflects data
  • Supporting knowledge claims with evidence
  • Elaborating limits and open horizons of research
  • Accounting of procedure's transparently
  • Engaging reader intersubjectively

may be collected on the basis of analysis and used in iterative cycles of analysis and data collection. Although the five researchers in this project conducted their analyses alone, some of their traditions have developed and advocated doing qualitative analyses in collaborative groups. Finally, reflexivity of many different sorts can be developed and employed. These variations may be considered options rather than norms for all qualitative researchers, possible choices that can facilitate better analysis.

Our delineation of such potentially common variations in practice is by no means exhaustive. Our purpose here is only to demonstrate that procedures made explicit and employed routinely in some traditions need not be considered their exclusive possession. Many are compatible with and may be utilized without contradiction by other traditions and by individual qualitative researchers. The identification and study of potentially common variants of qualitative methods is important because it invites and encourages fruitful exchange among approaches with permeable boundaries. It also offers researchers who do not identify with any one approach broadly applicable methods drawn from various traditions that may well serve their particular research aims.

Determinants of Research Focus and Goals

The five researchers determined their research focus and goals in a number of ways. The sources included (1) topics in scholarly literature, (2) theory, (3) the study of the data, (4) the researcher's personal interests and sensitivities, and (5) the participant's emphases. All of these horizons of research play some role, whether explicitly or implicitly, in determining the focus of the analysis proper. All five analytic traditions can determine a focus centering on any one or any combination of these horizons. In this project (though not always previously), Fred's analysis made little use of theories, and he drew his analytic focus from literature topics, researchers' interests, and studying the data. Kathy decided to focus on the loss and regaining of self because this was emphasized by the participant as well as because this has been a theoretical focus in her past work on the experience of illness. Linda consulted the literature on resilience part way through her analysis and used the theoretically important concept of self-enhancement to guide her choice of discourse patterns on which she focused her analysis. Ruthellen's focus on Teresa's text as a story, containing multiple voices and involving internal work on the self, was informed by narrative and psychoanalytic theory. Rosemarie's approach emphasizes the importance of personal significance on the part of the researcher and the aim of transformation of self and society in the topic focus of analysis.

There were also variations in the content of subject matter that the five researchers took up in their analyses. Evidently human life is so complex that it admits of various aspects that can be addressed in different ways in the qualitative traditions. Phenomenology and grounded theory in this project focused broadly on Teresa's experience, though they are capable of researching specifically linguistic phenomena. Discourse analysis and narrative research typically focus on language. Although it is not possible for a researcher to develop knowledge of all the dimensions of human life in a given analysis, and some traditions have developed a focus on some more than others, all five traditions could include sustained analytic attention, each in its own way, to temporality, the body, intentionality, performance, instrumentality, emotionality, sociality, discourse, narrative, the unconscious, social positions and conditions, the self, and culture.

Use of Explicit Guidelines

As qualitative research has been established and has spread, there is an increasing emphasis on the need to identify explicit guidelines and steps. Giorgi (2009) has specified four basic steps of analysis. Glaser and Strauss (1967) delineated steps that have been modified by followers doing grounded theory. Anderson has found that five distinct cycles provide a crucial structure for intuitively oriented researchers. However, we have seen in the work of Freud, James, Maslow, and Kohlberg that excellent qualitative research has been and can be conducted without the use of these tools. Some researchers may feel constrained by stepwise procedure and might prefer to conduct an analysis in a more free-ranging way. Narrative researchers pride themselves on not establishing and imposing any requirement of a lockstep utilization of "method."

Recording Research Process

Some of the five researchers tracked and recorded their personal and scientific processes in the course of their analytic work, whereas others did so to a much lesser extent, if at all. Grounded theory (Glaser & Strauss, 1967) requires a meticulous recording as the researcher ascends from open coding to theory construction by organizing columns for data and the various levels of analysis as well as in writing research memos. Giorgi (2009) has also promoted methodical recording of reflections on each meaning unit. Similar accountability is seen in the meticulous documentation of discourse analysis, where lines of text are numbered for precise analytic references. Kindred processes of personal and scientific note taking can be and are sometimes employed in narrative research, even if strict forms of such accounts have not become routinized or viewed as mandatory. Such stepwise proceeding and record keeping are certainly not a requirement of good qualitative research, but they may provide a qualitative researcher in any orientation with a framework that guides analytic craft, encourages reflexivity, and promotes transparency in the scientific community.

Line-by-Line Analysis

In the actual practice of analysis, the five researchers carried out line-by-line analysis to varying degrees and in various ways. Each did so in accordance with their personal style and tradition, with various levels of documentation. Although some explicitly named or coded the themes of analytic units in the data, all conducted the work of conceptualizing the parts of the data as they worked through the analysis. Giorgi (2009) advocated meaning unit-by-unit analysis, although not all phenomenological psychologists use this procedure. Grounded theory researchers typically carry out line-by-line analyses, whereas discourse analysts work with features and segments of talk or text. In narrative research, line-by-line analysis is by no means a strict requirement, but it is a potentially compatible option.

Forms of Reasoning

Methodologies differentially emphasize eidetic, categorical, inductive, abductive, thematic, hermeneutic, structural, literary, and intuitive forms of reasoning. Although phenomenology makes explicit, systematic use of the *intuition* (in Husserl's sense) *of essences* in its eidetic analysis, other researchers practiced such intuition, perhaps even using some free imaginative variation when clarifying a pattern or a universal possibility that was exemplified in an individual experience or conduct on the part of Teresa. Kathy saw Teresa's loss of voice as an example of "losing a valued self." Linda saw excerpts from Teresa's discourse as examples of "enhancing oneself, diminishing others" and elaborated the qualities of this pattern that might be found and imagined in a variety of other examples. The five researchers developed *thematic analyses*, to various extents, detecting themes in the data and selecting some for extended focus and elaborate reflection. Ruthellen distinguished primary and secondary themes and considered how they were layered, raising this kind of analysis to a special height. In the phenomenological approach, thematic analysis—for instance, of spirituality—was not the main focus but was developed within the elaboration of the general structure of the experience. Some researchers, such as the narrative and intuitive analysts, used *intuition* in identifying unnamed, secret, highly implicit meanings in the data, and all five researchers had ways of developing such knowledge. Kathy, who was careful to stay close to the explicit expressions of the participant, was open to following up hunches about less explicit matters in the course of theoretical sampling and additional data collection and analysis. Although intuitive inquiry has drawn attention to and developed the practice of intuition as a research tool, all five researchers engaged their imagination and free associations, to varying extents, stretching beyond common sense and previous knowledge toward fresh insights, at first only vaguely grasped, in their encounters with the text. This is another potentially common practice that can be developed and formalized in various ways and to various extents by individuals and various approaches.

Comparative Analyses

A very important potentially common analytic procedure with many variants is the use of comparative analysis. This procedure is crucial for sharpening understanding and achieving generality of findings. Comparative analytic work may use different examples of the subject matter, different descriptions and/or interviews, and different participants' data. Although only Fred, Kathy, and Rosemarie used data from a second participant, all five *could* develop comparative analyses using additional participants and data. Linda's discourse analysis and Ruthellen's narrative analyses, which did not focus on the Gail texts, inform us of other kinds of comparative analyses in qualitative research. In Linda's analysis of both patterns of "enhancing oneself, diminishing others," she comparatively analyzed two excerpts from Teresa's text. Both Linda and Ruthellen compared Teresa's written description and interview, with informative findings. These analyses demonstrate the potential of comparative work not only between participants but within the data of each participant. The identification of multiple examples of phenomena and recurrent patterns requires intraprotocol comparisons. Comparative analysis, which is articulated quite explicitly in the phenomenological and grounded theory traditions, is a practice that is used in various ways by all qualitative researchers.

Collection of New Data for Analysis in Iterative Cycles

Another procedure that can be employed in all approaches is an iterative movement back and forth from data to analysis in cycles that can include the collection of new data. Although this procedure was first made explicit and formally emphasized in the writings of grounded theorists, the practice was later appropriated and reshaped in intuitive inquiry. A qualitative researcher in any tradition can extend analysis cyclically with fresh data.

Reflexivity Revealing Various Research Contexts

We noted above that all five analytic approaches are reflexive. All research traditions include potential for critical reflexivity and the capacity to develop it specifically in the course of every research project. The five traditions and the individual researchers in this project emphasize and develop, to varying extents, numerous directions and forms of such reflexivity. Some researchers paid special attention, before conducting the analysis, to their own presuppositions concerning the subject matter and definition of the topic. Reflexivity can also focus on the underlying philosophy, theory, the linguistic formulation of the research topic and problem, the social and political situatedness and implications of the research and the personal experiences, and the history of the researcher prior to and in the research process. The researchers' presuppositions and linguistic starting points can be explored prior to the analysis, as Ruthellen did; researchers can track their personal motivations and experiences connected with the research as intuitive inquiry requires; researchers can ask themselves how they are reading the text in the process of analysis, as Linda did; and researchers can monitor the ethical implications of their practices with regard to research participants and with regard to the research as a sociohistorical institution, as these researchers did together. Because qualitative researchers acknowledge that science is a human process, the assumptions, points of view, positions, and consequences of their analysis

TABLE 12.2. Potentially Common Constituents of Analytic Practice

♦ Sources and contexts of topics and goals: literature, theory, the data, researcher's personal sensitivities, participant's views
♦ Dimensional focus: temporality, the body, intentionality, performance, instrumentality, emotionality, sociality, discourse, narrative, the unconscious, social positions and conditions, the self, and culture
♦ Using procedural steps as a flexible guide for moments of analysis
♦ Tracking and recording personal and scientific research process
♦ Analyzing data line by line
♦ Naming or coding data constituents
♦ Analytical modes: eidetic, thematic, categorical, hermeneutic, inductive, abductive, structural, literary, intuitive
♦ Comparative analyses of examples, protocols, and various participants' data
♦ Collecting new data following analysis in iterative cycles
♦ Engaging a group of researchers in analysis
♦ Critical reflexivity: philosophical, disciplinary, linguistic, social, historical, personal

may be brought to light as part of its process. Qualitative research involves an expansive sense of critical accountability, which none of these five traditions would limit in principle. Table 12.2 summarizes the potentially common constituents of analytic practice.

Differences among Analytic Approaches: Specialization in Qualitative Research

Important as are the above common fundaments and potentially complementary variations of qualitative analytic practices and traditions, differences among approaches are also striking and significant. Each analytic tradition has developed special potentials for qualitative analysis. The differences among them are not so absolute as to render these traditions incommensurate; special procedures may be combined. Rather, they are occasions for fruitful conversation, mutual critique, and deepening methodological awareness within the family of qualitative traditions, even when dialogue may appear to be contentious.

Each Tradition Is Complex and Multifaceted

None of these five traditions has developed in a silo, and none has been static, univocal, or monolithic. In its more than 100 years, phenomenology has undertaken a series of "turns" motivated from within: the existential, the hermeneutic, the narrative, and the emancipatory. Similarly, grounded theory has developed along several lines, ranging from neopositivist to hermeneutic and constructivist forms. Discourse analysis is a nonspecific term encompassing linguistic, conversational, and critical varieties. Narrative psychology has almost innumerable variants and takes pride in resisting standardization of procedures and in embracing diverse traditions of psychoanalysis, feminism, and literary theory, to name only a few. Intuitive inquiry is explicitly pluralistic and inclusive of mainstream and transformative perspectives within psychology. Each of these traditions is still evolving in multiple directions. There are debates, in some cases similar debates, that take place within each of these traditions. And yet each tradition also has a certain distinctiveness and potential purity that may make it a particularly apt choice for certain research projects and researchers.

Philosophical Differences

Although the five analytic traditions we explore here define themselves in contrast to the naturalistic (objectivistic) ontology and epistemology that have dominated mainstream psychology, they draw on and embody different philosophical traditions that are also critical of each other. Following from this, each defines the subject matter of psychology in a unique way. Phenomenology raises questions about knowledge that assumes dualistic ontology, postulates hypothetical constructs, and utilizes inferences of matters external to lived experience. Phenomenology methodically engages eidetic analyses using imaginative free variation and emphasizes precise descriptive understanding of experiential processes. Phenomenology is able to analyze each of the other approaches.

Grounded theory research may be conducted from various philosophical standpoints ranging from neopositivist to constructivist. All are critical of the premature importation of theory and offer original methods for developing midlevel theory using inductive and abductive reasoning. Grounded theory is often used to bridge continental and hermeneutic orientations with neopositivist-based social science. Discourse analysis is critical of traditional terminology such as *experience* and *psychology* and challenges the idea that meaningful reality resides in objects of study. In this way it can subsume other approaches to psychology which, after all, are themselves patterns of discourse that beg for analysis.

Narrative psychology, which views experience as inexpressible until it is emplotted; locates meaning in language and storytelling; draws on the humanities and diverse traditions of social, critical thought; and is itself capable of subsuming and studying each of the other approaches. Intuitive inquiry emphasizes the intimacies, mysteries, and collective potentials of human life, which are placed above particular theories and methods, providing systematic ways of plumbing hidden personal depths and forging into the futures of our cultural history with transformative vision.

Within and between these traditions, we find debates about the extent to which meaning is given or constructed, discovered or created, and structured by language or nonverbal. These approaches debate the role and status of external variables in human science, the character and function of language in human life, the relation between the subjective and the objective in science, the role of theory, and even the nature of knowledge itself.

Directions of Inquiry

Each of the five approaches has a distinctive focus and goal of inquiry. Whereas phenomenology, grounded theory, and intuitive inquiry use verbal data to access nonverbal lived experience (unless the topic concerns language), discourse analysis and narrative psychology focus on written and verbal expressions with attention to their social contexts, ways of making meaning, and consequences, which are also examined by grounded theorists. Phenomenological psychologists tend to analyze all available and additional imagined data. Discourse analysis focuses explicitly on a part of the data and intensely analyzes a small number of extracts from the corpus of data. Narrative inquiry typically focuses on language in a holistic way that draws heuristically on diverse theoretical traditions chosen by individual researchers in the conceptual framing of research questions. Intuitive inquiry focuses inward on the personal life of the researcher to an extent unparalleled by the other approaches and undertakes the goal of transforming the researcher's life and culture with a deliberateness not found in the other approaches.

Diverse Scholarly Contexts and Concepts

Each approach has its own analytic literature that contains a distinctive stock of knowledge. Qualitative analytic concepts derive from various traditions, including the phenomenological, existential, European hermeneutic, heuristic, psychoanalytic, feminist, symbolic interactionist, speech act theory, humanities, and others. Conceptualizations therefore take different forms depending on the scholarly context assumed by the researcher. The role of theory varies across these approaches. Whereas phenomenology is atheoretical and asserts that the concrete description of "the things themselves" provides the best form of conceptual comprehension for human science, grounded theory and intuitive inquiry aim, through increasing levels of abstraction, at building a theory and hypothetical thought. Whereas phenomenology stays within the structures of experience, grounded theory considers such social positions as age, race, and gender and such environmental contexts as social institutions and culture, if they enter the situation of inquiry and can be established as relevant to the studied experience. Narrative inquiry uses concepts that highlight how language indicates the meanings and positioning of various selves, whereas discourse analysis uses concepts and a stock of knowledge that bring to light the social instrumentality and consequences of discursive practices. Concepts drawn from other disciplines can also enter the stock of knowledge used in these analyses, as we see in phenomenology's use of philosophy, discourse analysis's and grounded theory's use of sociology, narrative psychology's use of literary and psychological theory, and intuitive inquiry's use of language and values related to transpersonal and spiritual traditions.

Procedural Sets

Differences in procedures often concern emphasis and are not absolute. Personal engagement is very pronounced in intuitive inquiry, whereas in other approaches, researchers may (but do not necessarily) take a relatively disinterested stance. Phenomenologists aim to bracket prior knowledge, whereas narrative psychologists may deliberately begin with and consistently use guiding frameworks through the analytic process. Phenomenology and grounded theory begin analysis without theory and relate their findings to various theories at a late stage in analysis or after the analysis is complete. Narrative psychology approaches the data to ascertain multiple levels of meaning that are contained in the narration. Discourse analysis excerpts the data and compares fragments, whereas the phenomenological and narrative approaches attempt to encompass the whole and keep its overall organization in mind in interpreting its moments. Although phenomenology and grounded theorists use stepwise procedures, their practice is flexible and analytic moments may take place simultaneously. Narrative research and especially the first cycle of intuitive inquiry are comparatively free-ranging. Grounded theory and intuitive inquiry use abductive reasoning and form and test hypotheses. As we saw from the participant's responses, some analyses such as phenomenology and grounded theory appear to remain more participant-centered and closer to the life of the person, whereas the procedures of discourse analysis and intuitive inquiry decenter the knowledge from the person. Narrative approaches may take either stance or both. Table 12.3 summarizes the differences among analytic practices.

Complementary Findings: Multifaceted Knowledge

Some psychologists have questioned whether qualitative research is sufficiently cohesive and systematic to constitute a unified body of scientific knowledge. Even though the potential unity of multiple methods has been spelled out in principle (Wertz, 1999), we began this project without assuming that the findings of the various approaches would be compatible with each other, and we wondered if they would fail to form a coherent picture of the subject matter.

TABLE 12.3. Distinctiveness in Five Traditional Approaches

Phenomenological psychology

- ◆ Century-long, multifaceted movement with various turns (e.g., existential, hermeneutic)
- ◆ Critical of dualistic ontologies/epistemologies and hypothetical constructs
- ◆ Methodical use of epochés of science and existential positings (phenomenological reductions)
- ◆ Descriptive reflection on experiential processes and meanings (intentional analysis)
- ◆ Systematic study of essences using imaginative free variation (eidetic analysis)
- ◆ Holistic/relational explication of engagement in lifeworld situations (structural analysis)

Grounded theory

- ◆ Variants ranging from positivist to hermeneutic and constructivist
- ◆ Inductive and abductive reasoning
- ◆ Theoretical sampling of data
- ◆ Midlevel theory building and testing
- ◆ Use of status variables that earn their way into theory
- ◆ Bridging with traditional hypothetical science

Discourse analysis

- ◆ Problematization of traditional psychological concepts
- ◆ Radical attention to the instrumentality of talk
- ◆ Focus on practices rather than the person
- ◆ Extraction and conceptualization of patterns in fragments of talk
- ◆ Special tools of and procedures for linguistic analysis
- ◆ Knowledge of social contexts and consequences of conversation

Narrative research

- ◆ Foundations in humanities, literary studies, and ethnography
- ◆ Emphasis on the storied nature of life in creation of meaning
- ◆ Wide-ranging variants not limited by rigid procedural steps
- ◆ Conceptual stances from diverse disciplinary, theoretical, and social positions
- ◆ Use of layered thematic and structural analyses
- ◆ Focus on multiple voices and internal as well as sociocultural constructions of self

Intuitive inquiry

- ◆ Origins in investigation of spirituality and transformation
- ◆ Expansive researcher reflectivity and intimate engagement with data
- ◆ Articulation and transformation of researcher's understanding of the topic
- ◆ Active cultivation of intuition and imagination as research skills
- ◆ Goals of personal, cultural, historical transformation
- ◆ Affirmation of mystery

Although each yielded distinctive knowledge using Teresa's texts, there was considerable overlap—many of the knowledge terms converged. There were also significant differences. However, far from suggesting that the distinct qualitative analytic approaches splinter human science into incommensurate subjective relativities in which anything goes and in which contradictions are not resolvable, the findings from this demonstration allow movement toward a coherent and variegated body of knowledge.

Qualitative research methods, and their relationships, are understood through their findings. We now return to the findings of the five researchers, which, generated within the limited context of a study with primarily one participant, have begun to yield some general knowledge. Coherence among these findings is one way to demonstrate our claim of compatibility among diverse qualitative methods. In this section, one of us—Fred Wertz— explored the possibility of drawing together the findings from each of the five approaches in a beginning attempt at integrating some of the general knowledge generated in this project. As Allport (1942) long ago suggested, more recently developed by Churchill, Lowery, McNally, and Rao (1998), and Wertz (1986) in qualitative research, validity exceeds and takes priority over reliability. That is, diverse viewpoints and analytic findings enhance the truth of our knowledge rather than compromise it. The following brief attempt at a synthesis of some of the general knowledge gained from our diverse perspectives is itself limited in its perspective. In this demonstration, Fred used an existential framework and style, which is one among various ways that a synthesis of different qualitative findings may be sought. In such integrations of qualitative knowledge, as in qualitative analysis itself, pluralism is an epistemological and methodological virtue.

Traumatic Misfortune

Initially, traumatic misfortune is neither spoken nor constructed, but suffered. Antitheticality itself, trauma is not an object of consciousness but a destruction of the very intentionality of consciousness. An inimical Other, inflicted upon a person, disrupts that person's life as it is being lived. Relational life undergoes shock, a fall, a collapse, a disintegration, a vacuum of meaning, a kind of death. Primary are the uncanny emotions—terror, horror, dread, anxiety. Significant possibilities evaporate as relational life, the very core of the person, is undermined and thrown in question. Spellbound, one's practical activities come to a halt; one becomes isolated from others, and the previously sought future dims. Trauma is expressed not in words but in the cry, the scream, which is at once an isolated internality and a primitive stirring of transcendence—an inchoate protest of an anomic, suffering, embodied person, and a beginning revival of psychological life. Resilience is an extension of the transcendence of the cry in a restoration of intentionality, a life historical process of (re)engagement in which world relations with others are revived and the future is reopened.

Life Historical Process

The psychology of extreme misfortune is a life historical process that includes the past and future and changes through time. The misfortune of a traumatic event in part draws its significance from one's personal history of antithetical events whose meanings are retained and echoed in the current trauma, which is implicitly, in part, a repetition. Teresa's struggle for an adult identity was an attempt to rise up from the unfortunate subordination she had experienced in her family, and the cancer that undermined her efforts to become a professional singer echoed her father's previous interference with her independence and aspirations. Her cancer held the significance of a threat to her future, both a literal and existential death. The trauma sufferer is challenged to turn a tragic narrative into a tale of hope, courage, romance, even comedy in a triumphant reversal of fate. To this end one reengages previously developed ways of coping with adversity in the past. For Teresa, this involved a tempering of emotions, assuming independent initiative, rational problem solving, taking control, and using her talents and resources to eventually ascend to new, special, extraordinary heights. As a child, Teresa disliked the "emotionality" of her home, marked by her father's outbursts. Long before she was stricken with thyroid cancer, she had learned to come to terms with threat by setting aside disturbing and intense emotions in order to effectively engage in practical action that would lead to special success and distinction and broadening emotional fulfillment. A person may use various kinds of available psychological resources to rise from the occasion of trauma and to invent a new life, as Teresa did, or if possible and desirable, to restore one's former life, as Gail did. Misfortune is therefore also an opportunity, and a traumatized person can actualize old and new dreams and potentials through growth and development in the course of time.

Embodiment

The historical process of living through misfortune is an embodied one. The vulnerabilities and powers of the embodiment are at the heart of this experience. The body is the locus of emotionality and instrumental action, both a challenge one has to cope with and a way of being oneself. In coping with her cancer, Teresa overcame her initial "meltdown" by adopting a cool, even numb stance that allowed her to objectify her body as she learned about her disease, rationally planned to overcome it, and effectively carried out her strategy. As a singer, Teresa's teacher had helped her learn to meet the challenge of her body by employing meticulous technical control of emotionality and embodiment in the act of singing. This interplay between reason and feeling represents the intersection of important aspects of Teresa and teaches us about one means to cope with adversity and to transcend both bodily illness and emotional turmoil. A person may have a life-threatening disease and uncanny, disabling feelings and yet find a way to keep such emotions at bay in order vanquish the illness through technical rationality, thereby freeing oneself for a new life. This raises interesting questions about the role of suppression, denial, and dissociation in successful coping. The tension in Teresa's life between thinking and feeling, and how she balanced and interwove the two, informs us of important general psychological issues. How can logic and reason overcome dread, horror, agony? Perhaps the answer lies at a deeper, mysterious, unreflective level, that of "reverse mirroring"—an embodied way a person copes with potentially overwhelming aggression, as Teresa did in the face of her anaplastic cancer, by shutting down and numbing feelings and bodily sensations. Such calm inner peace mirrors, in reverse, a viciously spreading violence. This general possibility of reverse mirroring, and other typical forms of embodied emotionality and coping, require further study.

Sociality

One feels singled out by misfortune and trauma, which are individuating, isolating, and lonely. The inimical severs one's connections and threatens to disrupt one's solidarity with the beloved others who support one's well being. Teresa's relationships with her mother, her teacher, and her peers were severely tested. These relationships were shaken, became problematic, and while some offered life-saving help, others never returned to what they were prior to the cancer. In the experience of misfortune, the threatened person is attuned to other people's potential harmfulness, helpfulness, trustworthiness, and indifference. Others are scrutinized and gauged with regard to their tendencies to further traumatize, to withdraw, and to help the person restore relatively desired world relations. Stigma and shame (self-devaluation) are horizons of misfortune, for trauma involves a diminishment and failure of personal existence ("no one loves a loser"). Trauma carries with it the possibility of being rejected and abandoned, a loss of social admiration, and self-esteem. Teresa's doctors saved her life. Teresa's mother took over important executive functioning as mother and daughter steered clear of potentially disintegrating emotions. Teresa's father came through with gifts that were enjoyed but not sufficient to repair the long history of tense relations. Teresa was abandoned and became marginalized by peers. Her relationship with her teacher, who had been a "good father" in times of upward flourishing, poignantly and tearfully deteriorated. Trauma and misfortune reveal others as one's true friends (helpers, life savers) or enemies (uncaring, indifferent, betraying, antipathetic others).

Within this horizon of vulnerability, self-disclosure—the expression of the experience of trauma—is a significant issue for the sufferer because it both promises solidarity and can evoke help but also risks a deepening of misfortune and isolation. Sharing trauma with other people—disclosing private experience—is hopeful but dangerous and manifests in typical variations ranging from truth telling to concealing and deceiving others. In telling family and friends what happened, a person may protect his or her fragile feelings and the vulnerabilities of the relationship with them. Trust and fear structure interpersonal relationships, which may be enhanced or dissolved.

Moreover, others play a complex role in shoring up or assaulting a person's identity definitions, of carrying warded-off emotions, and of providing or dismantling the social context from which the person lives. Teresa resented, even as she understood, her fellow voice students, as well as her father, for not being solicitous or concerned enough. Posttrauma social engagement may initiate new forms of relationship, including deeper intimacies, dependencies, and mutuality. Teresa married and, in time, tentatively began to communicate more deeply, to expose her vulnerabilities with her husband, and to explore possibilities of being cared for. Valued qualities of supportive others include truthfulness, sharing, practical assistance, softness, recognition and understanding of personal goals and resources, alliance, care, encouragement, and accompaniment into the future. The successful quest for identity may be shored up by others.

Agency

Agency is involved in the making of a comeback, which requires planning and effort. The person engages in a battle against trauma in an attempt to resume a free life, one that is preferred to the unfortunately lost and reduced life of suffering. The person makes a concerted effort to transcend victimhood and reopen the future, sometimes developing new forms of empowerment. Teresa's ability to act decisively in response to a life-threatening diagnosis of anaplastic cancer was not only proactive but, in some moments, the opposite of her self-described pattern of shutting down feelings and bodily sensation. Perhaps, in part, her ability to distance herself from feelings and bodily sensations allowed her to accept and endure necessary surgery and treatments. It is possible that the postsurgery person manages emotions differently from the way done prior to the diagnosis. Personal agency involves overcoming disempowerment and can involve a creative determination of the future. The tension between Teresa's intense emotions and her preference to live with a cool head through logic and reason was embodied in one of her forms of agency, which forged the way by transforming her life into one that included new modes of enjoyment, exhilaration, and pride. Through reasoning and planning in a culture that affords many opportunities for self-invention and redefinition for people of her age, she created a new identity, recasting herself as an intellectual.

Part of personal agency is one's action on oneself. One may carry on internal dialogues in which self-talk both reflects on one's life and moves one's life forward. For instance, Teresa felt she had lost everything ("I had never been anything but my voice") and wished to move on "as though nothing had happened." Inner work on the self may involve coping strategies that distance a person from feelings and bodily sensations, reflecting a discourse of denial. Agency may work unreflectively, as anger Teresa may have felt in response to her diagnosis was projected onto or "voiced" by her cancer symptoms within her own life story. Important people in Teresa's life mirrored back uncomfortable emotions that she might have understandably felt herself.

Language

When we consider misfortune and the human order, language *is* the story. The "experiences" detailed above were gleaned through Teresa's written and conversational discourse, which both reflects and shapes her life with consequences to listeners, herself, and analysts. Teresa's strength and emotional stoicism came through in her speech, which claimed the independent agency described above. In staunch refusal to speak in terms of the interviewer's narrative of social support, Teresa offered a counternarrative to one that has become more or less canonical in our culture and in psychology: No person is an island—on each other we depend. Her claim of self-determination is itself embedded in both individual history and her culture. Teresa resisted the interviewer's emphasis on others, as she had opposed her father in a culture that promotes tales of self-made persons with unique individualities. A compelling American cultural narrative features coping with adversity on one's own and thriving after tragedy. Our linguistic culture and performances, at the point of trauma and recovery, turn in various, sometimes contradictory, directions of social support and rugged individuality.

Any one of us may "do resilience" through talk by enhancing ourselves and diminishing others. In such a general pattern of discourse, one articulates detailed claims to being an accomplished, in-charge agent and diminishes others by constructing them as unable to cope, rendering them peripheral to the account of "resilience." Presence and absence of detail in language bestow reality and value accordingly. Glossing over the details of other people and speaking of them as passive, as avoidant, as having adverse consequences, and as lacking in agency, effectiveness, and value may be instrumental in setting oneself apart and in fashioning a new life of action, productivity, independence, positive value, and high status. Language is instrumental in "doing self." "Doing agency" by enhancing oneself and diminishing others is one discursive strategy patterned through detailed description, lots of action, temporal extension, and great feats.

The language of "misfortune" and "resiliency" is complex, for one may not only claim but may deny agency on the part of self and construct oneself as a sufferer, with emphasis on external forces, in one's talk. Both agentic and patient positions may be patterned in discourse. Other people too—for instance, Teresa's voice teacher—could be spoken of as agents as well as patients. The instrumentality of discourse is embedded in context, for instance, in the freedom and control of writing in which Teresa articulated her extraordinarily promising rise in the opera world and her heroic battle against cancer in a race against death replete with expansive expeditions in mountain climbing and motorcycling. The talk-in-interaction of the research interview is dynamically coconstructed, less under a person's control than the written word. With her classmate, Teresa "did herself" as a psychologist. Conversation has social consequences and a history of practice. Teresa began to introduce herself to new people as a "psychology major" rather than as a singer, which she says was "odd" but "strangely refreshing." She used this new speech pattern to distance herself from her loss, to turn uncanny emotions into positive ones, and to take up new social relations and consequential activities. The interviewer praised the interviewee as "smart," "strong," and "courageous." The lack of acknowledgment of social support in the written narrative led the interviewer to proclaim admiration and sympathy as well as to question the completeness of the account. Linguistic performances are instrumental in producing specific ends and have a variety of social consequences in the particular contexts.

Language actively constructs reality and is important to understand in its instrumentality both within the research context and in everyday life. Narrative telling involves *internal* reworkings of a person's experience of self, including personal agency in overcoming adversity. Teresa's story is a tale of having lost everything that anchors the person in the world, of coming to terms with this calamity, and of making oneself a more expansive person with a set of worldly engagements that are richer than ever—a powerful, inspiring story.

Spirituality

Spirituality may reside at the heart of a person's acceptance of destruction, loss, and suffering by affording assurance of an ultimate horizon of well-being. A person's openness to transcendent meaning and value profoundly counters the destructiveness and nihilism of trauma. Connection with the transcendent may be lived via prayer, a sense of humility, thankfulness, an experience of receiving grace and/or healing, and a sense of the possibility of completion. The spiritual dimension of resilience is lived through the acceptance of suffering and fallibility through multifaceted, life-affirming intentionalities called *faith*. The person secures a renewed sense of congruence with and gratitude for life. Teresa's courage may be seen as a raw form of spirituality, which she lived even without a belief in God or involvement in communal religious rituals. Perhaps "reverse mirroring"—equanimity and peace in the face of devastating aggression, at bottom, is a spiritual mystery. This kind of faith is not abstract or ceremonious but is deeply embodied in nitty-gritty ways of taking on life as it is, engaging the worst of it, affirming the intrinsic and special value of the life one has been given, and making the most out of the precarious gift of life.

Selfhood

Selfhood is profoundly challenged and remains at issue in the experience of traumatic misfortune. The singing voice she lost was Teresa's life, her identity, her self. Existentially, the loss of voice was a death of self. The later reappearance of her voice was a rebirth of self, but in the irreversibility of time, a different voice and self. In traumatic misfortune, there is a general continuum ranging from the loss to the regaining of a valuable self. In some cases such as that of Gail, the self is temporarily disrupted, whereas in others, such as that of Teresa, there is an irreversible loss and transformation of self. Teresa lost the central anchor of her existence—of her identity and of her most important relationships—and yet she found the internal capacity to come to terms with herself and to reinvent herself, deliberately, by forming new goals and new ways of being with others in the world. It appears that facing and accepting loss are preconditions for the reconstruction of self, whether one recovers one's previous self or invents a new self.

Social relations, language, and culture are crucial in the process of self-recovery and transformation. For instance, Teresa doggedly resisted the attempts on the part of the interviewer to reframe her experience in the categories of a person reliant on social support. Teresa's ways of defining her selfhood as self-made underlie the central motif of her story. However, in the dynamic and ambiguous layering of selfhood, she also began to tell a new chapter of her story, the romantic tale of her marriage. Here, from the ashes of her mother-in-law's death, and from the poem that testified to the deep meanings of tragic death and loss, Teresa appealed to her husband and began to receive a caring response to her uncomfortable emotions and vulnerabilities. Human selfhood cannot be conceived in a final way as long as a person is alive, for it remains a work in progress, a story whose indeterminate ending cannot yet be told.

Lessons Learned: Individual Voices

Fred Wertz

First, my colleagues. It has been a pleasure and an honor to work with Kathy, Linda, Ruthellen, Rosemarie, and Emily. Their openness, courage in entering the unknown, sharp intelligence, strength in holding their positions, and excellent research will remain an inspiration to me. They taught me that scholars from different traditions can put competition and self-interest aside and, by engaging in conversation, can gain deeper mutual understanding and appreciation. Respectful boundary crossing is a good antidote to the inevitable narrowness of our specializations.

Second, the history of qualitative research. Qualitative research has had a significant place in psychology long before it had a name. The brilliant work of such researchers as Freud, James, Kohlberg, and Maslow is a veritable gold mine for the study of research methods and the development of qualitative methodology. Dedicated scholarship in this largely unexplored area has much to offer historians and methodologists of the qualitative movement as well as general psychology.

Third, the qualitative explosion that is sweeping psychology. When, as an undergraduate student in 1972, I undertook my first qualitative research project—an investigation of "the experience of time" with a single subject—my little sister, using interviews and her paintings—I was convinced that psychology could gain much from qualitative research. As I looked for educational opportunities, there were very few. Now almost 40 years later, the recent spread of qualitative research in psychology provides a rich opportunity for learning—a challenging and hopeful sign for the future.

Fourth, the exploration of trauma and resilience. There were too many surprising and illuminating findings in the research to enumerate here. In my own research, I was moved by the stark realization that trauma is an annihilation of intentionality itself, a kind of death in life. This gave me a new compassion for the victims of trauma and a new appreciation for the possibilities of post-traumatic growth, especially the integration of opposites—independence and interdependence, power and vulnerability, reason and emotion. In the synthesis of findings from the various analyses, I was fascinated by the dialectical relations of prelinguistic and linguistic processes, especially the ways in which language is involved in one's internal workings and transformations of self and in one's worldly relations with others. The general insights gained can be related to situations ranging from war and natural disasters to verbal abuse and the loss of a loved one, from injuries that verge on literal death to the passing mini-traumas of everyday life.

Fifth, the methodological insights. I learned about the unity and heterogeneity of qualitative research methods in psychology. The strong foundation of common practices across qualitative traditions was a powerful lesson for me. This project also encouraged me to respect the diverse contributions that can be made by different methods when rigorously grounded in this unitary foundation. Knowing a subject matter in different ways extends and enhances rather than undermines the truth of our knowledge. This project also reaffirmed my conviction that phenomenology can make important contributions to the basic foundation of psychological research methods as well as to the integration of knowledge from many traditions previously assumed to be mutually exclusive. Procedures articulated by phenomenology are implicit in the work of my colleagues even without their necessarily knowing it. The distinctive constituents of phenomenological method—the epochés (of science and of the natural attitude) and the procedures of intentional and eidetic analysis—provide the necessary core psychological method that ensures grounding in reality, freedom from prejudice, explication of meaning, and understanding of what psychological life is—its essential constitution. Finally, I learned how phenomenology can also be informed by and combined with methods developed in other traditions, as I will urge and guide my students to do.

Kathy Charmaz

This project has expanded my knowledge of qualitative methods and their status in psychology. I have gained much from my fellow researchers and Emily and very much appreciate having had the opportunity to work with them. Qualitative research is often transformative—for the researcher as well as the researched. In this case, our collaborative project has transformed how I view grounded theory as a distinctive method and as a method in relation to other methods.

Before embarking on this project, I viewed constructivist grounded theory as an inherently interpretive method. But this project has caused me to rethink what it means to remain close to the data and when to invoke interpretive license about the data. Grounded theory looks to the empirical world to define what is happening in the data. Yet this method also encourages making conjectures about these data and about the analytic categories we develop from them. My analysis here remains close to the data in part because the limited data restricted the iterative, comparative analysis that fosters theory construction. Nonetheless, I learned that being able to use the method might depend less on the number of cases and more on the richness of the data.

Our collaborative efforts have sharpened my awareness of what is intrinsic to grounded method and what researchers bring to their methods and the worlds they study. The bare bones of grounded theory consist of its particular strategies—coding, memo writing, constructing categories, theoretical sampling, saturating and integrating categories, and using comparative methods throughout. But how and to what extent researchers use these strategies may vary considerably. The content of inquiry and the unit of analysis also count. I had earlier viewed myself as a social psychologist who focused on individuals. Fred, Rosemarie, and Ruthellen's analyses, however, led me to conclude that they give greater emphasis to individuals than I do and that my focus on individuals extends to their situations and beyond.

During the past 3 years, I have broadened my definition of method. Grounded theory is more than its fundamental strategies. Rather method, content, and the presentation of the analysis blur. The lines are not so distinct. The substantive content of a grounded theory study informs which methods we use and how we use them. My analysis of losing and regaining a valued self suggests questions about those attributes of self that stay the same and those that change. If I were to conduct a full study, I would need to construct methods that could address these questions. Presentation of the written report matters. Like Ruthellen, I use literary devices, and many grounded theorists gravitate toward narratives. The study of a process has basic elements of narrative: a story line, characters and scenes, and direction. Literary devices are not part of grounded theory, but using them may make our written reports clearer and more accessible.

Last, our discussions and decisions about anonymity raised new questions about tensions between autonomy and paternalism in qualitative research. Our project made explicit what some ethicists and ethnographers have long understood: Anonymity and confidentiality are relative terms and cannot be guaranteed in practice. However unwittingly, researchers may offer false promises of anonymity and confidentiality. As we wrestled with ethical questions about anonymity, I felt that tacit assumptions about risk came into play. For me, our discussions belied notions of a set of ethical principles that, once identified, researchers could apply with confidence of having made the "right," that is, ethical decision. Such notions rely on unchanging and uncontested definitions of risk and imply that the subsequent ethical decisions are fixed and stable. Instead, our ethical decisions became fluid, conditional, contested, and open-ended, and may be questioned anew again. Ethics in research practice challenge textbook guidelines for conducting ethical inquiry.

Linda McMullen

I have learned a great deal from this project—much more than I could ever have anticipated at its outset. I am deeply grateful for the opportunity to have worked with all of my collaborators—Fred, Kathy, Ruthellen, Rosemarie, and Emily. I often tell my students to take advantage of opportunities that present themselves, even if (and, often, *particularly* if) they seem a bit risky and the outcomes are unknown. With this project, I, once again, have learned this lesson myself: What began as a "cold call" from Fred Wertz with an invitation to be part of a symposium on teaching qualitative research at the 2006 conference of the American Psychological Association turned into a 4-year project that has culminated in this book.

One of the most humbling lessons I have learned from this project is how little I (and perhaps other discourse analysts, with the exception of some who adopt a critical perspective) talk about the consequences of our analyses for those whose words we analyze. (One of the members of my research team recently assisted me in checking texts on discourse analysis for material on ethics. Only a very small number included a reference to ethics in the index and even fewer included more substantive coverage in the body of the text.) Because discourse analysts often work from naturally occurring sources of data (e.g., media interviews, magazine articles, blogs, message boards, archival transcripts) that are in the public domain, taking our analyses back to our participants is not a standard practice. In addition, because our analysis is not of the person(s) whose language/talk is being analyzed but rather of (often) culturally and historically relative discursive patterns and how these patterns are used to achieve particular ends, sharing one's analysis of data even with someone who participated in a research interview would not be common. Engaging in this practice in the present project has raised many questions for me: Should I inform participants in research interviews of the nature of my analytic practices? Is not informing them that our talk will be closely analyzed and that they might not feel understood by the analysis or perhaps even embarrassed by such close scrutiny of our talk a form of deception? If I choose to invite the participants to engage with the analysis, what form of engagement would I have in mind? Some critical discourse analysts (e.g., Willig, 2004) have argued that using a discursive psychology perspective to analyze accounts of personal struggles or stories of suffering generated from empathic, facilitative interviewing is not ethically justifiable because the interviewee is expecting that his or her experience will be the focus of inquiry and that his or her words will be taken at face value. While I resist the notion that certain topics or subject matter should be outside the scope of a particular methodology, I continue to think about these questions.

A lesson that has been reinforced and nuanced for me is the importance of knowing about the range of qualitative research methodologies and how they are and can be used. Although I stress to my students the importance of having the research question drive one's choice of methodology, I also tell them that they will most likely find themselves gravitating to (or developing) a methodology that suits their analytic strengths, their passions, and perhaps their political stance. I have learned, for example, that I could not do the kind of detailed descriptive work at which Fred is so gifted or the exhaustive line-by-line coding at which Kathy is so expert. I have also learned that the transformation of the researcher through qualitative work is not as important for me as it is for Rosemarie, and that, contrary to Ruthellen, I find myself thinking less and less in psychological terms. Getting up close to these methodologies and seeing how they are used with the same data has enabled me to develop a better understanding of each of them. And it is this increased awareness and appreciation that I now pass on to my students in the hope that their methodological choices will also be more informed.

Ruthellen Josselson

I am very grateful to have had the opportunity to work together with such a thoughtful and able group of colleagues from whom I have learned much. As the careful reader has no doubt gleaned, I am perhaps less interested in defining the boundaries of narrative methods than in exploring what one can do with a careful analysis of content and discursive process within a narrative account. Undoubtedly, another narrative researcher might have come up with a different set of emphases; narrative analysis is only a tool, not a procedure that guarantees particular results. In the end, the success of the work rests on the credibility and persuasiveness of the interpretive reading and on the contribution such an account may make to scholarly understanding. In other words, I am more likely to ask of a qualitative research paper, What did I learn that is interesting, that teaches me something beyond the text itself?, than to be concerned with whether the right steps were followed. The main principle of method is to document one's interpretations with reference to the text, to establish one's credibility through making the interpretive process transparent.

Although I have always thought of narrative research as employing phenomenology, grounded theory, discourse analysis, and intuition as part of our "toolbox," I have learned and now see that these methods are somewhat stricter in their pure forms. In effect, then, narrative researchers use only some of the basic principles of these other methods as ways of trying to look at narrative texts through different lenses and to do comprehensive readings in order to derive meanings.

I think that the primary scholarly implications of the analysis I have done is to raise questions about the management of intense emotions following trauma. How are emotion and rationality balanced? How are others, and others' emotions, employed in the process of coping? How does the availability of alternative identity possibilities have impact on trauma that shatters identity? The findings raise interesting questions about the use of internal representations of others in response to trauma that go far beyond the literature on resilience and social support and add richness to the understanding of what may constitute the experience of social support. These, then, become avenues for further investigation. If this were part of an actual research project, this analysis of Teresa would alert me to track these themes in the other interviews—to compare and contrast how others manage thinking versus feeling, how they enlist other people to help manage their internal states, and how they revise identity. I would also turn to the theoretical literature to see how these themes are understood in various conceptual frameworks. Narrative research is aimed at understanding processes, and Teresa's interview, or at least my analysis of it, offers some clues about some of the disintegrative and reintegrative processes that may occur following major trauma.

The experience of having Emily read our analyses was transformative for me personally in terms of my thinking about the ethics of qualitative research. Who, in the final analysis, "owns" the narrative? Working through the conundrums that arose from including Emily in our presentation helped me to understand better the issues of interpretive authority and the complexities of what we sometimes construct as "giving voice" to our participants.

Rosemarie Anderson

Because intuitive inquiry was originally developed to study transformative experiences, I was somewhat surprised to find how readily I was able to adapt the method to a topic that did not initially present itself as a topic related to transformation. During development of the method over the last dozen years, I have always considered intuitive inquiry a minority, qualitative method that is useful for topics that *required* intuitive insights to study them fully (Braud & Anderson, 1998). Topics of individual, social, and communal transformation often fall into this category. However, now I am beginning to think that intuitive inquiry and its procedures have broader application in psychological research. Therefore, I would like to make the following recommendations:

1. Integrate procedures within intuitive inquiry into other research approaches, qualitative or quantitative, that help you to integrate intuitive ways of knowing in the research design. Of course, researchers have always plumbed the depths of their intuitive insights in the conduct of research. However, intuitive inquiry offers unique procedures that specifically invite and discern intuitive insights in a rigorous manner. For researchers ordinarily not intuitive by nature, intuitive inquiry also provides a plan, that is, a hermeneutical structure with which to document and discern intuitive ways of knowing. For researchers who are more artistic by nature, intuitive inquiry also gives a means to integrate artistic and imaginal ways of knowing with scholarly and scientific discovery.

2. Use the analytic procedures of a preferred method as the descriptive analysis required by intuitive inquiry in Cycle 3. In this way, researchers would use the hermeneutic framework of intuitive inquiry and still retain the intellectual integrity of other qualitative and quantitative approaches. Because intuitive inquiry offers a postmodern perspective, final interpretation of the

findings in Cycles 4 and 5 may follow either a postmodern or more conventional perspective, as desired and appropriate to the audience receiving the scientific report.

3. Continue to employ intuitive inquiry as a "stand-alone" method to study those topics that by their nature require intuitive insights in order to study them well. Aside from topics within transpersonal and humanistic psychology, topics related to Jungian psychology, imaginal psychology, art, and art therapy are particularly aligned with intuitive inquiry.

In conclusion, many of us tend to think that science is the discovery of the principles for how the objective world "out there" works. Instead, intuitive inquiry avers a world reality that we create through new insights and understandings, which ever change. What I have discovered in this project is that my four qualitative research colleagues share this view, to various degrees, while nonetheless using different terms and metaphors. Therefore, I conclude this project feeling less lonely as a researcher. Mainstream psychological research—or at least qualitative research—has certainly changed since I was actively involved some years ago, and that knowledge comes as a welcome relief. Contemporary psychological researchers may be in a situation analogous to scholars and artists in the European Middle Ages who "saw" the world and "mapped" their cities from a flat-world perspective, which at least had the advantage of experiencing time and space as dynamic properties of the natural world and human perception. The Enlightenment and science have moved us into a more chronological, linear, and spatial depth perspective. Yet, the medieval dimensional perspective is valuable from another vantage point. Perhaps psychologists are now willing to imagine the world with dynamic realities, a world that we create and amplify through our hard-wrought research findings and theories.

Take-Home Messages

Here we list what we feel are the important general findings that have come to light along our journey. These conclusions, however, are only a beginning, rather than the end, of a journey. Each begs for further exploration.

1. Although psychology is a latecomer as a discipline to formally embrace qualitative research methods, it has a long and significant, though still largely unrecognized, tradition of practicing qualitative research. These pioneering works have much to offer contemporary methodologies.

2. There is a strong common foundation for qualitative research analyses in psychology, despite philosophical, theoretical, and specific procedural and methodological differences.

3. Qualitative research, given its unique goals and methods, makes several important contributions to the production of knowledge in the study of lived experience.

a. Ethical procedures and practices cannot be established, once and for all, prior to conducting qualitative research. Qualitative research requires not only the application of principles and standards of conduct but also the crafting of ethically‛ sensitive and *ongoing* relationships that extend from researchers to participants and beyond, to the participants' families and communities, as well as the scientific audiences and consumers of research. Researchers are responsible for taking leadership roles in a continual process of collaborative reevaluation and revision of research projects with various stakeholders.

b. Validity, or what many qualitative researchers prefer to call "credibility" or "trustworthiness," is established at each phase of research. It involves an infusion of science with what is outside science—human life as lived, as well as a conversation among multiple, mutually critical perspectives from different subjectivities, and between psychologists and nonscientists (including participants). In these relationships, no one set of interests and values is exclusively privileged.

c. Data that are qualitatively analyzed from various vantage points, multiple times, and using multiple methods can yield complementary findings that enhance science. Critical, dialogical pluralism is a generative principle implying that different goals, theoretical backgrounds, methodological traditions, and individual researcher sensibilities are to be encouraged and invited in human science. From this it follows that qualitative meta-analysis is a viable and valuable praxis that requires expert knowledge of multiple traditions and historically extended investigations.

4. In contrast to the traditional received methodological hierarchy, on one hand, and an unprincipled relativism, on the other, a well-grounded, evidence-based science utilizing multiple approaches is possible and desirable. Different approaches can relate to each other not as strangers or rivals but as respectful friends, even family members, unified by our common interests in the subject matter and the demands it makes on our study. In adopting and exploring this communal paradigm, we have recognized our shared foundations and celebrated the uniqueness of each approach. Our answer to the challenges of methodological pluralism, to the fractious proliferation of methods in psychology, is not a struggle for dominance, which will only lead to a science dispersed in separate silos, but a unity of mutual respect and enrichment in striving for more complex understandings.

5. Although qualitative research has a capability to be faithful to the human order, there nevertheless remains a tension between the inevitably

limited and objectifying nature of knowledge and the lives of nonscientists. Although researchers have special expertise that inevitably places them in a position of power and knowledge, scientists' ethical obligations are primary in their vocation. Psychological researchers are accountable to nonpsychologists and nonscientists, regardless of their level of understanding of psychology and the commonality or divergence of their interests. The human sciences are enhanced by a dialogue with those whom they serve.

6. The qualitative research movement is shifting the disciplinary identity of psychology and its interdisciplinary relations. Historically, by identifying itself as primarily a natural science, psychology has had limited contact and interchange with such sister disciplines as cultural anthropology, history, sociology, economics, political science, literary studies, fine arts, theology, and philosophy. Qualitative researchers in psychology, from its early years as an independent discipline through the present, have understood and conducted psychology as a uniquely *human* science closely allied with the arts, humanities, other cultural sciences, and with service professions such as education, health, and social work. Qualitative psychologists and scholars from these disciplines have learned much from each other about research methodology and about their common human subject matter. One of the most exciting, challenging, and promising dimensions of the qualitative research movement is its interdisciplinarity.

The approaches to qualitative research that we have explored in this project are by no means homogeneous. Although each tradition is distinct, all share common roots, have historically informed each other, and continue to draw on each others' offerings. Phenomenology, the oldest tradition, forged inroads into hermeneutics, emancipatory practice, critical thought, narrative, and other traditions that took on lives of their own and challenged traditional assumptions. Constructivist grounded theory, narrative psychology, and intuitive inquiry draw on phenomenology and have carved out distinct contributions of their own. The linguistic turn in the social sciences has engendered such powerful new approaches to psychology as discourse analysis. Narrative researchers may use the strategies of discourse analysts, who in turn use the concept of narrative, to develop original ways of understanding and telling the human story. Hermeneutic traditions are integrally important in narrative and intuitive inquiry, both of which delve into the depth and height dimensions of human life. Intuitive inquiry can integrate virtually all the other traditions and yet gives them, within its context, a distinctly transformative and visionary character. These analytic traditions and practices, even in their differences, are by no means mutually exclusive. It is to be expected that, just as qualitative researchers have developed through exchange with each other, with mainstream psychology, and with other social sciences, humanities, and artistic disciplines, they will continue their generative conversation and cross-fertilization in the future.

References

Allport, G. W. (1942). *The use of personal documents in psychological science* (prepared for the Committee on the Appraisal of Research, Bulletin #49). New York: Social Science Council.

American Psychological Association. (2002). APA ethical principles of psychologists and code of conduct. Retrieved January 10, 2010, from *APA.org.*

Braud, W., & Anderson, R. (1998). *Transpersonal research methods for the social sciences: Honoring human experience.* Thousand Oaks, CA: Sage.

Churchill, S. D., Lowery, J. E., McNally, O., & Rao, A. (1998). The question of reliability in interpretive psychological research: A comparison of three phenomenologically based protocol analyses. In R. Valle (Ed.), *Phenomenological inquiry in psychology: Existential and transpersonal dimensions* (pp. 63–85). New York: Plenum Press.

Dilthey, W. (1977). Ideas concerning a descriptive and analytical psychology (1894). In *Descriptive psychology and historical understanding* (R. M. Zaner & K. L. Heiges, Trans.). The Hague: Martinus Nijhoff.

Freud, S. (1965). *The interpretation of dreams.* New York: Basic Books. (Original work published 1900)

Gergen, K. J. (1992). Social construction and moral action. In D. N. Robinson (Ed.), *Social discourse and moral judgment* (pp. 9–27). London: Academic Press.

Giorgi, A. (2009). *The descriptive phenomenological method in psychology: A modified Husserlian approach.* Pittsburgh, PA: Duquesne University Press.

Glaser, B. G., & Strauss, A. L. (1967). *The discovery of grounded theory.* Chicago: Aldine.

Husserl, E. (1977). *Phenomenological psychology: Lectures, summer semester, 1925* (J. Scanlon, Trans.). Boston: Martinus Nijhoff. (Original work published 1962)

Josselson, R. (2007). The ethical attitude in narrative research: Principles and practicalities. In J. Clandinnin (Ed.), *The handbook of narrative inquiry* (pp. 537–567). Thousand Oaks, CA: Sage.

Kahneman, D. (2003). Experiences of collaborative research. *American Psychologist, 58*(9), 723–730.

Kvale, S., & Brinkmann, S. (2009). *InterViews: Learning the craft of qualitative research interviewing* (2nd ed.). Thousand Oaks, CA: Sage.

Wertz, F. J. (1986). The question of reliability in psychological research. *Journal of Phenomenological Psychology, 17*(2), 181–205.

Wertz, F. J. (1999). Multiple methods in psychology: Epistemological grounding and the possibility of unity. *Journal of Theoretical and Philosophical Psychology, 19*(2), 131–166.

Willig, C. (2004). Discourse analysis and health psychology. In M. Murray (Ed.), *Critical health psychology* (pp. 155–169). London: Palgrave Macmillan.

Gail's Texts

B elow is the second data set used in comparative analyses by three researchers—Fred Wertz (Chapter 5), Kathy Charmaz (Chapter 6), and Rosemarie Anderson (Chapter 9). These data arose from the same context as the Teresa texts in Chapter 4—a graduate class on qualitative methods—and parallel them, including both a written description of "misfortune" and a follow-up interview. Although the researchers did not have this demographic information when they conducted their analyses, the participant we call "Gail" subsequently reported, for our readers' information, that she was 24 years old at the time of her participation and that her mother, who was born in the United States, traces her roots to Europe (England, Scotland-Ireland, France, Germany, and Wales). Her father was born and raised in Africa (Tanzania) and is Indian by ethnicity. The interviewer was a female student in an applied developmental psychology doctoral program. This appendix offers readers the opportunity to consider the researchers' analyses in light of the raw data on which they were based. Also, given that none of the five researchers analyzed these texts in full detail, this appendix gives readers the opportunity to apply each and all of the five analytic approaches to this data in their own ways. Such original analyses of this data can be compared with the limited analyses of these texts offered by those researchers who used them and also with the analyses of the Teresa texts.

Written Description

Instructions: *Describe in writing a situation when something **very** unfortunate happened to you. Please begin your description prior to the unfortunate event. Share in detail what happened, what you felt and did, and what happened after, including how you responded and what came of this event in your life.*

Written Protocol

It was my junior year at XXXXX University. It was December 2001, and I was at gymnastics practice. I was in the best physical shape of my life at the time. We were having a "mock meet" because the competition season was on its way. Half of us began to warm up on the uneven bars. I felt confident and secure. Bars was my best event. I had a good feeling about this day. I felt good about my routine and knew this was my year to shine. It was tough in the years past; I had to constantly prove myself to my coaches, by showing them that I could compete well under pressure, and that they could count on me to do well in a big competition. But this was the year where things would change. My training was leading me up to a better and better standing with my coaches and myself. My confidence improved by each practice.

It was a Tuesday. Or was it a Thursday? It's almost time for us to begin competing, but we get a brief warm-up period beforehand. I get on the bar for my third warm-up turn. I successfully complete the difficult release move combination in the beginning half of my bar routine. "Great!" I think. This is going smoothly. Just as I expected. I continue my transition from the high bar to the low bar, and now my signature move right up to the high bar again. This was the tricky part in my routine because it was a new sequence, but it was all the more exciting because it was *my* own sequence, and I was ready to signature it in competitions. As I come up from the low bar to the high bar I feel suspended in the air for what felt like a second or two. "Great!" I think again. I'm high enough this time to get enough momentum to continue the rest of my routine.

All of a sudden, with the blink of an eye, I feel my body coming down quickly . . . instantly . . . toward the ground. I'm going fast. I'm almost head first, going like a torpedo on to the mat underneath the bar. Somehow I managed to miss the bar. I was so high, but too far away from the high bar to catch it. I'm coming down fast. Even though it was so fast, I felt that moment take forever. All of a sudden I hear a crack. Or was it a tear? It sounded like the Velcro that holds the mats together ripping apart. I almost turned to see what it was. Wait. Something feels funny. Wait. Something doesn't feel right. I was on the floor kneeling down underneath the high bar. I feel my right elbow with my left hand. Something feels very, very wrong. There was no elbow anymore, my arm was contorted. I couldn't feel that bony part of my arm. It was bent the wrong way. I panicked. *That Velcro sound was from my elbow?* I'm holding my arm, feeling the new bend created by the fall to the floor. Then it hits me. Look at what happened to me, in a split second. I thought about my competitive season . . . going down the drain. I thought about sitting out all those meets . . . again. I thought about the doctor. I thought about surgery. I panicked more when I thought about surgery. I remember the shock. When I felt my elbow, I said "Oh my God! Oh my God!" in panic and disbelief that something so intense could happen in a split second. Then, as it all started to sink in and the panic came over me, I kept saying, "No!! No!! No!!", first in denial and passionately, then through sobs and a feeling of defeat and frustration. I remember that at first I didn't cry. Then, I realized that it hurt. Of course it did. Look at what I did to my elbow. It was backwards, my forearm was facing outwards. This has GOT to hurt, I thought. That probably made it hurt more.

Kristen, my teammate, comes over first. Then Ben, my assistant coach. I remember asking how this could have happened, and I remember Kristen's "Oh my God!" when she saw my arm. I don't remember who came over next, but I know the athletic trainer, Kathy, was there because she was asking me important questions like if I could move and feel my finger tips. There was so much chaos I didn't even know how to answer these questions. I was praying that I would be able to do this. Somehow my fingers started moving, and I'm pretty sure I was able to feel them. I wondered if being able to feel and move my fingers meant that I didn't need to have surgery. Things got a little foggy after that because it felt like the entire team was crowded around me and everyone had something to say. In my head I was still slowly coming to terms with what had happened. Something really wrong happened to my right elbow! Kathy started to wrap my arm. The pain got more intense as I watched her wrap my contorted arm with ace bandage onto a foam board. How was I even going to hold this arm up? Then things started to get dark; all I wanted to do was close my eyes. I got very dizzy, and I couldn't answer any questions any more. I remember my teammates trying to help get me up. It must have taken three girls to stand me up because at that point, I felt like I had lost all strength. It took me a while to get my bare foot into a sandal. My foot kept slipping out of it because I had no strength or intention to place it in the sandal and keep it in. I was finally on my feet as someone draped a zipper-up sweatshirt around my shoulders. I walked outside into the snow with my leotard, shorts, sandals, a zipper-up sweatshirt, and my carefully wrapped-up arm into the car to go to the sports doctor.

Ben took me in his car. I was happy it was him because through all the chaos, somehow it felt like he was there listening to me and really feeling for me. The next thing that really stands out in my mind is the doctor taking a look at my swollen arm. I didn't look, but I felt him move my arm around a few times and somehow it came back into place. It's funny that I can't remember if that process hurt. I'm sure it did. I was actually impressed with how easily he put my arm back in place, considering he had a reputation for being a pretty lousy doctor. I was put in a cast and told that I dislocated my elbow (pretty obvious!) and chipped a piece of a bone in the process. The cast would heal the bone chip, and the good news was that I would be casted for only 3 weeks. When I got home that evening, although I was glad I had missed an exam scheduled for that evening, I felt like my life lost some of its purpose. I felt handicapped and I really felt the physical pain. I received a lot of attention that night from my roommates, and from my teammates who came to visit. It was nice that a lot of the girls came over, but I felt really horrible. I was upset, I was disappointed, and I was still a little shocked. I finally cried that night in bed when I was by myself. I cried because I was really, really down. The worst physical pain and discomfort came when I awoke the next morning to find my right hand had severely swelled up overnight. I somehow dragged myself to class even though I was unable to take notes.

In the days following the injury, my mind vacillated between the positive and negative outlook of the situation. On the one hand, it was just a bone chip and dislocation. I did not have to get surgery, and after 3 weeks, rehabilitation could start because my cast would come off. The coaches were optimistic that I'd be able to condition myself back to shape in a few months and still be able to compete this season. Their hope kept my hopes up, because it seemed as though they hadn't given up on me yet. On the other hand, I had been in such great shape before the injury. This was supposed to be my year. And there I was . . . handicapped. These thoughts kept running through my head.

The rehabilitation stage was longer than I thought it would take. Once I got my cast removed, I had this vision that I'd be able to start working out again. I wanted to lift weights right away to get my strength back, I wanted to start doing balance beam to maintain my tricks while minimizing tricks done using my arm. I knew it would take a while to get back on the uneven bars, but there *had* to be something I could do. I thought it would be a matter of weeks before I was back to competing. I did not want to sit on the sidelines and watch the girls practice day after day. I needed a purpose. I was in for a reality check when I happily came into the gym with my little uncasted bare arm (which I couldn't really move). I wasn't completely healed yet. The bone still had to form, but I got the cast removed to begin gaining back range of motion in my arm. This was a set-back I wasn't prepared for. I spent the next month and a half impatiently getting movement back in my arm, doing simple conditioning exercises without weights, and eventually getting back on the beam to do simple leaps and jumps. At this point, competition season had started without me. I was determined to get back as fast as I could, but it was as if my body wasn't prepared to.

It took another two doctor visits until I was cleared to put pressure on my right arm. By this time, it was halfway through the competitive season. I had my work cut out for me. I was *so* focused at this time. I was determined to make the fastest comeback ever. As I refined my skills on the balance beam, I began to put pressure on the existing beam lineup. At the same time, I began to get my floor routine back in action. The team needed me most on vault, and I was determined to step in. My proudest moment was returning to the beam lineup in early March at Michigan State. Although I didn't turn in my best performance at my first meet back, my teammates and coaches congratulated me one by one upon my finish.

The next week at Cornell, I did the best beam routine of my life. By the end of the season I had competed floor exercise, the vault, and the balance beam to help my team in our conference championship. During these few meets, I truly enjoyed every moment of competition. Even though I had been competitive for 13 years, never did my performance feel so significant. Upon completion of the season, I received the most amounts of votes from my teammates and coaches to be elected team captain for the following year. It seemed as though my hard work and motivation had not just gotten me back on the apparatus.

The following competitive year was my best to date. My strongest event was the uneven bars, which was the event where my injury occurred just a year before. I proved to be a very consistent and reliable competitor on the event, scoring marks as high as 9.825 out of a perfect 10.0. This was the year I realized that I had fully redeemed myself. What had once been my weakness now became my legacy. Three years later, I continue to strive for excellence on the uneven bars, as my focus carries me closer to my dreams of athletic success than ever before.

Introduction to the Interview

The purpose of the interview was to look at the role of personal agency and social support in dealing with a traumatic or very unfortunate event. The written protocol was used as a guide in developing the interview questions. The interview was conducted face to face and tape recorded to ensure accuracy of its transcription. One of the primary goals was to examine how and when each type of support was manifested in the participant's experience of the event. Initially, the interviewer tries to determine the participant's definition of an unfortunate event. Throughout the interview the focus is on understanding the participant's intrinsic motivation as well as her definition of support and how they were instrumental in dealing with or overcoming the unfortunate event. The participant was able to elaborate on her experience of the event in regards to its effect on her and how internal and external motivation aided in her recovery. Furthermore, the interview elaborated on thematic elements of the participant's experience that appeared in the written protocol. In addition to describing internal and relational support, the interview discusses the themes of disbelief or shock, shame, having a sense of personal responsibility, control or lack thereof, disability, fear, process of recovery, and resiliency. The participant's willingness and ability to thoroughly describe her experience in the written protocol and during the interview tremendously aided in the fluency of the interview process. In retrospect, the interviewer may have asked less structured questions to acquire more experiential data.

Interview Transcript

INTERVIEWER: We are looking at the role of personal agency and social relations or support in dealing with trauma, the how and the when. So my first question for you is, why did you choose to describe this event?

PARTICIPANT: When I think of unfortunate circumstance, I think of something obviously negative, something kind of instantaneous, something unplanned, something that went very much against what I wanted. I was so much headed in one direction—then all of sudden this huge, huge upset that happened with the blink of an eye. It happened so quickly. There are different things like I didn't get accepted into this one grad school. Do I want to talk about that? This felt like it was more, more instant. I thought it would be more rich if I was able to talk about everything that happened; the exact specifics of the whole incident.

INTERVIEWER: You said that you wanted to make this year better than previous years. Can you talk a little bit more about that?

PARTICIPANT: It was very frustrating being part of a Division One team. When they recruit you, obviously they want you to be on the team so they talk you up . . . oh, you can help us here, you can help us there, you are going to be a key player . . . and then you get there freshman year and you don't really do as much; sort of a bench warmer. I didn't expect that to happen just because in gymnastics, sort of the younger you are, kinda the better you are physically. So why would you be benched your first year? So I guess my mind was then so in the realm of, I am going to be so good for the team, I am going to score high, and I am going to really be out there. It was disappointing after my freshman year because I wasn't out there as much as I wanted to be. I got a little taste . . . but it wasn't enough for me. I felt like I needed to be in there more. I still needed to compete more. It was very, very competitive. It was this competition between the team almost to make it to the lineup. If you didn't make it to the top six, then you couldn't compete. To answer your question . . . I hadn't done as well . . . competitively and I hadn't impressed my coaches enough for them to have enough faith in me. I still had to prove myself. I needed to be in there more.

INTERVIEWER: You were away at college so . . . after the accident, was your family involved?

PARTICIPANT: Actually, not so much because of the physical distance. When I got home I called my mom, and I didn't really want to do that because, you know . . . "Hi, Mom, guess what? I broke my arm." How do you say it lightly? She knew how much this sport was a part of my life. She knew how much this meant to me, and to report this to her, I didn't want her to be disappointed in me, not in me. I didn't want her to be disappointed for me. I didn't want her to worry. I didn't want her to get upset. I was upset too. I tried to hold the tears back. If she heard me cry, that would be really bad too. I told my sister too. She really felt for me too. She had also been a competitive gymnast for many years so she was able to really relate . . . almost like a teammate and also a sister. I don't really remember that much more of my family being involved . . . because it was a lot of, how am I going to get back? I was always thinking in the future . . . so I have a cast on my arm . . . let's just move on. It was right before Christmas and I remember sitting at the Christmas dinner table with my mom's side of the family, and I actually covered my arm the entire time. It was kind of foolish to hide it from my family, but at the same time I guess I must have been so ashamed . . . I didn't want people to feel bad for me. I didn't want people to ask what happened . . . It's not so much that it was traumatic, it was just depressing. I just didn't want to come to terms that it happened.

INTERVIEWER: Did they [her family members] have any involvement in the recovery process?

PARTICIPANT: My athletic trainer had probably the strongest role in my recovery process—she was there everyday in the gym. My mom and the rest of my family were not really around so much. I guess I didn't really need so much emotional support and psychological support from my family because I guess in some way I would say that my mind was very strong. Of course, I was upset . . . but at the same time I knew that my career wasn't over. It wasn't like, what am I going to do? It was, just how do I *move on*? I don't think I needed so much from my family, but I do remember my mom did come up. She took me around to do some food shopping and helped me to do some different things. I felt a little helpless at that point. So, I would say they were kind of in the background. I think my mom was able to tell that I was so focused that I didn't even need her in some respects. Of course, I needed her, but she almost took like a passive view to it. She didn't make me do the dishes . . . so that was good.

INTERVIEWER: I was going to ask you about how you dealt with disclosure . . . you talked about how you were hiding your arm.

PARTICIPANT: I do have another thing to say about that. My gymnastics coach at home. He is sort of like a father, a mentor. I am very, very close to him. He is from, like, my home gym. Telling him I broke my arm—he was completely shocked. He was mad at the situation. He was mad because he was my coach for so many years. He sent me off to college and then this happens to me. It hurt me to tell him because I didn't want to let him down. He was like my gymnastics God. It was kind of painful telling him because I didn't want to show my emotional side.

INTERVIEWER: So would you say it was more difficult to tell him or your family?

PARTICIPANT: Um, I would say it was the same. Then there is Dad. My dad is like the protective person so I wanted to show him it's okay . . . Here I am, this happened, but I am okay, trust me. Your little girl is okay. I didn't want him to be worried. You know, it's that whole—you don't want your parents to do any extra worrying for you. Between my coach and my parents it was just different because my coach was more frustrated with the situation and my mom was more protective.

INTERVIEWER: You said that you felt "handicapped." Can you describe what that means to you and how long you felt that way?

PARTICIPANT: I went to class the next day, and I couldn't write. I was frustrated because it hurt to write, and it took me a long time to write. So that was sort of a handicap, something so simple. I couldn't wash my face. I couldn't do my hair. Little things the day before that were just nothing . . . I wasn't able to do. My mind was so focused in getting better and what would happen afterwards. I wanted to just get rid of the pain. I was just very frustrated that the cast was there. The cast was a very visual thing. I was covering it. I didn't want people to see it. I didn't want people to see that I was handicapped. If I covered it, I was eventually able to straighten my arm a little bit more in the cast—which I don't think people should really do—then it was invisible. I'm okay. There were things I couldn't do, little taking-care-of-myself things that frustrated me.

INTERVIEWER: How long would you say you felt that way?

PARTICIPANT: Definitely throughout my cast being on. It reminded me everyday. So at least for 3 weeks. After that probably still on and off for another couple of months.

INTERVIEWER: You said you had to "drag" yourself to class. What do you think pushed you?

PARTICIPANT: When I say *drag*, I mean I literally had to drag myself out of bed. I was the type who always had to go to class. I didn't like the idea of being behind. I was like that since elementary school. I was in an immense amount of pain. I could not do the normal things . . . but I still had to get to class. If I sat in bed, I felt like I was feeling sorry for myself. I felt like it would give me a chance to kind of accept this instead. I literally had to push myself so much . . . push my body against my will in a way.

INTERVIEWER: It sounds like you got support from your teammates, your roommates, and your coaches. Tell me about your support in terms of each of these components.

PARTICIPANT: My teammates were able to relate a lot. My closer teammates . . . knew what I wanted, my goals, my frustrations, everything. They could tell that I wanted it so badly. They could really empathize with me and really push me to go further. So they were really, really helpful in that mostly because they could see where I was. My coaches . . . were very supportive. One of the coaches said "She's going to be back." That was so motivating. I did feel like they did support me. My roommates . . . took me out. We did tons of different things. They got me distracted and got my mind off feeling bad for myself. They were helpful with cooking for me and bringing food home for me. They were very motherly . . . nurturing. So, I think every group of people had their own role.

INTERVIEWER: How did you feel about the length of the recovery process?

PARTICIPANT: I thought after the cast would come off, I would be much more in control. I had this vision that I would start real slow. Of course, I was afraid too, but at least I would be in control of my recovery process. But they told me I couldn't lift weights. It was very frustrating because every time I would go to the doctor he would tell me . . . come back again in a month. I felt like the doctors were holding me back. I'd get my hopes up, and then I'd go to the doctor and—setback again. Looking back now I am really glad I didn't rush back into it. It was too long for me. In terms of any injury process it was actually very short—very, very short—but since my mind was so focused on *this is where I should be*, when I kept getting setbacks, it was so frustrating.

INTERVIEWER: You talked about the doctors holding you back. Do you feel like your body was holding you back also?

PARTICIPANT: It was definitely—[it] wasn't just the doctors holding me back. That is such a wrong thing to say. It was my X-rays holding me back. It was my physical bone, I guess. My bone wasn't growing so fast. It was about halfway fused when the cast came off. It took longer than I expected for my bone to actually heal. So it was easy for me to blame it on the doctors. It was almost like, don't you know how determined I am? If my brain could heal my arm, it would. It's like, don't you have more faith in me? You're looking at this X-ray, but what does that say? I had this kind of attitude.

INTERVIEWER: You talked about being "so focused" after being "cleared" by the doctor. Can you describe that?

PARTICIPANT: I remember being so eager. I had been focused for what felt like a very long time before that, so I felt like I was more than ready to go, especially since I said I was held back. When I was cleared, I was ready to go. I do believe, looking back, that I did push it a little too much. I remember I was careful for my arm, but my legs would be so sore after a certain point.

INTERVIEWER: It sounded like you got all that support before you were cleared. During your training, were you getting support outside of yourself?

PARTICIPANT: I don't know if the support was as much when I started doing things, maybe because I put on this sort of attitude that I was okay. I so wanted to be okay and not handicapped anymore that maybe I made it seem like I didn't need any help in a way. What I remember the most is the support when I was clearly handicapped. I got the most support from my closest teammate. She was really there throughout. I am surprised I haven't mentioned her yet. When I was cleared, it was probably less support because I probably didn't need it as much.

INTERVIEWER: The support you did get was in what way?

PARTICIPANT: She was training with me, but we would have talks about it. She would encourage me to get things back. She knew how much I wanted it, so she would kind of push me more. Not too much but she would be like "this is what you have to do tomorrow . . . this is where the team needs you, look at how far you have come." If I'd get frustrated, then she would kind of give me perspective.

INTERVIEWER: After your recovery, you said your performances felt "so significant," and I think you even said you enjoyed it more. Can you describe that?

PARTICIPANT: My first competition back I went on the balance beam. That was one of my weakest events, but it soon became my strongest event. That was the only one I could do for a while. I managed to do a whole beam routine without using my arms at all. My first meet back I looked at the sport differently. At that point I really appreciated the sport. I was just happy that I was on the event. I felt part of the team. I never felt like much a part of the team. I felt a lot of support that day . . . when I competed. Everyone had something to say. It was very, very moving. The next year following . . . when I did get back on the bars, there was definite fear going on at some points, but I felt very much [that] I appreciated the sport and it was significant to me.

INTERVIEWER: You say that you felt "fully redeemed." Tell me what you mean by that.

PARTICIPANT: This was by the time senior year came and I think that the fact that uneven bars was my main event—bars was always my best event beforehand—and the fact that I had gotten it back, and that was my main event, that was the event I competed in every meet, that was my best season on that event. . . . It wasn't just, great, I am getting good scores, or great, I am contributing. It wasn't just that kind of thing, but it was, wow, look at how far I came! Last year this was the last event I could do. Obviously I fell from that event. I hurt my arm so I couldn't swing. So I think fully redeeming myself was to get my bar team back, and that's what I had done. The three other events I was able to get back the year before but bars, there was just no way. The next year the whole thing turned around. Bars was the event for me. That's why I felt like I fully redeemed myself.

INTERVIEWER: Is there anything else you wanted to tell me about the experience?

PARTICIPANT: I realized that I never talked about fear. It took me a long time to get back on the bars. When I finally got on, I would just swing. I knew that would take me a while but I was afraid because in one of the tricks I do, I would contort my arm around like this, very unnatural to the body. It was my right arm too. A couple days after what happened, I was watching a teammate do that same transition from the high bar to the low bar, and she pretty much fell the same way I did. I just balled. I was so afraid. It just all came back, do you know what I mean? I was afraid for her. For me, it all came back. In terms of that trick, I felt my arm hyperextend . . . so quick . . . and I got so worried. I definitely had some experiences where I was set back a little bit, where I was afraid. This isn't the easiest thing in the world. That was the thing I didn't mention.

Author Index

Subject Index

f following a page number indicates a figure; *n* following a page number indicates a note; *t* following a page number indicates a table.

Abductive reasoning, 166–167, 296, 381, 383, 384*t*
   analytic methods and, 92
   compared to theoretical agnosticism, 166–167
Action research, 4, 207, 292, 297–298, 328, 334, 359
Agency, 95, 133, 143, 149, 157, 210–213, 216, 230, 238–239, 283, 284–285, 300, 305, 308, 310, 313, 319, 320, 388–390, 407, 408
Aim of research, 50–51, 89, 150, 359, 364, 368, 375
Allport, Gordon, 42–45
Analytic methods, 91–92. *see also* Data analysis
Anderson, Rosemarie, 66–69, 289–291, 303–304, 312–314, 320–329, 397–398
Anonymity
   ethical issues and, 356–358
   norms in our culture and, 5–6
   participant involvement and, 8
   participant's experience of the analyses and, 337–341
Anthropology, 11, 63, 64, 92, 400
Archival data, 18, 23, 26, 34, 89, 90, 93, 249, 252, 395
Art, 16, 18, 24, 34, 67, 90, 99, 110, 117, 130, 160, 184, 251, 253, 289, 398
   data collection and, 90
Assumptions, 2, 51, 54, 57, 59, 79, 80, 81, 83, 168, 251, 265, 271, 286, 292, 305, 308, 311, 319, 363, 379, 400

Attitude, researcher's, 22, 23, 28, 95, 125, 130, 132, 135, 136, 279, 307, 317, 369, 370, 373, 325

B

Bartlett, Frederic, 17
Benet, Alfred, 17
Best practices, 10, 24, 50, 86–87, 88
Bodily sensations, 258–259, 261, 263–265, 312–314, 327–328, 387–389
Body
   awareness, 257
   discourse and the, 326
   illness and the, 136, 141–142, 153–154, 182–183, 185–186, 188, 190, 192, 197, 200, 258–261, 265, 300, 328, 370, 386–387, 282
   injured, 371, 404, 406, 410–413
   intuition and the, 247, 257–259, 312–313
   lived experience and the, 257, 320
   mind–body relations, 128
   music making and the, 111, 141, 177, 182, 259–260, 291, 386
   objectified, 192, 320
   of the other, 187
   phenomenology and the, 128, 282, 290, 307
   qualitative research and the, 376, 380, 386
   self and, 178, 182, 185, 196–197, 200
   size, 245
Body Intelligence Scale, 257, 273

N

Narrative research
  discourse analysis and, 310–312, 319–320
  grounded theory and, 301–303, 318–319
  intuitive inquiry and, 320–321, 326–327
  Jerome Bruner, Ted Sarbin, and Donald
    Polkinghorne and, 63–66, 70–71
  narrative analysis and, 228
  overview, 4, 21, 63–66, 224–228, 238–240,
    314–321, 381, 384t, 400
  participant's experience of the analyses
    and, 345–346
  phenomenological psychology and,
    285–289, 317–318
  philosophical differences from other
    specializations and, 381
  Teresa's texts, 228–240
Neopositivism, 82, 84, 134, 381
Nobel Prize, 1, 17
Nonverbal expression/experience, 89, 285,
    286, 363, 382
Normal science, 76–78, 79
Norms, 5–6, 10, 16, 25, 43–44, 87, 207, 217,
    366, 368, 375

O

Ontology, 80–81, 95, 129, 381
Open reading step, 131–132, 283, 330, 369
Organization of the qualitative research
    project, 87–94
Organizations, professional, 77–78
Ownership of the data, 10, 334, 353, 355–356

P

Paradigmatic knowing, 65
Parapsychological experiences, 247
Participants, 50–51, 89–91. see also Gail's
    texts; Participant's experience of the
    analyses; Teresa's texts
Participant's experience of the analyses.
    see also Involvement of the research
    participant
  discourse analysis and, 346–348
  grounded theory and, 344–345
  intuitive inquiry and, 342–344
  narrative research and, 345–346
  overview, 331, 334–352, 364–365
  phenomenological psychology and,
    348–350

Participatory research, 4, 84, 85, 328, 359
Partnerships, 8–9, 84, 88, 297, 358, 361
Personality, 29–36
Phenomenological movement, 128–130
Phenomenological psychology
  Amedeo Giorgi and, 52–56, 70
  analytic methods and, 91–92
  bracketing, 125–126, 282, 288, 293
  discourse analysis and, 283–285, 305–308
  emergent ideation and, 371
  general psychology of trauma and
    resilience and, 150–156
  grounded theory and, 280–282, 293–297
  intentional and eidetic analysis, 70, 126–128
  intuitive inquiry and, 289–291, 322–323
  journals, 76
  lifeworld descriptions and, 131–136
  narrative research and, 285–289, 317–318
  overview, 4, 124–128, 129–130, 280–291,
    380, 384t, 400
  participant's experience of the analyses
    and, 348–350
  philosophical differences from other
    specializations and, 381
  reductions, 125, 127, 384
  Teresa's texts, 136–156
Phenomenological reduction, 125–126, 127,
    384
Phenomenology, 4, 52–53, 55, 71–72, 76, 78,
    82, 91, 124–127, 129–131, 133, 135, 225,
    281, 283, 285, 286, 288–290, 292–297,
    305–306, 314, 317, 333, 376, 378,
    380–383, 393, 396, 400
Philosophy, 52, 54, 66, 68, 79–81, 82–84, 95,
    124, 128–130, 283, 292, 379, 383
Photography, 90
Piaget, Jean, 17
Pluralism, 10, 48, 75, 82–83, 95–96, 126, 385,
    399
Polkinghorne, Donald, 63–66, 71
Positioning, 84, 178, 187, 207, 209, 214,
    216–217, 221–223, 284, 310, 318, 382
Positivism, 49, 82, 83, 130, 134, 303, 305
Postmodern perspective, 66, 82, 83, 324, 398
Posttraumatic stress disorder (PTSD), 159
Potter, Jonathan, 60–63, 70
Power, 5, 9, 10, 84–85, 205, 220, 221, 353,
    360–361, 367, 400
Practical aims of research, 43, 50, 51, 53, 83,
    84, 88, 94, 129, 288, 289, 358
Pragmatism, 58–59, 82
Praxis, 1, 10, 86, 246, 328, 364, 374, 399
Presentation of findings, 93–94, 245, 258. see
    also Reporting of findings

About the Authors

Frederick J. Wertz, PhD, is Professor of Psychology at Fordham University, where he served as department chair, received the Distinguished Teaching Award in the Sciences, and is a member of the Institutional Review Board. His scholarship focuses on the philosophy, methodology, theory, and cultural context of psychology. He served as editor of the *Journal of Phenomenological Psychology* and the *Bulletin of Theoretical and Philosophical Psychology;* coedited *Advances in Qualitative Research in Psychology: Themes and Variations;* and edited *The Humanistic Movement: Recovering the Person in Psychology.* Dr. Wertz has served as president of the American Psychological Association's Society for Theoretical and Philosophical Psychology and Society for Humanistic Psychology and is president-elect of the Interdisciplinary Coalition of North American Phenomenologists.

Kathy Charmaz, PhD, is Professor of Sociology and Director of the Faculty Writing Program at Sonoma State University. Much of her scholarship has either used or developed grounded theory methods. Her books include the award-winning *Good Days, Bad Days: The Self in Chronic Illness and Time* and *Constructing Grounded Theory: A Practical Guide Through Qualitative Analysis.* Dr. Charmaz has published numerous works on the experience of chronic illness, the social psychology of suffering, writing for publication, and grounded theory and qualitative research, and has served as president of the Pacific Sociological Association. She has received mentoring and lifetime achievement awards from the Society for the Study of Symbolic Interaction.

Linda M. McMullen, PhD, is Professor of Psychology at the University of Saskatchewan, where she served as department head and elected faculty member on the Board of Governors. Her research, supported by the Social Sciences and Humanities Research Council of Canada, is qualitative and discursive in form. It is focused on how people use language to do things and on how language shapes, and is shaped by, social and cultural contexts. Dr. McMullen has published several articles and book chapters and, along with Janet Stoppard, is editor of *Situating Sadness: Women and*

433

Depression in Social Context. She is a Fellow of the Canadian Psychological Association and has received the Jillings Award from the Saskatchewan Psychological Association for outstanding and longstanding service to the profession and the University of Saskatchewan Faculty Association Academic Freedom Award.

Ruthellen Josselson, PhD, is Professor of Psychology at the Fielding Graduate University. Her work uses narrative approaches to investigate a variety of topics. Her books include *Revising Herself: The Story of Women's Identity from College to Midlife, The Space Between Us: Exploring the Dimensions of Human Relationships, Playing Pygmalion: How People Create One Another, Best Friends: The Pleasures and Perils of Girls' and Women's Friendships* (coauthored with Terri Apter). She coedited, with Amia Lieblich, six volumes of *The Narrative Study of Lives,* and five volumes of narrative studies, with Amia Lieblich and Dan McAdams: *Turns in the Road, Up Close and Personal, Identity and Story, Healing Plots,* and *The Meaning of Others.* Dr. Josselson is a recipient of the American Psychological Association's Henry A. Murray Award and Theodore R. Sarbin Award, and is a cofounder of the Society for Qualitative Inquiry.

Rosemarie Anderson, PhD, is Professor of Transpersonal Psychology at the Institute of Transpersonal Psychology and an Episcopal priest. She is coauthor, with William Braud, of *Transpersonal Research Methods for the Social Sciences* and *Transforming Self and Others Through Research,* and is author of *Celtic Oracles.* In addition to intuitive inquiry, Dr. Anderson has developed the Body Intelligence Scale, which measures three types of body awareness; embodied writing; and a model of human development, which describes development from the perspective of the body.

Emalinda McSpadden, MA, is a PhD candidate in the Applied Developmental Psychology program at Fordham University, where she has also taught various psychology courses and chaired numerous conferences. She is a psychology instructor at Hunter College and Bronx Community College, and works as a group therapy moderator for cancer patients through the Albert Einstein School of Medicine. Ms. McSpadden's current academic work focuses on employing mixed methodologies in developmental and lifespan research.